Tuberculosis Treatment:
The Search For New Drugs

Author

Marcus V.N. de Souza

Instituto de Tecnologia em Fármacos – Farmanguinhos
FioCruz – Fundação Oswaldo Cruz
R. Sizenando Nabuco, 100
Manguinhos, 21041-250
Rio de Janeiro, RJ
Brazil

Bentham Science Publishers
Executive Suite Y - 2
PO Box 7917, Saif Zone
Sharjah, U.A.E.
subscriptions@benthamscience.org

Bentham Science Publishers
P.O. Box 446
Oak Park, IL 60301-0446
USA
subscriptions@benthamscience.org

Bentham Science Publishers
P.O. Box 294
1400 AG Bussum
THE NETHERLANDS
subscriptions@benthamscience.org

CONTENTS

FOREWORD

Tuberculosis has been present in humans since antiquity at the latest. The earliest unambiguous detection of *M. tuberculosis* was in the remains of bison dated to approximately 17,000 years ago. Skeletal remains show prehistoric humans (4000 BC) had TB, and researchers have found tubercular decay in the spines of Egyptian mummies dating from 3000-2400 BC.

The ready aerial transmission of TB results in high infection rates. One third of the world's population is thought to have been infected with *M. tuberculosis*, with new infections occurring in about 1% of the population each year. In 2007, there were an estimated 13.7 million chronic active cases globally, while in 2010, there were an estimated 8.8 million new cases and 1.5 million associated deaths, mostly occurring in developing countries. The distribution of tuberculosis is not uniform across the globe, with by far the majority of TB cases occurring in the developing world, *i.e.,* Africa, Asia, and South and Central America. Compromised immunity, largely due to high rates of HIV infection and the corresponding development of AIDS have been significant factors in the recent high numbers of infections. Widespread dissemination of multidrug-resistant tuberculosis and extensively drug-resistant is one of the major health issues faced by a number of countries.

A eBook on such a worrying disease, indicating new research and treatment will always be timely, especially one written by an active researcher. Dr. de Souza's interest in TB is reflected in his many efforts and publications to find new active anti-TB compounds.

The eBook is divided into chapters, dealing with aspects ranging from historical factors and treatments, to surveys of drugs actually in current trials and to studies on potentially active compounds, either currently used in treatment of other diseases, synthesized or found in nature.

One aim of the author in writing this eBook at this time was to generate and foster new researches and efforts into tackling this major disease. An aim, which reached, will have an important impact on the disease.

Dr. J.L. Wardell
Department of Chemistry
University of Aberdeen
Old Aberdeen
AB 24 3UE
Scotland

PREFACE

Tuberculosis (TB) is a chronic bacterial infection, spread through the air, and caused by a bacterium called *Mycobacterium tuberculosis*. This disease is one of the oldest infectious diseases known by man being present since antiquity and responsible for uncountless deaths. However, in despite of this problem only in twentieth century, the cure and control of tuberculosis were finally found. For example, the first drug used in TB treatment appeared in 1946 with the introduction of the antibiotic streptomycin, 64 years after the discovery of the etiologic agent of tuberculosis, the *Mycobacterium tuberculosis* by R. Koch in 1882. After that, the period known as the gold era of TB research (1940-70) was responsible for the introduction of synthetic and semisynthetic drugs. Due to these and other achievements, in the 1960s, 1970s and 1980s, the scientific community believed that the disease would be finally eradicated. However, in 1981, a new disease, known as AIDS (Acquired Immune Deficiency Syndrome) was identified, a contagious disease that caused specific damage to the immunological system. This disease is one of the major causes of the resurgence of TB. For example, the deadly combination between TB and HIV has led to a quadrupling of TB cases in several African and Asian countries. In the case of patients with AIDS, TB is the most common opportunistic infection and cause of death, killing 1 in every 3 patients. In addition, patients living with AIDS and contaminated with latent TB are 30 times more likely to develop active TB than no infected patients. There are also different factors which are responsible for the resurgence of TB, such as immigration, war, famine, homelessness, the lack of new drugs and multi-drug-resistant tuberculosis (MDR TB) due to inconsistent or partial treatment. Considering TB problems, the World Health Organization (WHO) declared this disease a global health emergency in 1993. Recently, another important factor in TB treatment worldwide is the advent of XDR (Extensive Drug Resistant or Extreme Drug Resistance), which is commonly defined as strains resistance to all the current first-line drugs, as well as any fluoroquinolone and, at least, to 1 of 3 injectable second-line drugs (capreomycin, kanamycin or amikacin), which like MDR-TB can be transmitted from an infectious patient to other people.

In spite of the high impact caused by tuberculosis worldwide nowadays, nearly 45 years have passed since a novel drug was introduced into the market to treat TB, except for rifapentine (1998), a very close analogue of rifampin and more recently bedaquiline, a diarylquinoline approved by FDA for multidrug-resistant tuberculosis in December 2012. Due to the increase of MDR and XDR-TB in the world, we need new strategies and drugs to face this new problem or no available treatment will be distributed. In this context, different kinds of organizations, such as academic institutions, government research laboratories, non-governmental organizations, pharmaceutical industry and contract research houses. Considering that, the purpose of this eBook is describe several aspects of research in TB drug discovery, such synthetic and natural drugs in advanced clinical trials, drugs used in other kind of diseases evaluated against tuberculosis, fixed dose combinations, basic research, promising synthetic class of compounds, natural products from different sources, combinatorial chemistry, and mechanism of action. These subjects are organized on eight chapters, four of them dedicated to TB synthetic drugs and the others four to natural products. Chapter one was devoted to the TB treatment and the development of TB drug discovery, chapters two is described TB drugs candidates that are in advanced clinical trials, the third one is related to drugs already used in other kind of diseases evaluated against tuberculosis. Finally, chapter four highlights synthetic compounds from different chemical classes, which were evaluated against *M. tuberculosis* in the last fifteen years. Chapters 5-8 were dedicated to TB drug discovery based on natural products separated on natural products on advanced clinical trials, plants, fungus and marine natural products, respectively. I hope that this eBook will provide a contribution for researcher in industry and universities working in medicinal chemistry, drug discovery, biochemistry, pharmacology, and biology area who are involving in the fight against this disease.

ACKNOWLEDGEMENTS

I would like to thank very much all the people that supported and contributed to making this eBook a reality. Several people read and reread the manuscript giving important contributions in different aspects improving the text and the quality of this eBook. A special thanks for my students Adriana Ferreira Faria, Alessandra Campbell Pinheiro, Camilo Henrique da Silva Lima, Karla Ceodaro Paes,

Cristiane França, Laura Nogueira de Faria Cardoso, Marcelle de Lima Ferreira Bispo, Marcele Moreth, Pedro Santos Mello de Oliveira, Raoni Schroeder Borges Gonçalves, Silvia Helena Cardoso and Thaís Cristina Mendonça Nogueira for they outsdanding work in TB field and help in several aspects of the research. I would like also to thank the professors Adilson D. da Silva, James Lewis and Solange M.S.V. Wardell, Marcone A. L. de Oliveira, Maria C. da S. Lourenço, Mauro V. de Almeida, Robert H. Dood, Thatyana R. A. Vasconcelos and Wilson J. C. Filho for their collaboration, support and encouragement during the entire process. I appreciated very much the opportunity that professor Clifton E. Barry III gave to me to work in his TB research laboratory at National Health Institute (NIH) I learned a lot from him. Thanks also for his team and Helena Boshoff for the very good moments and scientific discussions.

CONFLICT OF INTEREST

Marcus V.N. de Souza

Instituto de Tecnologia em Fármacos – Farmanguinhos

FioCruz – Fundação Oswaldo Cruz

R. Sizenando Nabuco, 100

Manguinhos, 21041-250

Rio de Janeiro, RJ

Brazil

Email: marcos_souza@far.fiocruz.br

ABBREVIATIONS

Ac	=	acetyl
AD	=	Annum Domini
ADME	=	absorption, distribution, metabolism and elimination
AG	=	arabiongalactan
AIDS	=	Acquired Immune Deficiency Syndrome
Am	=	amikacin
Ar	=	aromatic
BC	=	Before Christ
BCG	=	Bacillus Calmette-Guérin
BTZs	=	1,3-benzothiazin-4-ones
Cbz	=	carbobenzoxy
CFM	=	clofazimine
CFU	=	quantification of colony forming units
Cm	=	capreomycin
CM2	=	cyclodextrin/lecitin
CMN	=	*Corynebacteria, Mycobacteria and Nocardia*
Cp	=	ciprofloxacin
Cs	=	cycloserine

DBU	=	1,8-Diazabicycloundec-7-ene
Dc	=	drug combination
DMF	=	dimethylformamide
Dnd	=	deazaflavin-dependent nitroreductase
DOT	=	Directly Observed Therapy
DP	=	decaprenol phosphate
DPA	=	β-D-arabinofuranosyl-1-monophosphoryldecaprenol
EmbA and *EmbB*	=	arabinofuranosyl transferases
Et	=	ethyl
ETH	=	ethambutol
Eti	=	ethionamide
FAS	=	enzyme fatty acid synthase
FDA	=	US food and drug administration
FDC	=	fixed-dose combination
FQ	=	fluoroquinolone
GATB	=	Global Alliance for TB Drug Development
GFP	=	green fluorescent protein microplate assay
GTX	=	gatifloxacin
GLC	=	Green Light Committee
HIV	=	Human Immunodeficiency Virus

HPLC	=	high-performance liquid chromatography
HTS	=	High-Throughput Screening
INH	=	Isoniazid
Km	=	kanamycin
LDA	=	diisopropylamine lithium
LORA	=	low oxygen recovery assay – luciferase readout
LVX	=	levofloxacin
M.	=	*Mycobacterium*
M. tb.	=	*Mycobacterium tuberculosis*
MABA	=	microplate alamar blue assay
MAC	=	*Mycobacterium avium* infections
(mAGP) complex	=	mycolyl-arabinogalactan–peptidoglycan
MBC	=	minimal bactericidal concentration
MBD	=	minimal bacterial dose
MCA	=	mycothiol S-conjugate amidase
MDR	=	multi-drug-resistant tuberculosis
Me	=	Methyl
MED	=	minimal effective dose
MET	=	metronidazole
MIC	=	minimal inhibitory concentration

NRP-TB	=	nonreplicating persistant
MCPBA	=	*meta*-chloroperoxybenzoic acid
Ms	=	Mesyl
MST	=	median survival time
MTBC	=	*Mycobacterium tuberculosis* complex
MXF	=	moxifloxacin
NIAID	=	National Institute of Allergy and Infectious Diseases
NNRTIs	=	Non Nucleoside Reverse Transcriptase Inhibitors
Of	=	ofloxacin
PAS	=	*p*-aminosalicylic acid
PDF	=	Peptide Deformylase
Ph	=	phenyl
PIs	=	Protease inhibitors
Prt	=	protionamide
PTPs	=	Protein Tyrosine Phosphatases
Py	=	piridine
PYZ	=	Pyrazinamide
QSAR	=	quantitative structure activity relationship
RIF	=	rifampicin
rpoB	=	ribosomal polymerase gene

SAR	=	structure-activity relationship
SI	=	selective index
Sm	=	streptomycin
STD	=	Sexually Transmitted Disease
STX	=	sparfloxacin
TAACF	=	Tuberculosis Antimicrobial Acquisition and Coordinating Facility
TB	=	tuberculosis
TDR-TB	=	totally drug-resistance tuberculosis
TLM	=	thiolactomycin
TUBs	=	tuberactinomycins TUBs
TVC	=	*Tuberculosis verrucosa cutis*
TVX	=	trovafloxacin
XDR	=	extensive-drug-resistant or extreme-drug-resistance
XXDR	=	totally drug-resistance tuberculosis
WHO	=	World Health Organization

2

CHAPTER 1

Important Historical Facts of Tuberculosis Treatment and Drug Development

Marcus V.N. de Souza[*]

Instituto de Tecnologia em Fármacos - Farmanguinhos, FioCruz - Fundação Oswaldo Cruz, R. Sizenando Nabuco, 100, Manguinhos, 21041-250, Rio de Janeiro, RJ, Brazil

Abstract: In this chapter will be highlight some important historical facts of tuberculosis treatment and drug development, such as theories, studies and treatment of TB between 17-20th Century, historical aspects of TB drug discovery, side effects, fixed-dose combinations, causes of the resurgence of TB, AIDS, multi-drug-resistant tuberculosis (MDR TB) and extensive-drug- resistant (XDR).

Keywords: Tuberculosis, *Mycobacterium tuberculosis*, drugs, treatment, fixed-dose combinations, multi-drug-resistant tuberculosis (MDR TB), extensive-drug-resistant tuberculosis (XDR TB), natural products, synthesis, AIDS, theories, historical aspects.

INTRODUCTION

Tuberculosis (TB) is one of the oldest infectious diseases known by man, being transmitted through the air and caused by the bacterium *Mycobacterium tuberculosis*. This disease affects mainly the lungs (pulmonary TB), but in over 15% of the patients this bacteria also enters the blood and infects different parts of the body, such as the brain, stomach, bones, skin, intestine, liver, kidneys, spinal cord and breasts. TB has been present since antiquity and there are some evidences that indicate this fact. For example, TB was found in spinal column fragments of Egyptian mummies dated back to 2400-3400 BC [1-5]. Another evidence were the 92 mummies discovery in the Early Bronze Age in the site of

*Adress correspondence to Marcus V.N. de Souza: Instituto de Tecnologia em Fármacos - Farmanguinhos, FioCruz - Fundação Oswaldo Cruz, R. Sizenando Nabuco, 100, Manguinhos, 21041-250, Rio de Janeiro, RJ, Brazil; E-mail: marcos_souza@far.fiocruz.br

Bab edh-Dhra in Jordan, which indicates two cases of tuberculosis [6], and also in India around 2000 BC, which indicates TB cases in preserved bodies [7]. The code of Hamurabi (1948-1905 BC), which was written in Babylon, supposedly mentioned this disease, however, the first time that the symptoms of pulmonary TB such as expectoration, cough, hemoptysis and wasting were well documented was in the library of Assurbanipal (668-626 BC), king of Assyria [8]. In Greece, from 460 to 370 BC, the father of medicine, Hippocrates observed that the disease was able to affect and kill who was in contact with the sick person, and prevented the doctors from visiting patients in terminal stages. Probably, was Hippocrates, who gave the name of ''Phthisis'', a Greek term (Φθίω), which means ''I waste away'' to indicate the wasting which accompanied the disease [8]. The name *consumption* was derived from this Greek term and it was also used. TB was common in The Roman Empire and there are medical texts, which describe the disease. In 130-200 AD, Claudius Galen acknowledged consumption as a not curable disease, exhorted people to avoid contact with sick people and prescribed a treatment based on rest, healthy food and fresh air [8]. In the middle age, the most known fact about TB is the scrofula from Latin "scrofulae", which means "sow" also named *morbus regius*, *mal de roi* and *king's evil* [9,10]. This disease is defined as a form of tuberculosis that affects the skin on the neck. At that time, people believed that scrofula could be cured by the touch of the Kings, being Clovis of France (481-511) and Edward the Confessor (1042-66) of England, the two alleged kings that started this practice, which took place in England, for instance, until the beginning of the 18th Century with Queen Anne (1702-14) [9,10]. In South America, there are also evidences of TB, which were found in a Pre-Colombian mummy from Peru and northern Chile over 900 years old, indicating the presence of the disease before the colonization of the Europeans [11,12]. Unfortunately, TB was one of the biggest killers in human history, responsible for around one billion deaths in the world between the 18th and 19th centuries. For instance, the number of deaths worldwide in the 19th Century was around 7 million per year, and Paris, London and New York were the most affected cities. In Paris, for example, TB was responsible for 30% of the deaths [13]. Due to the tragic TB statistics studies predicted the end of European civilization by the end of the 19th Century. For a better understanding of this disease it is necessary some historical facts, concepts, theories, studies and TB treatment until the discovery of TB chemotherapy and his development. In this context, the next five sections will be highlights these points.

ORIGIN OF THE BACTERIA

Mycobacterium is a member of the family *Mycobacteriaceae,* which are Gram-positive and part of the CMN group (*Corynebacteria, Mycobacteria and Nocardia*). In this context, there are several hypotheses and studies about the origin of this bacterium, which is responsible for TB on Earth [14,15]. Normally, the agents responsible for TB are defined as *Mycobacterium tuberculosis* complex (MTBC), comprising *M. tuberculosis, M. bovis, M. bovis* BCG, *M. africanum, M. canetti, M. microti, M. pinnipedii.* and *M. caprae* species, which possess about 99, 9% genetic sequence similarity [16]. A known theory about the origin of *M. tuberculosis* was evaluated between 15.000 to 35.000 years ago, when the ancestral bacteria arose from soil and first infected animals (*M. bovis* bovine TB bacterium) by inhaling or eating grass, further contaminating humans through the milk and animals' flesh [17-19]. This theory was based on the genetic differences in gene DNA sequences from different groups of *M. tuberculosis* and *M. bovis*. However, genomic studies of both bacteria contradict the theory that *M. bovis* is the progenitor of *M. tuberculosis*. Another theory is that there was a more primitive germ belonging to the same genus *Mycobacterium*, for example, *M. ulcerans*, which is estimated to be 150 million years old, indicating that the genus is far older than, for example, the primates [20]. It is also important to mention that the genome of the tuberculosis bacillus was entirely sequenced in 1998, which gave valuable information about this disease and its origin [21]. For instance, when the genome sequence of *M. tuberculosis* was compared to the bacillus *Mycobacterium leprae*, which causes leprosy, there was a great similarity between the genetic make-ups of these two bacilli, which indicated a common progenitor [21]. Leprosy, like TB is an old disease, which was also known as Hanson's disease, in homage to the Norwegian physician Gerhard Armauer Hansen, who, in 1873, was the first to identify the Gram-positive bacteria *Mycobacterium leprae* [22]. According to statistics, at present, there are more than two million people affected by this disease, with over 800 000 new cases every year worldwide [23].

TUBERCULOSIS NAMES

The name Tuberculosis comes from the word *'tuber'*, derived from the verb *'tumesco'*, which means, in Latin, all kinds of degenerative protuberances or tubercles. It was developed and coined by Gaspard Laurent Bayle (1774-1816), Josef Leopold Auenbrugger (1722-1809), René Théophile Hyacinthe Laënnec (1781-1826), Johann Lucas Schonlein (1793-1864) and Rudolf Virchow (1821-1902). However, this term only became widely adopted at the beginning of the twentieth century [24].

Due to the fact that TB is one of the oldest infectious diseases in the world and it can affect almost any tissue or organ of the body, it has received different names throughout human history, such as wasting disease, white swelling (TB of the bone), gastric fever, bronchitis and inflammation of the lungs, delicacy of the lungs hectic fever, lung weakness, pleural abscess, debility, graveyard cough, hectic fever, decline, swollen glands, complaint in the chest, pleural abscess, miliary TB (X-ray lesions look like millet seeds), lupus vulgaris (TB of the skin), prosector's wart or tuberculosis verrucosa cutis (TVC), also a kind of TB of the skin, transmitted by contact with contaminated cadavers, in professionals, such as surgeons, anatomists, veterinarians and butchers, and mesenteric disease (TB of the abdomen), which was a common children disease caused by milk from TB infected cows, which is a rare disease now due to pasteurized milk. In Table **1**, some important TB names in human history are described.

Table 1: Some important TB names in human history.

Date	Name	Who used the name and where
460-370 BC	Phthisis (Consumptions) the name is because this disease consumes people from within with its symptoms of bloody cough, fever, pallor, and long relentless wasting	Greek term used for Hippocrates, in Greece
1st AD	Tuberculum or tubercula	Pliny and Aurelius Celsus, in Rome
2st AD	Phthisis (Consumptions)	Claudius Galen, in Rome
Middle Age	Scrofula (swollen neck glands) or King´s evil due to the belief that a king's touch would cure scrofula	In Europe
16th Century	Tubercula or scirrhositates	In Europe
17th Century	Tubercles	Named in Holland by Franciscus de la Boe, also known as Dr. Silvius.
Mid of 17th Century	The disease was known as the "White Plague" because it makes patients look pale	In Europe and The United States
18th Century	Vampirism	Industrial Revolution in England
18th Century	Pott´s disease (TB of the bones)	Percivall Pott in England

THEORIES, STUDIES AND TREATMENT OF TB BETWEEN 17-20th CENTURY

Since Antiquity, there are registries of TB symptoms, as well as some theories based on observation, *e.g.*, to avoid contact with sick people or treatment based on rest, healthy food and fresh air. However, in the Middle Ages (450-1450), the period of History between Classical Antiquity and the Renaissance, especially in the period known as The Dark Age (476-1000), no progress in science was done. After this period, the Renaissance (from the early 14th to the late 16th century) appeared in the European History, more specifically in Italy, making an effort to restore the values and artistic styles of classical antiquity. In this context, an important study about TB was made by the Italian Girolamo Frascastorius (1478-1553) in his book *De Morbis Contagiosis* in 1546, which described theories to explain how TB infected people, based on contagious particles (invisible particles) present in air, bed sheets and clothing [25].

17th Century

More detailed studies began in the 17th century, when scientists of different fields started to build theories and hypothesize about how people contracted the disease, starting to search for a means of fighting against it (Table **2**). In this context, in 1672, the English Thomas Willians (1621-1675), one of the greatest physicians in the 17th century, who died from tuberculosis, believed that this disease was one of the hardest to be cured, as well as other chest diseases responsible for leading to TB [26]. In that century, the Dutchman Anton van Leeuwenhoek (1632-1723), also known as the father of microbiology and microscopy, made great advances in the development of microscopes with important discoveries, such as the identification of bacteria for the first time (1674), red blood cells (1675), human spermatozoa (1677) and others [27]. An important study in the TB field was made by the Dutchman physician Franciscus de la Boe, commonly named Dr. Silvius, which, in 1679, published the book *Opera Medica*, describing by help of dissection, the evolution of the disease, named by him tubercles. It was characterized by deterioration of the lungs, as well as others areas of the body [28]. He also presented a clear description of cavities and nodes caused by TB. The English physician Thomas Sydenham (1624-1689), was also known as the

British Hippocrates, as well as the father of English medicine, since his studies were based on the Hippocratic methods, which are observation and experience. Responsible for several contributions in the medicine field, Sydenham also gave an important contribution to the understanding of the disease, based on the relation between TB in cattle and humans, and suggested that before consuming meat, the chest or diaphragm of a carcass had to be examined and avoided, if nodules were found on the wall of its organs. Sydenham also believed that pollution and fume were responsible for causing TB [29]. In 1689, the English preacher and physician Richard Morton (1637-1698) was the first to report eating disorders, named by him as "A Nervous Consumption", at present known as anorexia nervosa. In 1694, in his book Phthisiologia or a Treatise of Consumptions (Latin version -1698), Morton described two cases of anorexia nervosa, as well as related symptoms, which were associated with pulmonary TB, such as fever, coughing, difficulty in breathing and enlargement of the tracheal and bronchial glands. Besides, he believed that pulmonary TB often healed spontaneously [30]. In 1699, the Republic of Lucca, in Italy, was the first government to create regulations to fight against the spread of TB, which was based on a report made by doctors and sent to authorities, with all the names of the deceased by the disease. This report was published, and measures for disinfection, taken, such as the burning of corpse and possessions of the victim to avoid the contamination of others [31]. The doctors also were required to perform autopsies in the victims of TB, however, due to the fear of catching it, they were not made. For example, the Italian anatomist Antonio Maria Valsalva (1666-1723) and his disciples avoided autopsies in people who had died of TB [32].

18th Century

In the 18th Century, pulmonary Tuberculosis took a great proportion in Europe, due to the beginning of the Industrial Revolution, which was responsible for the migration of people from rural to urban areas, into crowded cities. Unfortunately, in that century, the causes of TB were still an unsolved puzzle for the scientists, but breakthroughs toward the comprehension of this disease were achieved (Table **3**). For instance, in 1702, John Jacobus Manget made a good description of the chronic and contagious disease known as miliary tuberculosis, which was characterized by a spread of the bacteria to the other organs of the body, using as transport the blood or the lymph system [33]. An important theory in the century was made by the English physician Benjamin Marten (1704-1782), who published in London, in 1720, a small book with 186 pages named: A New Theory of Consumptions: More Especially of a Phthisis or Consumption of the Lungs [34]. This theory was based on the actions of "minute living creatures", and after these organisms institute in the body, they are, according to Martin, able to create the symptoms of consumption. Marten also hypothesized that closer contact with people with TB, which comprises a close conversation, was enough to contract the disease, due to the presence of creatures inside the lung that could spread by the breath. In the end of the 17th century and the beginning of the 18th century, the Italian physician Giovanni Maria Lances (1654-1720) was the first to describe percussion of the chest bone, which was an important tool in pulmonary TB diagnosis. This diagnosis was applied by the Austrian physician Josef Leopold Auenbrugger (1722-1809), who, in 1754, invented the method of auscultating the patient's chest and applied it from 1758 to 1762 at The Spanish Hospital, where during this period he was chief physician. His study identified sounds, which were characteristic of several chest diseases and, in 1761, in Vienna, its results were published in a book entitled A New Discovery that Enables the Physician from the Percussion of the Human Thorax to Detect the Diseases Hidden Within the Chest [35]. Another important study was performed by William Stark (1741-1770), who examined the growth and development of tubercles proving the correlation with the evolution of the disease [36].

The 18th century was also marked by measures trying to stop the disease in Europe. In France, for example, in 1716, a butcher who had sold meat from contaminated cattle was sentenced to pay 5.000 pounds, banished for nine years and could not maintain his profession anymore. For example, in 1732, the ones who had sold meat without inspection in Germany were punished with corporal discipline. In 1782, the Department of Public Health of Naples, in Italy, created laws to avoid the spread of TB, such as the report of all TB cases, disinfection and the creation of separate places in the hospitals. The utilization of animals infected with tuberculosis for alimentation was not allowed in Prussia (1785) and Austria (1788), being punished with banishment [37].

Table 2: Important contributions in TB field in the 17th and 18th Century.

Date	Name	Contribution
1546	Girolamo Fracastorius	Wrote book: *De Morbis Contagiosis*, which described theories to explain how TB infected people.
1672	Thomas Willians	TB was one the hardest diseases to cure, as well as other chest diseases responsible for leading to TB.
1674	Anton van Leeuwenhoek	Made great advances in the development of microscopes with important discoveries, such as the identification of the bacteria for the first time.
1679	Franciscus de la Boe	TB was characterized for the deterioration of the lungs, as well as other areas of the body.
1683	Thomas Sydenham	Established relation between TB in cattle and humans, and that pollution and fume were responsible for causing TB.
1689	Richard Morton	Report on eating disorder, at present known as anorexia nervosa, named by him as "A Nervous Consumption".
1699	Unknown authors	The Republic of Lucca in Italy, was the first government to create regulations to fight against the spread of TB.
1702	John Jacobus Manget	Described the pathological features of miliary tuberculosis
1720	Benjamin Marten	Wrote a book named: A New Theory of Consumptions: More Especially of a Phthisis or Consumption of the Lungs.
1761	Josef L. Auenbrugger	Wrote a book named: A New Discovery that Enables the Physician from the Percussion of the Human Thorax to Detect the Diseases Hidden Within the Chest.

19th Century

In the beginning of the 19th century, TB still missed a sound comprehension and treatment; however, many important studies had been done toward the solution (Table **3**). For example, the French physician Gaspard Laurent Bayle (1774-1816) made an important contribution to the understanding of the disease by dissecting over nine hundred post mortem people who died of TB and defined six kinds of TB: tubercular, granular, ulcerous, calculous, cancerous and phthisis with melanosis. He also described and defended that not only did TB affect the lungs but also different organs, such as the heart, skin, intestines, bones, and the brain [38]. It is also important to mention that Bayle made relevant contributions in the cancer field and considered TB and cancer close diseases in his book: Traité des maladies cancéreuses, which has been published in 1833 by his niece. Another important study made in this century was produced by the English scientist Thomas Young (1773-1829), which in 1815 wrote a book entitled: A Practical and Historical Treatise on Consumptive Diseases that described the tremendous difficulty to save people infected by TB and stated that, only 1 in 1000 patients could be cured, demonstrating in his book how difficult and how far it was to find a treatment against TB [39]. Finally, in the middle of the 19th century, the puzzle was solved and TB was not anymore a mystery: a bacterium, a simple organism, was responsible for causing the disease and for killing billions of people. Due to this important discovery, the disease started to be seen as curable and treatments, suggested for the first time. In 1816, the French physician René Théophile Hyacinthe Laënnec (1781-1826) invented, at the Necker Hospital in Paris, the stethoscope, which was an important tool in the diagnosis of different chest diseases. Laënnec studies were published in 1819 in his important book: *De l'auscultation* mediate [40]. In 1836, the English physician George Bodington (1799-1882) recommended a regime based on mild exercise, special diet, fresh air in abundance and minimum use of medicaments to his patients with TB [41]. However, his ideas were very criticized in this period and his treatment was not adopted. In this context, during the period between 1839-1845, the physician Dr. John C. Croghan (1790-1849), the owner of Mammoth Cave in Kentucky, United States, brought people with tuberculosis into the cave, which according to Dr. Jonh could cure the disease, due to the constant temperature and purity of the air [42,43]. However, this form of treatment only started to be recognized as an important tool against TB, when the German botany student Gustav Adolf Robert Hermann Brehmer (1826-1889) who suffered from TB, was advised by his doctor to move to a place with a better climate. Following this piece of advice, Brehmer moved to the Himalayas, where he studied botany. Surprisingly, he returned in good health condition and cured to Germany, where he started studying medicine. In 1854, Brehmer presented his medical dissertation, with the touching title: Tuberculosis is a Curable Disease, which in that period of time was not well accepted. In spite of this problem, Brehmer opened a hospital in Sokołowsko (German: Gorbersdorf), in Poland, which is a village with altitude between 540-590 m above sea level, surrounded by mountains and valley. This first tuberculosis sanatorium was built in 1855, in the middle of the mountains, forests and gardens, providing an excellent quality of life, which was based on a combination of fresh air, good nutrition, moderate exercises and nature. Due to its excellent results, his work became a model for further sanatoriums. Brehmer's work continued with his patient Peter Dettweiler (1837-1904), who, after being cured, became his assistant. In 1876, he opened the Falkenstein sanatorium near Frankfurt [44]. In the same year, the first sanatorium was built in The United States by the American physician Edward Livingston Trudeau (1848-1915) [45] in the Adirondack Mountains of New York, at Saranac Lake. Trudeau developed TB by taking care of his brother, who suffered from the disease. After he had moved to Saranac Lake in 1873, he was cured. After that, he dedicated his life to helping other people with the disease and built the Adirondack Cottage Sanitarium, renamed the Trudeau Sanatorium in 1884 and opened it in 1885. He also dedicated his life to the search for new treatments to fight TB, and, in 1894, he built the first laboratory (Saranac Laboratory) in The United States devoted to the study of this disease. Due to the important results of sanatoriums from 1836 to 1890, they spread around Europe and the United States and became a fundamental treatment at the beginning of the twentieth century, besides being a powerful weapon to prevent the spread of the disease. In 1865, the French physician and military doctor Jean Antoine Villemin (1827-1892) demonstrated that TB was an infectious disease and could be transmitted by contact from humans to cattle and from cattle to rabbits, and also suggested a specific microorganism responsible for the transmission. In spite of the evidences of Villemin's experiments, his results were not well accepted and ignored until seventeen years later [46]. In this context, in one evening of March, in 1882, at Berlin Physiological Society, a German scientist and physician called Heinrich Hermann Robert Koch (1843-1910) demonstrated one of the most important discoveries in the TB field and also in the medical history, which had been published three weeks before in the Berliner Klinische Wochenscrift under the title of *"The Etiology of Tuberculosis"*. This discovery was the identification of the etiologic agent of tuberculosis, the bacterium called by him tuberculosis bacillus, the *Mycobacterium tuberculosis* also named bacillus of Koch in his homage. Koch, additionally, did not believe in the similarity between human and bovine tuberculosis, which also contributed to a better understanding of the disease [47]. In 1883-1884, Koch formulated some postulates, which were refined by him in 1890. These postulates, known as Koch´s postulates or Henle-Koch postulates for the contribution of his professor Friedrich Gustav Jakob Henle, (1809-1885), described that for a bacteria to be the cause of a disease it had to be present in all cases of the disease; the bacteria must be isolated and grown in a pure culture from the host with the disease; the culture of the respective bacteria must cause disease when inoculated into a healthy host and the bacteria must be isolated again from the experimentally infected host [48].

In 1890, during the Tenth International Medical Congress in Berlin, Koch reported a "cure" for tuberculosis, a glycerin extract of the tubercle bacilli named by him tuberculin, which had cured guinea pigs infected by *Mycobacterium tuberculosis*, although its therapeutic benefits were not effective [49]. This discovery enabled an outstanding application in the next century, "a diagnostic test for tuberculosis", which, in 1907, was first studied and adapted by the Austrian pediatrician and scientist Clemens Peter Freiherr von Pirquet (1874-1929) and expanded, in 1908, by the German physician Felix Mendel (1862-1925) and the French physician Charles Mantoux (1877-1947). This test commonly known as Mendel-Mantoux, Mantoux screening test, Tuberculin Sensitivity Test, Pirquet test, or PPD test, which stands for Purified Protein Derivative was based on the application of tuberculin under the skin, causing, in the case of positive reaction, swelling at the injection site. For their discoveries in TB field, Koch was awarded with the Nobel Prize in Physiology in 1905. Koch also made outstanding discoveries in other fields and changed medical history, such as the discovery of *Bacillus anthracis* (1876), the etiologic agent of anthrax, the discovery of *Vibrio cholerae* (1883-1884), the etiologic agent of cholera. For his achievements, together with the French scientist Louis Pasteur (1827-1892), Koch is considered one of the founders of modern bacteriology and microbiology. In the same year that Robert Koch identified the etiologic agent of tuberculosis (1882), the artificial pneumothorax began to be described, probably the most important treatment against TB, before the advent of the antitubercular drugs in the middle of the 20th Century. Pneumothorax is defined as the collapse of a lung, with the escape of air into the pleural cavity between the lung and the chest wall. At the beginning of the 19th Century (1822-1832) the English physician, James Carson, demonstrated a possible application of pneumothorax in the TB field by using infected animals and introducing an injection of air into the pleural space, allowing it to heal and survive with a single functioning lung. Carson has tried this treatment without success in two patients, because their lungs refused to collapse. However, from

1882 to 1912, the Italian physician Carlo Forlanini (1847-1918) developed successfully the artificial pneumothorax, also called collapse therapy, which was based on inducing a collapse, submitting the lung to rest and making it temporarily inactive so that it could heal with scar formation. Forlanini's method consisted of injecting nitrogen into the pleural cavity, through a hypodermic needle and his apparatus had a portable design and a system of glass, basically with a graduated reservoir for nitrogen or filtered air, a control reservoir, hand pump, filter and chest needle [50].

In 1895, the German physician Professor Wilhelm Conrad Roentgen (1845-1923) discovered X-rays [51], an important tool that has been used up to nowadays, which allowed a precise diagnosis of pulmonary TB and its stage. For this outstanding discovery Roentgen was laureate with the first Nobel Prize in physics in 1901.

Table 3: Important contributions in TB field in the 17th and 18th Century.

Date	Name	Contribution
1810	Gaspard Laurent Bayle	Defended that not only did TB affect the lungs but also different organs, such as heart, skin, intestines, bones, including the brain.
1815	Thomas Young	Wrote a book entitled: A Practical and Historical Treatise on Consumptive Diseases, which described the difficulty to save people infected with TB.
1816	René T. H. Laënnec	Invented at the Necker Hospital in Paris, the stethoscope.
1836	George Bodington	Recommended to his patients with TB a regime based on mild exercise, special diet, fresh air in abundance and minimum of medicaments.
1839 - 1845	John C. Croghan	Brought people with tuberculosis into the cave.
1854	Gustav Adolf Robert Hermann Brehmer	Presented his medical dissertation with the touching title Tuberculosis is a Curable Disease and built the first sanatorium.
1865	Jean Antoine Villemin	Demonstrated that TB was an infectious disease and could be transmitted by contact from humans to cattle and from cattle to rabbits and also suggested a specific microorganism responsible for the transmission.
1882	Robert Koch	Identified the etiologic agent of tuberculosis, the bacterium called by him tuberculosis bacillus, the *Mycobacterium tuberculosis* also named bacillus of Koch in his homage.
1882-1912	Carlo Forlanini	Developed successfully the artificial pneumothorax
1895	Wilhelm C. Roentgen	Discovered the X-rays.

20th Century

In this century, several outstanding breakthroughs towards the cure and control of tuberculosis were finally found, saving billions of human lives. Due to these achievements, in the 1960s, 1970s and 1980s, the scientific community believed that the disease would be finally eradicated. For example, in the first thirty years of the century, immunotherapy was the focus of treatment for infective diseases. In spite of immunizating the non contaminated people, it was not effective against infected people, because they did not have time to produce immunity. The immunization could be defined as the introduction of the attenuated bacteria in the human body by injection, which stimulated antibody formation. In this condition, the bacteria would be too weak to provoke the infection disease. Based on this principle, in 1908, an efficient diagnostic test for tuberculosis was developed by the German physician Felix Mendel (1862-1925) and the French physician Charles Mantoux (1877-1947). This test, which continues to be used nowadays, is commonly known as Mantoux test, and it was based on the application of tuberculin under skin, which causes in the case of positive reaction, a swelling at the injection site. Between 1908-1919 in Pasteur Institute Lille - France, the bacteriologist Albert Calmette and the veterinarian Camille Guérin, both French, developed the vaccine against TB named BCG in their homage (bacillus Calmette-Guérin), which was prepared from a strain of the attenuated live bovine tuberculosis bacillus, *Mycobacterium bovis* that had lost its virulence in humans through special culture in artificial medium for years. In 1921, the vaccine BCG was developed in humans and it is still being used nowadays in childhood vaccination [52-54].

HISTORY OF TB DRUG DISCOVERY

The Magic Bullet

The Twentieth Century was marked by a new approach in the treatment of infectious diseases, the chemotherapy, which was based on destroying pathogenic microorganisms by using chemical compounds without affecting the host cells. This term was first used by the great German-Jewish physician and microbiologist Paul Ehrlich (1854-1915), Nobel Prize in medicine in 1908, who was also the first to coin the term ''magic bullet'', the perfect drug, able to fight against the disease efficiently and selectively without side effects [55-57]. The use of chemical compounds against diseases was based on the theory known as "the germ theory", which proposed that microorganisms were responsible for many diseases, and several scientists have contributed to confirm this theory throughout human history (Table **4**).

Table 4: Important contributions for germ theory.

Date	Name	Contribution
1546	Girolamo Frascastorius	The first to propose that infectious diseases were caused by contagious invisible particles (in English "germ").
1668	Francesco Redi	One of the first to refute the spontaneous generation.
1674	Anton van Leeuwenhoek	Made great advances in the development of microscopes with important discoveries, such as the identification of bacteria for the first time.
1844	Agostino Bassi	Proposed that living microorganisms were responsible for human and animal disease.
1847	Ignaz P. Semmelweis	Discovered the importance of the hygiene to combat diseases.
1856	Louis Pasteur	Refuted the spontaneous generation and proved that fermentation process occurred by growth of microorganisms, which reproduced in nutrient broths.
1860	Joseph Lister	Developed the principles of "antiseptic surgery".
1873	Gerhard A. Hansen	Identified the etiologic agent of leprosy, *Mycobacterium leprae*.
1876	Robert Koch	Identified the etiologic agent of anthrax, *Bacillus anthracis*.

Basically, the history of modern chemotherapy started in 1859, when the French biologist Antoine Béchamp (1816-1908) synthesized the compound called atoxyl (Fig. **1**), which was used by Paul Ehrlich's group as the starting point for the synthesis of new atoxyl analogues, by using aniline and arsenic acid to treat skin disease. This German scientist made outstanding discoveries in hematology, immunology and chemotherapy fields, and, in 1904, in collaboration with the German chemist Alfred Bertheim (1879-1914) and the Japanese bacteriologist Sahachiro Hata (1873-1938) began the synthesis and evaluation of different analogues of atoxyl in the search for a cure for syphilis [58,59]. This sexual transmitted disease is caused by bacteria called *Treponema pallidum,* and it was a serious world health problem, compared to AIDS (Acquired Immune Deficiency Syndrome) nowadays, especially in Europe and The United States. For example, in the beginning of the Twentieth Century about 10% of American males had syphilis. Unfortunately, the treatment used at that time was based on mercury and its salts, which were administrated by different *via*, such as rubbing mercury on the skin and through mouth. According to the majority of the patients, this treatment was terrible and worse than the disease itself with several side-effects, such as abdominal pain, mouth ulcers and tooth and hair loss. The cure for the disease started between 1904 and 1909 with more than six hundred atoxyl analogues prepared and evaluated for Ehrilch team. In 1909, the compound number 606 (dihyroxydiamino-arsenobenzene-dihydrochlooride), also called dioxydiaminoarsenobenzol, arsphenamine and Ehrilich 606, found excellent results *in vivo*, and after clinical studies, this compound was marketed in 1910 with the trade name of "Salvarsan" (Fig. **1**). The production of this drug was developed by Hoechst, a German chemical company, becoming a powerful drug against this disease, saving millions of lives [58,59]. It is important to point out that the right structure of salvarsan was only solved in 2005 by Nicholson and co-workers as a mixture of cyclic As-As of three and five member rings [60].

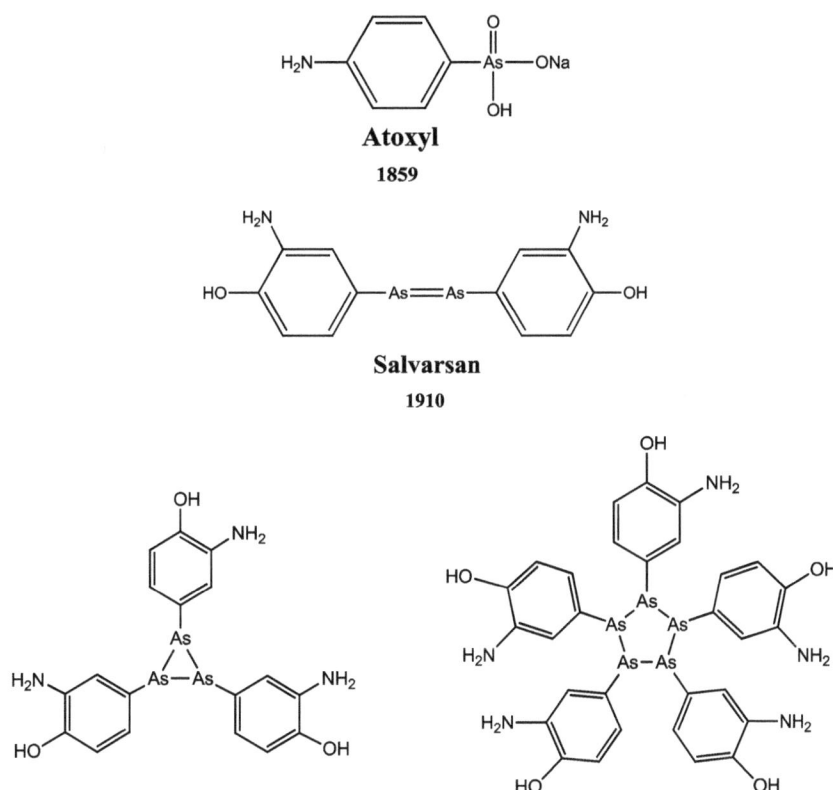

Figure 1: Structures of atoxyl and salvarsan.

Gold Therapy

In the search for new treatments against TB, the gold compounds were introduced at the beginning of the Twentieth Century against tuberculosis bacteria, influenced by Robert Koch, who, in 1890, at International Medical Congress in Berlin, reported that gold-cyanide complexes were effective against *Mycobacterium tuberculosis* in cultures, but not in guinea pigs. In the mid-1920s, the gold therapy was popularized, especially by Danish physicians, such as Holger Mollgaard (1885-1973), who, in 1925, introduced sanocrysin (sodium aurothiosulphate) $Na_3[O_3S-S-SO_3]$, being extensively used until 1934, mainly in Europe [61].

The Penicillin Era

After the gold therapy, many other classes of compounds have been tested against TB without success. However, in 1928, an important era started, changing the medical history: the discovery of the antibiotics. The first compound of this class was fortunately discovered in 1928, from the *Penicillium* mold by the Scottish scientist Alexander Fleming and named Penicillin by him (Fig. **2**). In spite of the failure of Penicillin in TB treatment, this outstanding discovery launched a new era for the treatment of infectious diseases and was the key in the search for new compounds of this class and other ones [62,63].

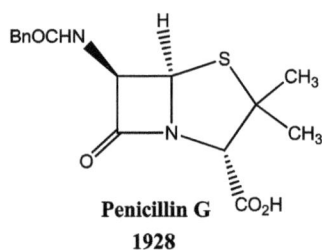

Figure 2: Structure of penicillin G.

Sulfonamide, A Synthetic Antimicrobial Agent

The synthetic chemical compounds were of great importance in the fight against the infectious diseases and brought hope for the cure of TB. In this context, one the first synthetic classes of antibacterial agents was the sulfonamides, which was discovered by the German scientist, Gerhard Domagk (1895-1964), in December 1932.

Domagk, who graduated in medicine and had a high opinion about Ehrilch's theory "the magic bullets", believed that the dyes could be used as drug. This class of compounds had been chosen by Domagk, because at that time, he worked at Bayer Company, which discovered a series of aniline dyes. His work brought the first sulfonamide, named Prontosil, (Fig. **3**) in 1932, which had an antibacterial action against streptococci in mice. It is important to point out that Prontosil was active only in living animals and no effects had been observed *in vitro*. The answer for this question was produced in 1936, with the discovery that Prontosil was a prodrug producing the active compound *p*-aminobenzenesulfonamide (Fig. **3**). Due to the great relevance of this class of compounds, which had a fundamental importance in preventing infections during World War II, Domagk was awarded with the Nobel Prize in 1939. However, the Nazi regime forbade him to accept it,

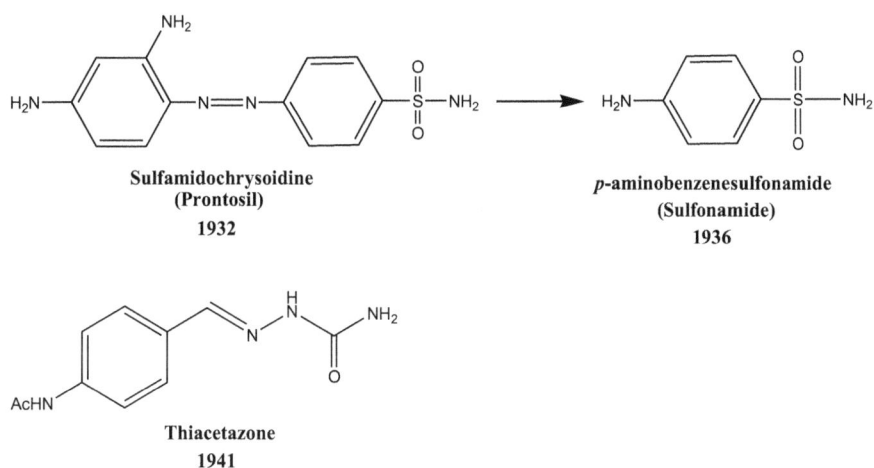

Sulfamidochrysoidine
(Prontosil)
1932

p-aminobenzenesulfonamide
(Sulfonamide)
1936

Thiacetazone
1941

Figure 3: Structures of prontosil, *p*-aminobenzenesulfonamide and thiacetazone.

and only after the war was over, he was able to receive the prize in Sweden. In spite of the outstanding contribution of this class of compounds in the chemotherapy, sulfonamides were tested *in vivo* by Rich and Follis at Jonh Hopkins Hospital in 1938, with weak activity against TB. It was nevertheless a fundamental step for the discovery of new compounds against TB and other infectious diseases. In 1939, Domagk identified sulphathiazole and sulphadithiazole with more anti-TB activity than the related sulfonamides. Considering that, and continuing his work, in 1941, Domagk sent a series of thiosemicarbazides to be tested, which furnished as result an important piece of information: this class of compounds was much more active than sulfonamide class, and, in 1946, one compound, named thiacetazone, specially showed promising perspectives, (Fig. **3**). However, due to problems with clinical trials and toxicity this compound was only introduced in the market in 1962 [64,65].

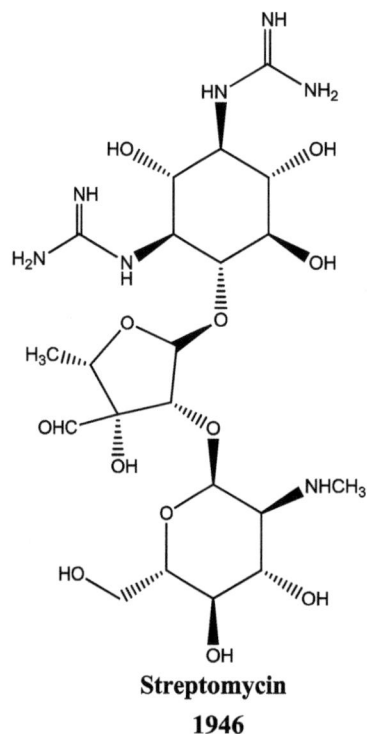

Streptomycin
1946

Figure 4: Structure of Streptomycin.

Streptomycin, The First Antibiotic Against TB

The first drug used in TB treatment appeared in 1946 with the introduction of the antibiotic streptomycin (Fig. **4**), 64 years after the discovery of the etiologic agent of tuberculosis, the *Mycobacterium tuberculosis* by R. Koch in 1882. The story of streptomicyn, which was extracted from the soil from *Streptomyces griseus*, began in 1943, when the biochemist and microbilogist Selman Abraham Waksman (1888-1973) and his co-workers Albert Schatz and Elizabeth Bugie discovered, at Rutgers University, that streptomycin was active against certain pathogens, especially the bacteria *Mycobacterium tuberculosis*. In 1944, in colaboration with two medical researchers at the Mayo Clinic, William H. Feldman and H. Corwin Hinshaw, the test *in vivo* started in guinea pigs, and in 1945, the clinical trials began with thirty-three patients, confirming the animal results and becoming the first drug to be used to treat TB. Due to their outstanding work Waskman, who also claimed having coined the word antibiotic, was awarded with the Nobel Prize in medicine in 1952. The discovery of streptomycin was also marked by a long debate between Waskman and Schatz, who claimed the co-invention of this antibiotic. The debate resulted in litigation, which ended in court with the official decision that Waksman and Schatz would be considered co-discoverers of streptomycin [66]. The importance of streptomycin to TB treatment and to other diseases, such as bubonic plague, urinary tract infection, typhoid fever, cholera and tularemia was tremendous, saving lives and bringing hope to humankind. However, after its introduction in the market, streptomycin became resistant in some patients, indicating that the cure for TB was just beginning.

The Importance of Nature in TB Drug Discovery

After the discovery of streptomycin, the period known as the gold era of TB research (1940-70) was responsible for the introduction of synthetic drugs. However, nature still has playing a crucial role in drug discovery until nowadays. For example, other aminoglicosides as kanamycin from *Streptomyces capreolus*, and the semisynthetic amikacin produce from kanamycin A are still being used in TB treatment as second-line drugs (Fig. **5**) [67]. Another important class of second-line anti-drugs from nature is known as tuberactinomycins (TUBs), which possessed into its structure cyclic petides being represented by viomycin and capreomycins, which have close structural similarities. Viomycin (tuberactinomycin B) is produced by the actinomycete *Streptomyces vinaceus* being discovery by Ciba in 1953 and marketed in 1960´s by both Ciba and Pfizer as TB drug. Capreomycins, which are less toxic and more effective than viomycin as TB second-line drugs were patented by Lilly in 1959-60 from fermentation of *Streptomyces* capreolus [67]. Another example of the importance of nature in TB-drug discovery is D-cycloserine obtained from *Streptomyces sps* and until nowadays used as TB second-line drug [67].

Kanamycin
A R = H; R_1 = OH; R_2 =NH$_2$
B R = H; R_1 = R_2 = NH$_2$
C R = H; R_1 = NH$_2$; R_2 = OH

Amikacin
  R = COCH(OH)CH$_2$NH$_2$; R_1 = OH; R_2 = NH$_2$

1960s

Tuberactinomycin A   R = OH; R^1 = OH; R^2 = CONH$_2$
Tuberactinomycin B (Viomycin)   R = H; R^1 = OH; R^2 = CONH$_2$
Tuberactinomycin N   R = OH; R^1 = H; R^2 = CONH$_2$
Tuberactinomycin O   R = H; R^1 = H; R^2 = CONH$_2$

D-Cicloserine
1955

1959-60

Capreomycin IA   R = OH; R^1 =

Capreomycin IB   R = H; R^1 =

Capreomycin IIA   R = OH; R^1 =   -NH$_2$

Capreomycin IIB   R = H; R^1 =   -NH$_2$

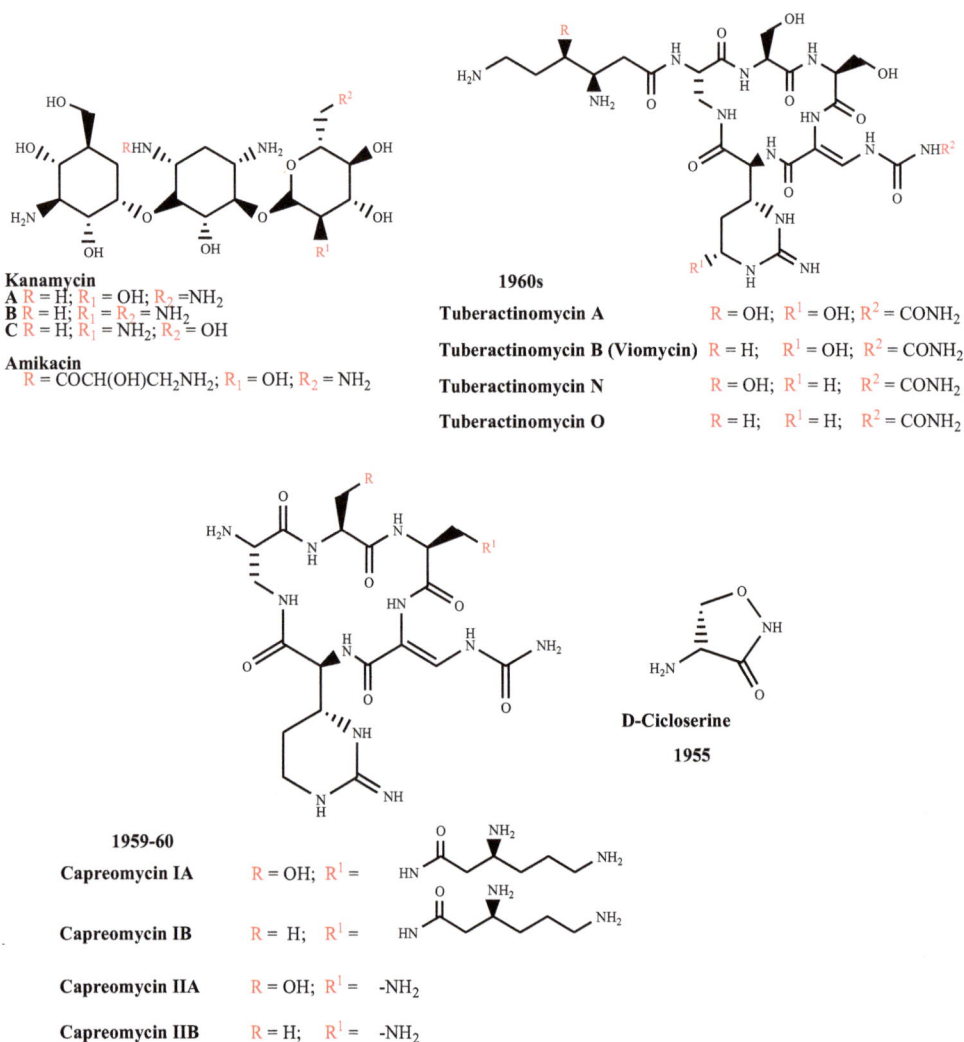

Figure 5: Structure of kanamycin, amikacin and D-cicloserine.

Rifamycyns

Another outstanding example of the importance of mother-nature in TB chemotherapy is the semisynthetic compound named rifampicin or rifampin (Fig. **6**). This compound belongs to the family of ansamycins antibiotics named rifamycins, first isolated in 1957 from fermentation broths of *Streptomyces mediterranei* from a soil sample, collected from a pine arboretum near Saint Raphaël, France. The procedure was performed at Dow-Lepetit Research Laboratories in Milan, Italy by the scientists Piero Sensi (Italian) and Pinhas Margalith (Israeli) with a broad spectrum of bacteria. The rifamycins were identified and named Rifamycin A, B, C, D, E, S and SV, and Rifamycin B was the first rifamycin to be introduced commercially. In search of new oral anti-bacterial agents, Dow-Lepetit Research Laboratories made modifications of the rifamycins leading to the discovery of rifamycin SV, which was introduced in some countries for infections of the biliary tract. Dow-Lepetit Research Laboratories continued to make structural modifications in the rifamycin system, producing a good understanding of the structure-activity relationship of this class, which led to the discovery of rifampin (USAN) or rifampicin (INN) (Scheme **1**). From 1965 to 1970, this semisynthetic antibiotic was developed and introduced in the market and, due to its potent oral activity; it became one of the most important drugs in TB treatment and in other infectious diseases. For example, in TB rifampin is responsible for the reduction of the duration of therapy, from 12 to 6 months when combined with other drugs, as well as the reduction from 9 to 2 or 3 months in latent infection. Its mechanism of action is based on the inhibition of bacterial DNA-dependent RNA polymerase, which produces essential proteins and is responsible for copying their own genetic information, the DNA [68,69].

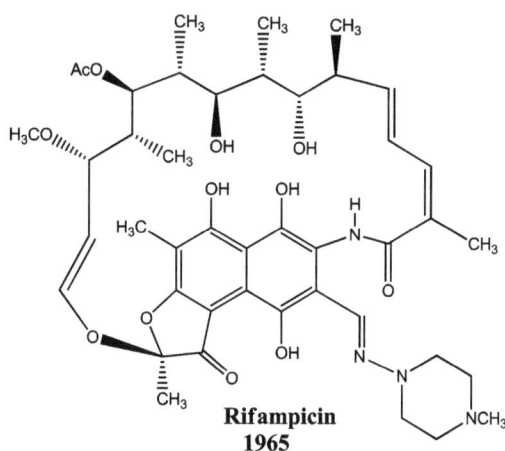

Figure 6: Structure of rifampicin.

The Second Drug Against TB

In 1946, three years after the discovery of streptomycin, the compound *p*-aminosalicylic acid (PAS) (Fig. **7**) was successfully used against TB, being in 1948, the second drug and the first synthetic compound to be used in TB treatment.

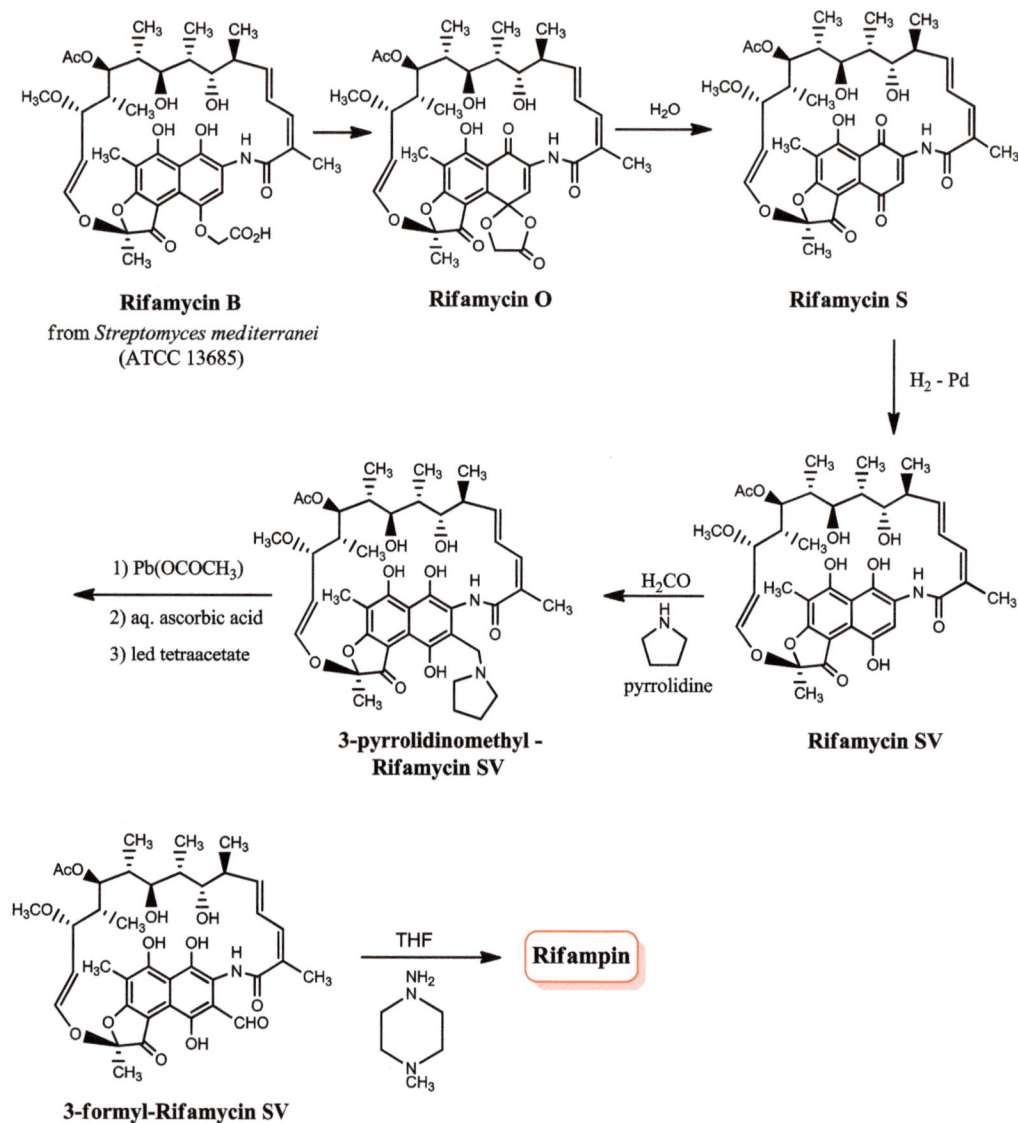

Rifamycin B
from *Streptomyces mediterranei*
(ATCC 13685)

Rifamycin O

Rifamycin S

1) Pb(OCOCH₃)
2) aq. ascorbic acid
3) led tetraacetate

**3-pyrrolidinomethyl -
Rifamycin SV**

pyrrolidine

Rifamycin SV

3-formyl-Rifamycin SV

Rifampin

Scheme 1: Semisynthesis of rifampin [67].

The Danish Jorgen Lehman started the discovery of PAS as a TB drug in 1943 at the Sahlgrenska Hospital in Gothenburg, Sweden. Its discovery was based on the observations described by Frederick Bernheim in 1940. Bernhein observed that salicylate and benzoate stimulated the oxygen consumption of *Mycobacterium tuberculosis*, indicating its growth and virulence. In this context, Lehman conceived the idea that a biochemical inhibition of these compounds could be effective in blocking or retarding the growth of the *M. tuberculosis*, testing PAS in animals with good results. In 1946, a small clinical trial with 12 patients was reported with promising perspectives, and in 1948, the trials began demonstrating that PAS was effective against TB and resistant strains emerging during the streptomycin therapy, contributing for a better efficacy of streptomycin [70].

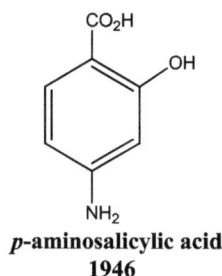

p-aminosalicylic acid
1946

Figure 7: Structure of *p*-aminosalicylic acid (PAS).

The Golden Era

After the discovery of streptomycin and PAS, the golden era of TB drug discovery started (1950 to 1970), with the discovery of many important drugs in TB treatment, anticipating the eradication of the disease [67]. In this context, many companies started to search for new compounds in the fight against TB. For example, in 1952, three companies Hoffman LaRoche, E.R. Squibb & Sons and Bayer discovered independently and almost simultaneously, a potent drug named isoniazid (Fig. **8**), which would change the TB history. This discovery was based on previous studies about the anti-TB properties of nicotinamide (Fig. **8**) made independently by Huant and Cover in 1945 and, McKenzie, in 1948. Another interesting fact in the isoniazid discovery was that, when the dispute about the brand name and patent rights were in advanced stage, the companies found out that this compound could not be patented. This molecule had already been discovered and described in 1912 by two Prague chemists, Hans Meyer and Josef Mally, as part of their Doctor of Philosophy (PhD), which synthesized this compound from ethyl isonicotinate and hydrazine, without knowing that they had in hand one of the most powerful anti TB drugs ever produced. The clinical trials of isoniazid were made by Robitzek and Selikoff at the Sea View Hospital, in New York in 1952 and it was soon introduced in the market. The benefits with its introduction were tremendous, due to its efficacy and low cost. For instance, before isoniazid, the price for treatment per patient in America was around $3.500 and after it, the price went down to less than $100, making TB treatment accessible to everybody and not only to rich people [71].

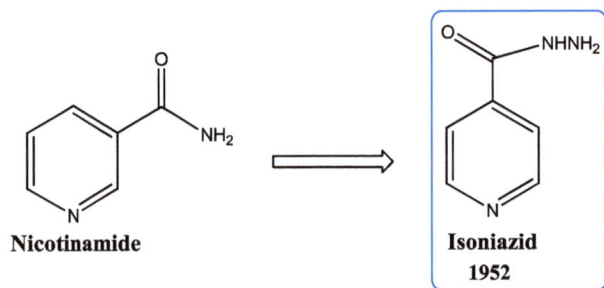

Figure 8: Structure of isoniazid and nicotinamide.

The discovery based on the anti-TB proprieties of nicotinamide also brought other important TB drugs into the fight against the disease, such as pyrazinamide (1952), ethionamide and prothionamide (1956) (Fig. **9**). Pyrazinamide synthesis was made independently in the same year by both Kushner at Lederle Research Laboratories and Solotorovski at the Merck laboratories. In the case of ethionamide and consequently, its analogue prothionamide, discovered by Lederle Research Laboratories, the synthesis was based on the work of Gardner and co-workers in 1951, which identified and declared that thioisonicotinamide (Fig. **9**) possessed anti-TB activity comparable to thiosemicarbazones. In 1961, another important TB drug, named ethambutol, was discovered by Lederle Research Laboratories (Fig. **9**). Its discovery was based on the fact that diamines and poliamines had good activity against *M. tuberculosis* [67].

TB TREATMENT

At present, the first-line TB treatment is based on six drugs: isoniazid, rifampicin, pyrazinamide, streptomycin, ethambutol and thiacetazone, which are available in cheap generic forms and are very effective, if taken as prescribed, curing more than 95% of the cases. These drugs complement each other and are used in various combinations, which are very important to prevent the emergence of multiple drug-resistant organisms that could lead to an ineffective treatment.

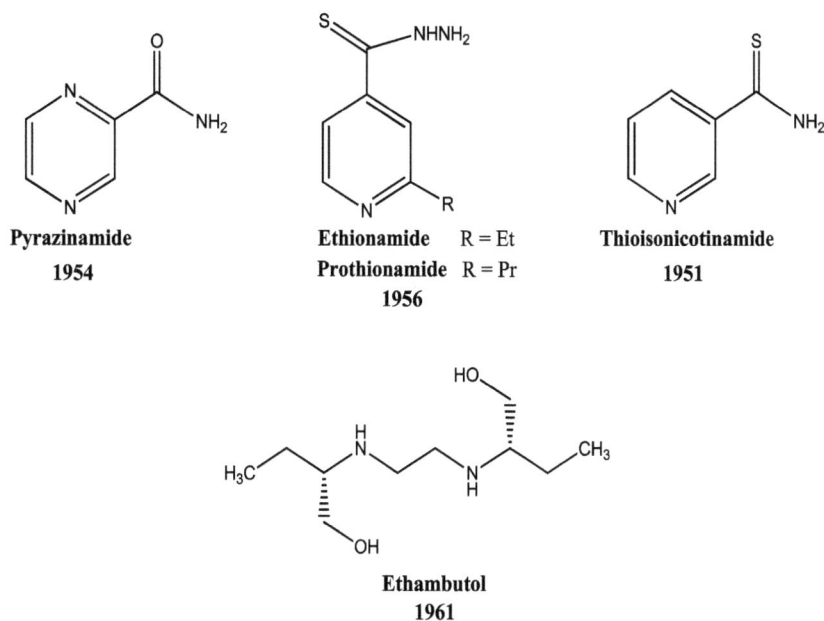

Figure 9: Structures of pyrazinamide, ethionamide, prothionamide, thioisonicotinamide and ethambutol.

A typical treatment for a non-drug resistant strain of TB is two months of isoniazid, pyrazinamide, ethambutol and rifampin, followed by four months of rifampin and isoniazid with the recommended dosage based on daily or thrice-weekly treatment (Table **5**) [72-79]. This TB treatment is called Directly Observed Treatment Short-Course (DOTS), which is a program internationally considered as the most cost-effective of all the health interventions, which started in 1990s. At that time, TB management was disorganized and ineffective. According to WHO, DOTS is based on five key principles: (1) government commitment to sustained TB control activities; (2) case detection by sputum smear microscopy among symptomatic patients self-reporting to health services; (3) standardized treatment regimen from six to eight months for, at least, all sputum smear-positive cases, with Directly Observed Therapy (DOT) for, at least, the initial two months; (4) a regular, uninterrupted supply of all essential anti TB drugs and (5) a standardized recording and reporting system, that allows assessment of treatment´s results for each patient and of overall TB control programme. This strategy, now covering 180 countries, is accessible for over 70% of the world population and DOTS has shown excellent results [72-79].

Table 5: Essential antituberculosis drugs.

Drugs Abreviations	MIC (µg/mL)	Mechanisms of Action	Dose Dorm
Isoniazid (INH)	0.01-0.2	Inhibition of mycolic acid synthesis (cell wall) and other mechanisms	Tablet 100, 300 mg
Rifampicin (RIF)	0.05-0.5	Inhibition of RNA synthesis	Tablet or capsule 150, 300 mg
Pyrazinamide (PYZ)	20-100 pH 5.5 or 6.0	Disruption of *M. tuberculosis* membrane transport and energetic	Tablet - 400 mg

Fixed-Dose Combination

The use of fixed-dose combination (FDC) tablets for TB treatment has been strongly recommended by WHO and The International Union Against Tuberculosis and Lung Disease since 1994 (Table **6**). This strategy can be defined as a formulation of two or more substances biologically active, combined in a single drug, available in certain fixed doses and it has a long history of development (Table **7**). For example, in the case of TB treatment history, after the introduction of streptomycin in the market, patients became resistant to this drug, and in 1948 it was administrated with PAS, contributing for a better efficacy of streptomycin. Nowadays, this strategy has been used successfully in different kinds of diseases, such as cancer, AIDS, malaria, infectious diseases, hypertension, neurological disorders and others. Several advantages can be seen in the employment of FDCs, including reduction in the risk of emergence of drug resistant strains and also, of medication errors, better patient compliance, reduction in the cost of treatment, dosages adjustment according to patients' needs and simplified drug supply management, shipping and distribution [72-79].

Table 6: Fixed-dose combination of drugs.

Drug	Dose Form	Strength for Daily Use	Strength for Use 3 Times Weekly
INH + RIF	tablet / tablet or pack or granules[a]	75 mg + 150 mg / 150 mg + 300 mg / 30 mg + 60 mg	150 mg + 150 mg / 60 mg + 60 mg
INH + ETH	tablet	150 mg + 400 mg	-
INH + RIF + PYZ	tablet / tablet or pack orgranules[a]	75 mg + 150 mg + 400 mg / 30 mg + 60 mg + 150 mg	150 mg +150 mg + 500 mg / -
INH + RIF + PYZ + ETH	tablet	75 mg + 150 mg + 400 mg + 275 mg	-

From essential drugs: WHO Model List (revised in December, 1999). In: *WHO drug information, 1999, 13(4):249-262.*
[a]For pediatric use.

Table 7: History of Fixed-dose combination in TB treatment.

Treatment	Specifications	Year of Introduction
Pediatric FDC	RIF + INH RIF + INH + PYZ RIF + INH + PYZ	1999 (WHO essential drug list) 13th WHO essential drug list
DOTS-Plus	MDR (Multidrug-resistant)-TB	1999 (WHO)
DOTS	Directly observed treatment, short course 4 drug FDC RIF + INH + ETH + PYZ	Early 1990s 1993 (available in market) 1999 (WHO essential drug list)
FDC	Thiacetazone + INH + ETH + INH RIF + INH + PYZ	1950s-1970's
DOT	Directly observed treatment	1958
Combination drug	Streptomycin + PAS INH + PAS INH + Streptomycin	1948 1952-1955 1952-1955

Causes of the Resurgence of TB

Due to the great progress made in TB treatment at the end of the 1970's, the scientific community believed that the disease would be finally eradicated. However, in 1981, a new disease, known as AIDS (Acquired Immune Deficiency Syndrome) was identified, a contagious disease that caused specific damage to the immunological system. The causative agent of AIDS, called Human Immunodeficiency Virus (HIV), is a retrovirus (RNA genome) that infects the cells and through enzymatic mechanisms incorporates its genome into human genome. AIDS is one of the major causes of the resurgence of TB. For example, the deadly combination between TB and HIV has led to a quadrupling of TB cases in several African and Asian countries. In the case of patients with AIDS, TB is the most common opportunistic infection and cause of death, killing 1 in every 3 patients. In addition, patients living with AIDS and contaminated with latent TB are 30 times more likely to develop active TB than no infected patients [80-82]. There are also different factors which are responsible for the resurgence of TB, such as immigration, war, famine, homelessness, the lack of new drugs and multi-drug-resistant tuberculosis (MDR TB) due to inconsistent or partial treatment. Considering TB problems, the World Health Organization (WHO) declared this disease a global health emergency in 1993.

Isoniazid or Rifampin Resistant Strain and MDR-TB

At present, it is difficult to estimate, but, at least, 4% of all TB patients worldwide are resistant to, at the minimum, one of the current first-line drugs. When standard treatments fail due to resistant strains to isoniazid or rifampin, there are some treatment plans (Table **8**). However, a more serious problem in TB treatment is the advent of MDR-TB (multidrug-resistant tuberculosis), which is defined as resistance to, at the minimum, rifampicin and isoniazid. It is estimated that, at least, 20 percent of all registered TB cases were caused by MDR-TB. Several elements are responsible for MDR-TB problem, such as poor social conditions, incorrect prescriptions, abandonment of treatment, immigration from countries with high rates of MDR-TB and no public health care system [78,79,83].

Table 8: Treatment plans for resistant TB.

Isoniazid-Resistant TB	Rifampin-Resistant TB
1) Rifampin/rifabutin, pyrazinamide and ethambutol daily for at least 2 weeks. **2)** The same three drugs twice a week for 6-9 months.	**1)** Isoniazid, streptomycin, pyrazinamide + ethambutol (daily for 8 weeks or daily for 2 weeks + twice a week for 6 weeks). **2)** Isoniazid, streptomycin + pyrazinamide 2-3 times a week for 7 months.

National HIV/AIDS (www.projectinform.org)

The treatment of MDR-TB is complex (Table **9**) and requires careful diagnosis, employing laboratories to follow drug-susceptibility, hospitalization, at least in the beginning of the treatment and the use of second line drugs, such as amikacin (Am), capreomycin (Cm), ciprofloxacin (Cp), cycloserine (Cs), ethionamide (Eti), kanamycin (Km), ofloxacin (Of), *p*-aminosalicylic acid (PAS) and protionamide (Prt), which are the last line of defense in the fight against TB. According to WHO, the re-treatment regimen should include at the minimum four drugs never used by the patient, including an injectable amikacin, capreomycin or kanamycin and a fluoroquinolone. Pyrazinamide and ethambutol can be added in the treatment because of lower probability of resistance than other essential drugs. However, the problem of second-line drugs are much lower efficacy and the requirement of even longer administration periods (18-24 months) with higher cost (from $19.000 to 50.000 per person). Depending on the complexity of the treatment, it can reach 1 million dollars per person, compared to only $10-20 of the standard treatment, higher rates of adverse effects (Tables **10** and **11**) and low cure rates (around 60%) compared to more than 95% in the current TB treatment [67,78,79]. Due to the MDR-TB problem, in 1999, WHO established the Working Group on DOTS-Plus for MDR-TB. DOTS-Plus is based on the five key elements of the DOTS strategy and its main goal is preventing the development and spread of drug resistance. In this context, WHO and co-workers have developed guidelines to treat, manage and survey MDR-TB, which is an important measure in the fight against drug resistance. Other actions have also helped the combat against MDR-TB, such as The Green Light Committee (GLC), based in the WHO Headquarters, in Geneva, which focuses on finding alternatives to provide second-line TB drugs at lower cost [72-79].

Table 9: Suggested treatment regimens [78].

Susceptibility to Essential Drugs	Initial Phase		Continuation Phase	
	Drug	**Duration**	**Drug**	**Duration**
Resistance to INH+RIF	Sm[a]+Eti+FQ[b]+PYZ+/-ETH at least 6 months		Eti+FQ+PYZ+/-ETH 12-18 months	
Resistence to all Essential drugs	1 injectable + 1 fluoroquinolone + 2 of these 3 oral drugs: PAS, Eti, Cs	at least 6 months	The same drug 18 months except injectable	

[a]if resistence to S is confirmed, replace this drug with Km, Am or Cm.
[b]Fluoroquinolone (FQ) (ciprofloxacin or ofloxacin).

WHO/CDS/TB/2003.313 Treatment of tuberculosis: guidelines for national programmes, third edition revision approved by STAG, June 2004.

Table 10: Side effects of first line anti-TB drugs.

Drug	Side Effects	Potential Drug Interations
Isoniazid	**Mild:** Rash, gut upset, headache, fever, loss of appetite, joint pain and mood changes. **Severe:** Hypersensitivity, anemia, peripheral, neuropathy and dizziness liver problems.	Antacids increased blood levels of phenytoin, psychotic episodes with disulfiram, alcohol and steroids.
Rifampin	**Mild:** Fever, abdominal distress, rash, gut upset, orange body fluids (urine, tears and saliva) and light sensitive. **Severe:** Exfoliative dermatitis in HIV positive cases, anemia, acute renal failure, and liver problems.	Oral contraceptives, oral anticoagulants, azole-anti-fungal drugs, dapsone, methadone, sulfonylureas and anti retroviral drugs (most PIs and NNRTIs).

Table 10: contd....

Pyrazinamide	**Mild:** fever, abdominal distress, arthralgia, fever, hepatitis and rash. **Severe:** Hepatitis, light sensitivity and skin flushing.	
Ethambutol	Eyesight problems, gut upset, rash, fever, headache and dizziness.	Antacids

Table 11: Side effects of second line anti-TB drugs.

Drug	Side Effects	Potential Drug Interations
Amikacin, Kanamycin and Streptomycin	Hypersensitivity, joint pain, kidney problems, inner ear damage, nausea and rash.	Some antibiotics and diuretics.
Ciprofloxacin, Ofloxacin and Levofloxacin	Rash, allergic reaction, sleep problems, abdominal distress, headache, anxiety, tremors, diarrhea, hepatitis, arthralgia.	Antacids.
Cycloserine	Dizziness, headache, mood and cognitive deterioration, psychosis, tremors, seizures and neuropathy.	Isoniazid, ethionamide and alcohol.
Ethionamide	Liver problems, nausea, anorexia, diarrhea, rash and gut upset.	
PAS	Liver problems, diarrhea, abdominal distress and hypothyroidism.	
Rifapentine	Fever, eye inflammation, hepatitis, joint pain, rash, gut upset, orange body fluids (urine, tears and saliva), light sensitivity, liver function changes and acute renal failure.	Oral contraceptives, steroids, fluconazole, alcohols, methadone and protease inhibitors.

XDR-TB

Recently, another important factor in TB treatment worldwide is the advent of XDR (Extensive Drug Resistant or Extreme Drug Resistance), which is commonly defined as strains resistance to all the current first-line drugs, as well as any fluoroquinolone and, at least, to 1 of 3 injectable second-line drugs (capreomycin, kanamycin or amikacin), which like MDR-TB can be transmitted from an infectious patient to other people. This definition of XDR-TB was agreed by the WHO Global Task Force on XDR-TB in October, 2006 [83-85].

The principles of the treatment for XDR-TB are the same for MDR and standard TB, however, due to the reduced number of drugs used in the treatment, the rate of mortality, cost, time of hospitalization and side effects are much higher when compared to MDR-TB. One important study in XDR-TB treatment was made by Keshavjee and co-workers in the Tomsk oblast of Russia, reporting that 14 out of 29 (48.3%) patients successfully completed the treatment [86]. Currently, another important problem of drug resistent tuberculosis is known as XXDR or TDR-TB (Totally drug-resistance tuberculosis) strains that are resistant to a wide variety of drugs used to treat tuberculosis.

ACKNOWLEDGEMENT

None Declare.

CONFLICT OF INTEREST

The author(s) confirm that this chapter content has no conflict of interest.

REFERENCES

[1]   Zink AR, Sola C, Reischl U, Grabner W, Rastogi N, Wolf H, Nerlich AG. Characterization of *Mycobacterium tuberculosis* complex DNAs from Egyptian Mummies by spoligotyping. *Journal of Clinical Microbiology* 2003;**41**:359-67.

[2]   Latour B. Did Ramses II die from tuberculosis? *Recherche* 1998;**307**:84-85.

[3]   Ziskind B, Halioua B. Tuberculosis in ancient Egypt. *Revue des maladies respiratoires* 2007;**24**:1277-83.

[4]   Nerlich AG, Haas CJ, Zink A, Szeimies U, Hagedorn HG. Molecular evidence for tuberculosis in an ancient Egyptian mummy. *Lancet* 1997;**350**:1404.

[5]   Zimmerman MR. Pulmonary and osseous tuberculosis in an Egyptian mummy. *Bulletin of the New York Academy of Medicine* 1979;**55**:604-8.

[6]   Ortner DJ. Disease and mortality in the Early Bronze Age people of Bab edh - Dhra, Jordan. *American journal of physical anthropology* 1979;**51**:589-97.

[7]   Subba RDV. Tuberculosis in ancient India. *Bulletin of the Indian Institute of History of Medicine (Hyderabad)* 1972;**2**:156-61.

[8]   Daniel TM. The History of tuberculosis. *Respiratory Medicine* 2006;**100**:1862-70.

[9]   Susan W. Henry IV of France touching for scrofula, by Pierre Firens. *Journal of the history of medicine and allied sciences* 2003;**58**:79-81.

[10]   Grzybowski S, Allen EA. History and importance of scrofula. *Lancet* 1995;**346**:1472-4.

[11]   Salo WL, Aufderheide AC, Buikstra JH, Todd A. Identification of Mycobacterium tuberculosis DNA in a pre-Columbian Peruvian mummy. *Proceedings of the National Academy of Sciences of the United States of America* 1994;**91**:2091-4.

[12]   Arriaza BT, Salo W, Aufderheide AC, Holcomb TA. Pre-Columbian tuberculosis in northern Chile:molecular and skeletal evidence. *American journal of physical anthropology* 1995;**98**:37-45.

[13]   Bernier J. The interpretation of pulmonary tuberculosis in the 18th century. *Canadian bulletin of medical history = Bulletin canadien d'histoire de la medicine* 2005;**22**:35-56.

[14]   Smith NH, Hewinson RG, Kremer K, Brosch R, Gordon SV. Myths and misconceptions:the origin and evolution of *Mycobacterium tuberculosis*. *Nature Reviews Microbiology* 2009;**7**:537-544.

[15]   Mostowy S, Behr MA. The origin and evolution of *Mycobacterium tuberculosis*. *Clin Chest Med* 2005;**26**:207-16,v-vi.

[16]   Cole ST. Learning from the genome sequence of *Mycobacterium tuberculosis* H37Rv. *FEBS Letters* 1999;**452**:7-10.

[17]   Rothschild BM, Martin LD, Lev G, Bercovier H, Bar-Gal GK, Greenblatt C, Donoghue H, Spigelman M, Brittain D. *Mycobacterium tuberculosis* complex DNA from an extinct bison dated 17,000 years before the present. *Clinical Infectious Diseases* 2001;**33**:305-11.

[18]   Kapur V, Whittam TS, Musser JM. Is *Mycobacterium tuberculosis* 15,000 years old? *J Infect Dis* 1994;**170**:1348-49.

[19]   Donoghue HD, Spigelman M, Greenblatt CL, Lev-Maor G, Bar-Gal, G K, Matheson C, Vernon K, Nerlich AG, Zink AR. Tuberculosis:from prehistory to Robert Koch, as revealed by ancient DNA. *Lancet Infectious Diseases* 2004;**4**:584-592.

[20]   Hayman J. *Mycobacterium ulcerans:*an infection from Jurassic time? *Lancet* 1984;**2**:1015-1016.

[21]   Philipp WJ, Nair S, Guglielmi G, Lagranderie M, Gicquel B, Cole ST. Physical mapping of *Mycobacterium bovis* BCG Pasteur reveals differences from the genome map of *Mycobacterium tuberculosis* H37Rv and from *M. bovis*. *Microbiology* 1996;**142**:3135-45.

[22]   Irgens L. The discovery of *Mycobacterium leprae*. A medical achievement in the light of evolving scientific methods. Am J Dermatopathol 1984;**6**:337-43.

[23]   Visschedijk JBJ, Eggens H, Lever P, Van Beers S, Klatser P. *Mycobacterium leprae* - millennium resistant ! Leprosy control on the threshold of a new era. *Tropical medicine & international health:TM & IH* 2000;**5**:388-99.

[24]   Dormandy T. The White Death. A History of Tuberculosis. Hambledon and London, 2001, p.28-39;131-32.

[25]   http://en.wikipedia.org/wiki/Girolamo_Fracastoro

[26]   Ustun C. Dr. Thomas Willis´ Famous Eponym:The Circle of Willis. *Turk J. Med. Sci.* 2004;**34**:271-4.

[27]   Baker RCJr. Leeuwenhoek, the short-focus lens and the history of optics;an experimental inquiry. *Microscope* 1993;**41**:1-6.

[28]   Morton LT. Le Boe, F. (SYLVIUS) - Opera medica, 1679. *In* MORTON, L.T.:A medical bibliography (Garrison and Morton). London, Butler & Tammer Ltd., 1983,p.300.

[29]   http://en.wikipedia.org/wiki/Thomas_Sydenham

[30]   Silverman JA. Richard Morton 1637 - 1698. Limner of anorexia nervosa:his life and times. A tercentenary essay. *JAMA:the journal of the American Medical Association* 1983;**250**:2830-2.

[31]   Dormandy T. The White Death. A History of Tuberculosis. Hambledon and London, 2001, p.52-3.

[32]   http://www.whonamedit.com/doctor.cfm/2053.html

[33]   Nicos PH, Doreen JAH. Cryptic miliary tuberculosis with a clinical prodrome resembling pancreatitis. *Respiratory Medicine Extra* 2006;**2**:95-97.

[34]   Doetsch, RN. Benjamin Marten and his "New Theory of Consumptions". *Microbiological reviews* 1978;**42**:521-8.

[35]   Fontanini F. Leopold Auenbrugger and chest percussion. *Giornale italiano di cardiologia* 1986;**16**:445-6.

[36]   Doyle L. William Stark (1740-1770):his life, manuscript and death. *Journal of Medical Biography* 2000;**8**:146-8.

[37]   Dormandy T. The White Death. A History of Tuberculosis. Hambledon and London, 2001, p.28-39;334-38.

[38]   Rousseau A. Gaspard - Laurent Bayle (1774-1816), the theorist of the Ecole de Paris. *Clio medica (Amsterdam, Netherlands)* 1971;**6**:205-11.

[39]   Gauger GE. The great mind of Thomas Young (1773-1829). *Documenta ophthalmologica. Advances in ophthalmology* 1997;**94**:113-21.

[40]   Roguin AR. Theophile Hyacinthe Laennec (1781-1826):the man behind the stethoscope. *Clinical medicine & research* 2006;**4**:230-5.

[41]   Dormandy T. The White Death. A History of Tuberculosis. Hambledon and London, 2001, p.57-59.

[42]   Thomas SW, Conner EH, Meloy HA. History of Mammoth Cave, emphasizing tourist development and medical experimentation under Dr. John Croghan. *Regist Ky Hist Soc.* 1970;**68**:319-40.

[43]   Cook GC. Early use of "open - air" treatment for "pulmonary phthisis" at the Dreadnought Hospital, Greenwich, 1900-1905. *Postgraduate medical journal* 1999;**75**:326-7.

[44]   Dormandy T. The White Death. A History of Tuberculosis. Hambledon and London, 2001, p.151-2.

[45]   Meade GM. Edward Livingston Trudeau, M.D. *Tubercle* 1972;**53**:229-50.

[46]   Chretien J. Commemoration of the hundredth anniversary of the death of Jean - Antoine Villemin (1827-1892). *Bulletin de l'Academie nationale de medicine* 1992;**176**:1017-22.

[47]   Munch R. Robert Koch. *Microbes and Infection* 2003;**5**:69-74.

[48]   Kaufmann SHE, Schaible UE.100th anniversary of Robert Koch's Nobel Prize for the discovery of the tubercle bacillus. *Trends in Microbiology* 2005;**13**:469-475.

[49]   Gradmann C. Robert Koch and the white death:from tuberculosis to tuberculin. *Microbes and Infection* 2006;**8**:294-301.

[50]   Sakula A. Carlo Forlanini, inventor of artificial pneumothorax for treatment of pulmonary tuberculosis. *Thorax* 1983;**38**:326-32.

[51]   Dunn PM. Wilhelm Conrad Roentgen (1845 - 1923), the discovery of X-rays and perinatal diagnosis. *Archives of disease in childhood. Fetal and neonatal edition* 2001;**84**:F138-9.

[52]   Crispen R. History of BCG and its substrains. *Progress in clinical and biological research* 1989;**310**:35-50.

[53]   Verhoef J. The BCG controversy. *International journal of antimicrobial agents* 1994;**44**:291-5.

[54]   Toida I. Development of the *Mycobacterium bovis* BCG vaccine:review of the historical and biochemical evidence for a genealogical tree. *Tubercle and lung disease:the official journal of the International Union against Tuberculosis and Lung Disease* 2000;**80**:291.

[55]   Bosch F, Rosich L. The contributions of Paul Ehrlich to pharmacology:a tribute on the occasion of the centenary of his Nobel Prize. *Pharmacology* 2008;**82**:171-179.

[56]   Strebhardt K, Ullrich A. Paul Ehrlich's magic bullet concept:100 years of progress. *Nature Reviews Cancer* 2008;**8**:473-480.

[57]   Winau F, Westphal O, Winau R. Paul Ehrlich - in search of the magic bullet. *Microbes and Infection* 2004;**6**:786-789

[58]   Kaufmann, SHE. Paul Ehrlich:founder of chemotherapy. *Nature Reviews Drug Discovery* 2008;**7**:373.

[59]   Riethmiller S. From Atoxyl to Salvarsan:Searching for the magic bullet. *Chemotherapy* 2005;**51**:234-242.

[60]   Lloyd NC, Morgan HW, Nicholson BK, Ronimus RS. The composition of Ehrlich's salvarsan:Resolution of a century-old debate. *Angewandte Chemie, International Edition* 2005;**44**:941-944.

[61]   Benedek TG. The history of gold therapy for tuberculosis. *Journal of the history of medicine and allied sciences* 2004;**59**:50-89.

[62]   Bennett JW, Chung KT. Alexander Fleming and the discovery of penicillin. *Advances in Applied Microbiology* 2001;**49**:163-184.

[63]   Chain, E. The early years of the penicillin discovery. *Trends in Pharmacological Sciences* 1979;**1**:6-11.

[64]   Kyle RA, Shampo MA. Gerhard Domagk. *JAMA:The journal of the American Medical Association* 1982;**247**:2581.

[65]   Raju TN. The Nobel chronicles 1939:Gerhard Domagk (1895-1964). *Lancet* 1999;**353**:681.

[66]   Streptomycin, Schatz v. Waksman, and the balance of credit for discovery;W. Kingston *Journal of the history of medicine and allied sciences* 2004;**59**:441-462.

[67]   Souza MVN. Promising Drugs Against Tuberculosis. *Recent Patents on Anti-Infective Drug Discovery* 2006;**1**:33-45.

[68]   Floss HG, Yu TW. Rifamycin - Mode of action, resistance, and Biosynthesis. *Chem. Rev.* 2005;**105**:621-632.

[69]   Sirgel FA, Fourie FA, Donald PR. The early bacterial activities of rifampin and rifapentine in pulmonary tuberculosis. *Am J Respir Crit Care Med* 2005;**172**:128-135.

[70]   Dormandy T. The White Death. A History of Tuberculosis. Hambledon and London, 2001, p.366-367.

[71]   Dormandy T. The White Death. A History of Tuberculosis. Hambledon and London, 2001, p.367-368.

[72]   Treatment of Tuberculosis:Guidelines for National Programs, Geneva, World Health Organization, 2003. WHO/CDS/TB/2003.313.

[73]   Extra-pulmonary TB. Extra-pulmonary TB and the Revised National Tuberculosis Control Programme India:diagnosis, treatment and outcomes [onlineresource]. http://www.sunmed.org/ep-paper.html. [Accessed:20 June 2013].

[74]   De Souza, MVN. Current Status and Future Prospects for New Therapies for Pulmonary Tuberculosis. *Current Opinion in Pulmonary Medicine*, 2006;**12**:167-171.

[75]   Humphries M. Tuberculosis:history of directly observed therapy. *Lancet* 1995;**346**:380.

[76]   Bayer R, Wilkinson D. Directly observed therapy for tuberculosis:history of an idea. *Lancet* 1995;**345**:1545-8.

[77]   Panchagnula R, Agrawal S, Ashokraj Y, Varma M, Sateesh K, Bhardwaj V, Bedi S, Gulati I, Parmar J, Kaul CL, Blomberg B, Fourie B, Roscigno G, Wire R, Laing R, vans P, Moore T. Fixed dose combinations for tuberculosis:Lessons learned from clinical formulation and regulatory perspective. *Methods and Findings in Experimental and Clinical Pharmacology* 2004;**26**:703-721.

[78]   De Souza MVN. *New Strategies Combating Bacterial Infection.* Iqbal A and Farrukh A. Ed.;Wiley-VCH Verlag GmbH and Co. KGaA:Weinheim **2008**;vol *3*,p.71-87.

[79]   De Souza MVN, Gonçalves RSB, Ferreira ML. *Frontiers in Anti-Infective Drug Discovery.* Atta-ur-Rahman FRS & Iqbal CM. Ed.;Bentham **2009**;vol *9*,p.176-201.

[80]   http://www.avert.org/globalstats.htm

[81]   De Souza MVN, De Almeida MV. Drugs anti-HIV:past, present and future perspectives. *Quim. Nova* 2003;**26**:366-372.

[82]   Sharma SK, Mohan AK. HIV-TB co-infection:Epidemiology, diagnosis & management. *Indian Journal Medicinal Research* 2005;**121**:550-567.

[83]   Mukherjee JS, Rich ML, Socci AR, Joseph JK, Viru FA, Shi SS, Furin JJ, Becerra MC, Barry DJ, Kim JY, Bayona J, Farmer P, Fawzi MCS, Seung KJ. Programs and principles in treatment of multidrug-resistant tuberculosis. *Lancet* 2004;**363**:474-81.

[84]   Raviglione, M. C. and Smith, I. M. XDR Tuberculosis - Implications for Global Public Health *N. Engl. J. Med.* 2007:356-57.

[85]   http://www.who.int/tb/challenges/xdr/xdrtb_sept06news.pdf

[86]   http://ghsm.hms.harvard.edu/uploads/pdf/Annals_NYAS_2007_Tomsk.pdf

CHAPTER 2

Promising Drug Candidates in Advanced Clinical Trials

Marcus V.N. de Souza[*]

Instituto de Tecnologia em Fármacos – Farmanguinhos, FioCruz – Fundação Oswaldo Cruz, R. Sizenando Nabuco, 100, Manguinhos, 21041-250, Rio de Janeiro, RJ, Brazil

Abstract: To overcome the problems with available treatments, new drugs to treat TB are urgently required, specifically more potent therapies, with fewer side effects, to be used in shorter treatment regimens and to be employed to treat MDR TB and latent disease. Unfortunately, after the introduction of rifampin in the market (1966-1970), no new classes of anti-TB drugs have been developed in the last forty-three year, excepted by rifapentine, a very close analog of rifampin, which was introduced by the FDA in 1998 and more recently bedaquiline, a diarylquinoline approved by FDA for multidrug-resistant tuberculosis in December 2012. In this context, different new initiatives have been created to obtain promising drug candidates. Considering that, this chapter will be highlights promising drugs in advanced clinical trials that may soon be introduced onto the market.

Keywords: Tuberculosis, *Mycobacterium tuberculosis*, drugs, drug development, treatment, clinical trials, multi-drug-resistant tuberculosis (MDR TB), extensive-drug-resistant tuberculosis (XDR TB), AIDS, target, mechanism of action, synthesis.

INTRODUCTION

In spite of the high impact caused by tuberculosis worldwide nowadays, nearly 41 years have passed since a novel drug was introduced into the market to treat TB, except for rifapentine (1998), a very close analogue of rifampin and more recently bedaquiline, a diarylquinoline approved by FDA for multidrug-resistant tuberculosis in December 2012. Due to the increase of MDR and XDR-TB in the world, we need desperately of new strategies, treatments and drugs to face this new problem or no available treatment will be distributed. In this context, we can

Adress correspondence to Marcus V.N. de Souza: Instituto de Tecnologia em Fármacos – Farmanguinhos, FioCruz – Fundação Oswaldo Cruz, R. Sizenando Nabuco, 100, Manguinhos, 21041-250, Rio de Janeiro, RJ, Brazil; E-mail: marcos_souza@far.fiocruz.br

go back into the past when people died of tuberculosis in the sanatorium without treatment. Considering this problem, several actions have been taken and, in 2000, the Global Alliance for TB Drug Development (GATB; www.tballiance.org) was established, being the TB drug development its main priority. In this context, GATB has been working in partnership with different kinds of organizations, such as academic institutions, government research laboratories, non-governmental organizations, pharmaceutical industry and contract research houses. Due to its important work, GATB has changed the perspective of TB drug discovery.

PROBLEMS AND GOALS IN THE DEVELOPMENT OF NEW ANTI-TB DRUGS

There are basic factors involved in the development of new anti-TB drugs, such as more effective treatment of latent tuberculosis infection, prevention and treatment of the MDR-TB and potent sterilizing activity, which is defined as the ability of a drug, such as pyrazinamide and rifampin to destroy the bacteria, known as persisters. The sterilizing activity is closely related to the time of the treatment. Other important factors can be mentioned, for instance, cost, new mechanisms of action, good pharmacokinetic distribution and permeation into cells and lung tissue, potent bactericidal and selective activity against *Mycobacterial* species. Another problem to be solved is the combined treatment TB/HIV, which has several disadvantages and problems, such as a large number of pills, patient adherence, prolonged treatment regimens, immune reconstitution inflammatory syndrome, drug resistance in both etiological agents, overlapping side effect profiles of anti-TB and anti-HIV drugs and drug-drug interactions. One example of drug-drug interactions is the co-administration between protease inhibitors and rifampicin, which induces cytochrome oxidases P450 and accelerated the metabolism of this class of anti-HIV drugs reducing its concentration. Another point to be considered is that protease inhibitors reduced the metabolism of rifampin decreasing its serum concentration leading a higher toxicity level. For that reasons, the co-administration of rifampin and protease inhibitors are contraindicated [1]. Despite of the complexity on the development of new anti-TB drugs, some compounds are in advanced clinical trials (Fig. **1** and Tables **1** and **2**) [2-4].

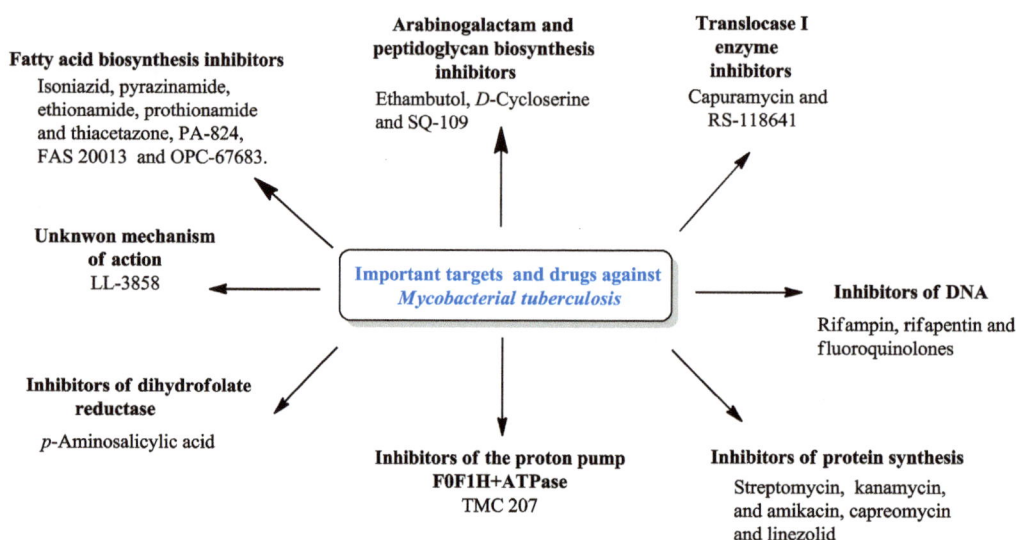

Figure 1: Important targets and drugs used or in development against tuberculosis.

Table 1: New promising drugs candidates in clinical trials against MDR-TB.

Compound	Class of Compound	Developer	Clinical Phase
Gatifloxacin	Fluoroquinolone	BMS	Phase III
Moxifloxacin	Fluoroquinolone	Bayer	Phase III
OPC-67683	Nitroimidazo oxazole	Otsuka Pharmaceutical	Phase III
PA-824	Nitroimidazol	PathoGenesis Inc	Phase II
SQ-109	Diamine	Sequella Inc.	Phase II
Linezolide	Oxazolidinone	Pharmacia Corporation	Phase II
Sutezolid	Oxazolidinone	Pfizer.Inc	Phase II
AZD-5847	Oxazolidinone	AstraZeneca	Phase II

Table 2: New promising drugs candidates in clinical trials against MDR-TB.

Compound	MIC (μg/mL)	Mechanism of Action	Sponsor/Coordinator
Gatifloxacin	0.03-0.12	Inhibition DNA replication transcription	European Comission; IRD; WHO/TDR; Lupin
Moxifloxacin	0.06-0.5	Inhibition DNA replication Transcription	Bayer; TB Alliance; CDC; University College London; John Hopk.U.
OPC-67683	0.006-0.012	Inhibition of cell wall biosynthesis	Otsuka Pharmaceutical
PA-824	0.015-0.25	Inhibition of protein synthesis Inhibition of cell wall lipids synthesis	TB Alliance

Table 2: contd...

SQ-109	0.16-0.32	Inhibition of cell wall Biosynthesis	Sequella Inc
Linezolid	0.125-0.50	Inhibition of protein synthesis	Pharmacia Corporation
Sutezolid	0.03-0.50	Inhibition of protein synthesis	Pfizer.Inc
AZD-5847	0.25-8.0	Inhibition of protein synthesis	AstraZeneca

PROMISING DRUG CANDIDATES IN ADVANCED CLINICAL TRIALS AGAINST TB

Fluoroquinolones

Fluoroquinolones is nowadays, an important class of synthetic antibacterial agents in modern arsenal against several bacterial infections, possessing a broad spectrum of activity against Gram-positive, Gram-negative and mycobacterial organisms as well as anaerobes [2,5-7]. For example, this new class of antibiotics is the first-line therapy for complicated urinary tract and bacterial diarrhea. They are also alternatives agents for the treatment of many sexually transmitted diseases, as well as osteomyelitis, some cases of wound infection and selected respiratory infections [5,7].

The history of fluoroquinolones began when Lescher, in 1962, discovered accidentally the nalidixic acid, 1-ethyl-4-oxo-1,8-naphthyridin-3-carboxylic acid as byproduct during the synthesis of the antimalarial compound chloroquine (Fig. **2**) [6]. In 1963 nalidixic acid was approved by the FDA for the treatment of urinary tract infection with a moderate activity on Gram-negative bacteria. In 1970´s the quinolones cinoxacin, oxolinic acid and pipemidic acid (Fig. **2**) were employed with a little improvement in comparison with nalidixic acid. However, it was only during the 1980´s with the combination of a fluorine atom at position 6 and piperazinyl group at position 7 in the norfloxacin (Fig. **2**) that the importance of quinolones started [6]. This combination produced a broad spectrum of activity and better pharmacokinetic profile against Gram-negatives and some Gram-positives bacteria with antibacterial activities 1000 times more potent that those observed in the nalidixic acid [6].

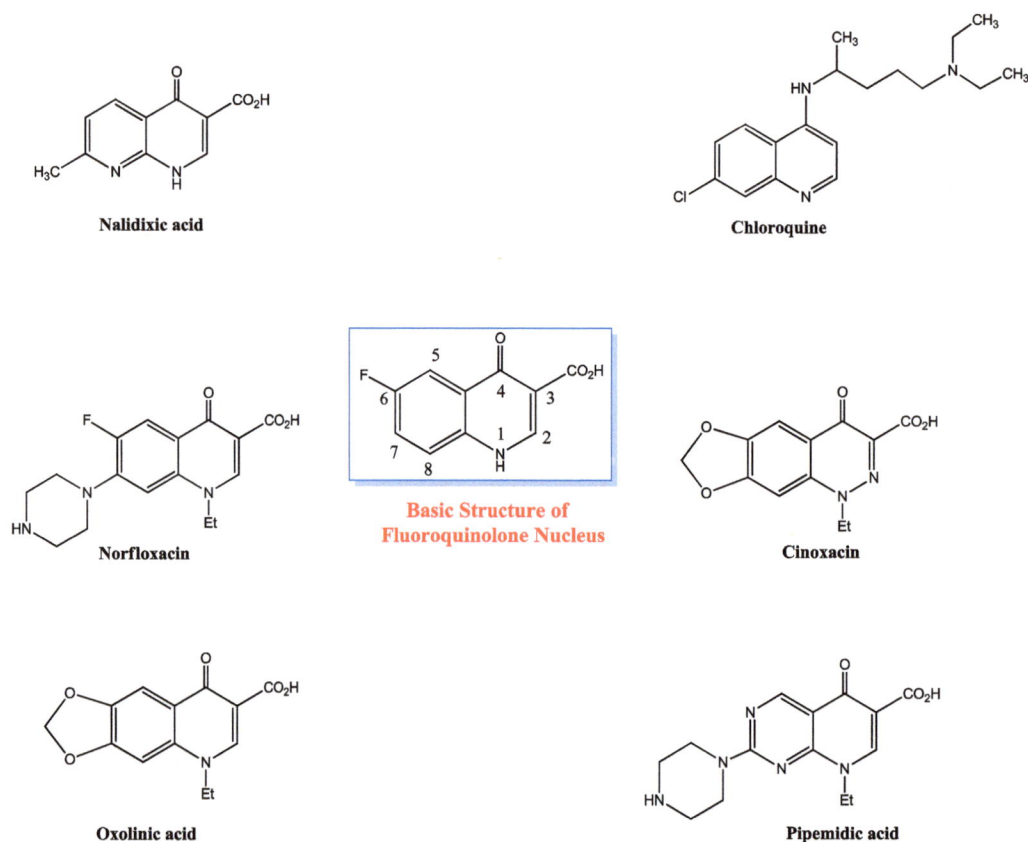

Figure 2: Fluoroquinolone drug development.

Quinolone Structure-Activity Relationship (SAR)

A number of structure-activity relationships (SAR) have been examined for the quinolones, but is mainly focused on C-6, C-7 and N-1 substituents [5-7]. These positional modifications of the parent structure showed that higher potency as well as broader bacterial coverage occurred with a fluorine atom at C-6 and the concomitant presence of the heterocyclic base of optimal size, preferentially a piperazine or a pyrrolidine moitey, at C-7. In general, optimum activity requires a substituent at the N-1 position and today the cyclopropyl group is recognized as one of the most effective substituents (Fig. **3**). The modifications of the positions C-5 and 8 could also provided improvement in the potency of this class being found in newer fluoroquinolone generations [5-7].

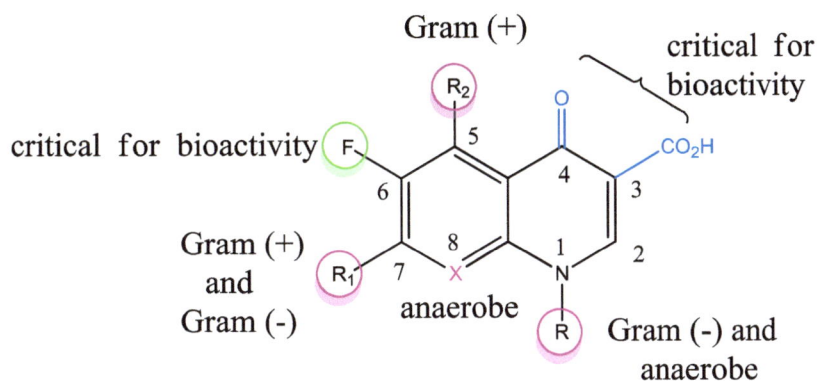

Fluoroquinolonic Nucleus

Figure 3: Structure-activity relationships (SAR) of fluoroquinolones [6].

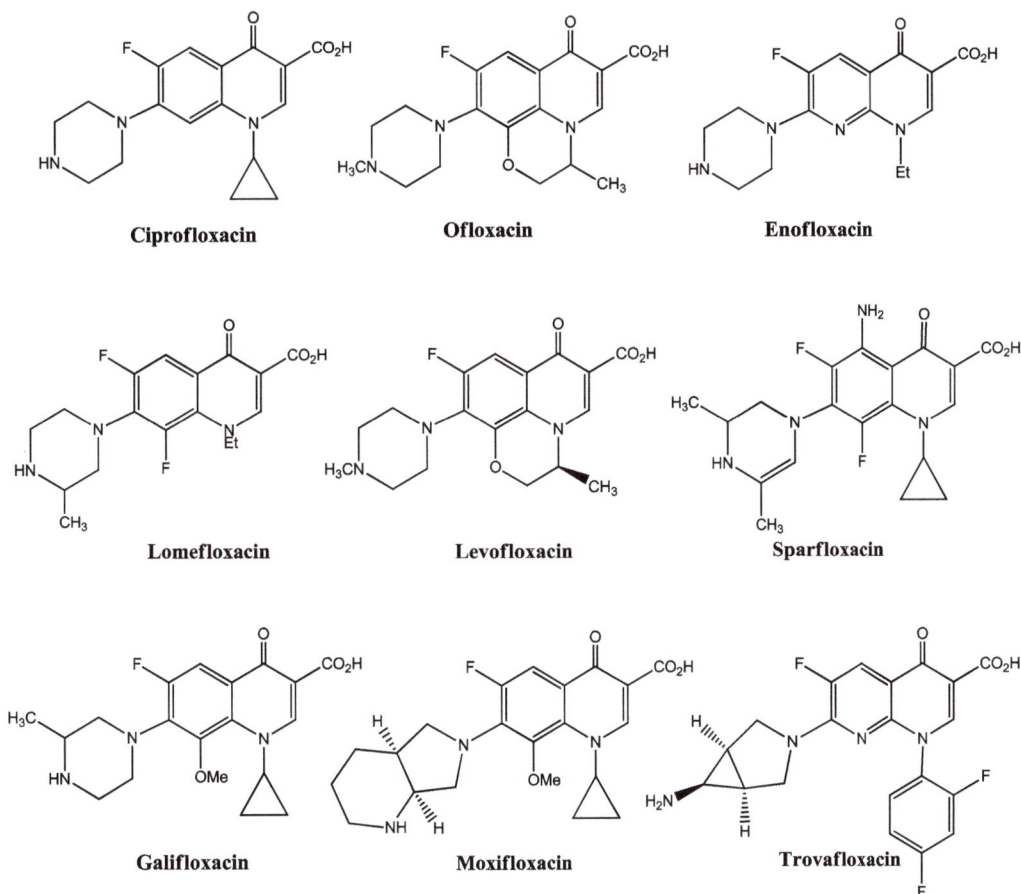

Figure 4: Second, third and fourth fluoroquinolone generations [7].

Basic the fluoroquinolones can be devised in four generations. The first generation is represented by nalidixic acid and cinoxacin, the second one by norfloxacin, ciprofloxacin (Cp), ofloxacin (Of), enoxacin and lomefloxacin, the third one by levofloxacin (LVX), sparfloxacin (STX) and gatifloxacin (GTX) and, finally, the fourth generation is represented by moxifloxacin (MFX) and trovafloxacin (TVX) (Fig. **4**) [7].

Mechanism of Action and Resistance

In 1975, Smith and workers showed that nalidixic acid act by inhibiting an important enzyme for bacterial multiplication. This enzyme was purified in 1976 by Gellert and workers and named DNA gyrase (topoisomerase II) an essential enzyme involved in the replication, transcription and reparation of the bacterials DNA [7]. DNA gyrase is composed of a tetramer of two GyrA and GyrB subunits each. Specifically, fluoroquinolones inhibit DNA gyrase bacterial type II and topoisomerase IV. Topoisomerase IV is composed of a tetramer of two ParC and ParE subunits each. Topoisomerase IV is responsible for decatenation, that is removing the interlinking of daughter chromosomes, thereby allowing segregation into two daughter cells at the end of the replication round. After the use of nalidixic acid in 1962, bacterials showed a fast resistance to the older fluoroquinolones whereas topoisomerase IV is basically the primary target in Gram-positive bacteria with important implications in the development of resistance [7]. The efficacy of the new fluoroquinolones against resistant strains is due to their dual activity inhibiting both DNA gyrase bacterial type II and topoisomerase IV that limit the emergence of fluoroquinolones resistance [6-8].

Recently, the fourth generation fluoroquinolones have attracted much attention due their fewer toxic effects, improved pharmacokinetic properties and extensive and potent activity against Gram-positive and Gram-negative bacteria, including resistant strains when compared with the earlier fluoroquinolones (Table **3**) because they attack both DNA gyrase and topoisomerase IV [6].

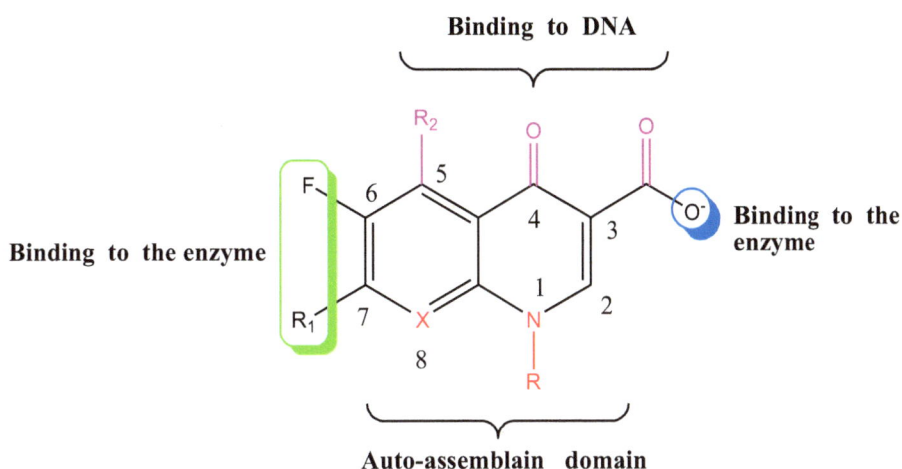

Figure 5: Biological interactions with fluoroquinolones [6].

Table 3: Spectrum of fluoroquinolones activity against several bacterial species [6].

Spectrum of Fluoroquinolones Activity					
Drug	Gram-Positive	Gram-Negative	Anaerobic Species	STD Organism	Pseudomonas Species
Ofloxacin	+	+++	0	+++	+++
Ciprofloxacin	+	++++	0	++	++++
Levofloxacin	++	+++	+	+++	+++
Sparfloxacin	++	+++	+	+++	0
Gatifloxacin	++	+++	+	+++	++
Moxifloxacin	++	+++	++	+++	++
Trovafloxacin	++	+++	+++	+++	++

Fluoroquinolones Against Tuberculosis

The use of fluoroquinolones in MDR organisms is increasing due to the follow advantages: fluoroquinolones have a broad and potent spectrum of activity and it can be administrated orally, with favorable pharmacokinetic profiles and good absorption, including proficient penetration into host macrophages.

The use of fluoroquinolones in clinical trials started in 1985 when Tsukamura and co-workers reported their study by treating nineteen patients with suffering from chronic drug resistant tuberculosis with ofloxacin (300mg/day), concomitantly with other drugs during 6-8 months [7,8]. After that, different studies have been made by different groups using ofloxacin, ciprofloxacin, levofloxacin, sparfloxacin and moxifloxacin (Fig. **4**) as mono therapy or in combination with first-line drugs against tuberculosis. However, when fluoroquinolones were combined with others different first-line tuberculosis drugs they have shown greater results than when used alone or in combination with second-line drugs in order to prevent the rapid emergence of fluoroquinolone resistance. For example, in two different clinical studies made by Kohno and Kennedy, they have used ofloxacin and ciprofloxacin respectively in combination with isoniazid and rifampicin with 100% culture conversion at 6 months [7,9]. It is important to mention that drug interactions are infrequent between fluoroquinolones and anti-tuberculosis drugs.

Nowadays, fluoroquinolones are approved as second-line agents by the WHO to treat tuberculosis in patients that have resistance or intolerance to first-line anti-tuberculosis therapy. However, the potential of fluoroquinolones in first-line therapy and against XDR is still under investigation. In this context, Moxi and Gatifloxacin are under Phase III clinical trials.

Moxifloxacin

Moxifloxacin (BAY12-8039) is a fluoroquinolone of fourth generation, developed by Bayer and marketed as Avelox (moxifloxacin hydrochloride), which possesses excellent activity against a variety of different types of Gram-negative, Gram-positive, and anaerobic bacteria, such as pneumonia, brochitis and sinusitis. Their excellent activity against *M. tuberculosis in vivo* and *in vitro* in different studies can be compared with other known fluoroquinolones (Table **4**) [2]. For example, in comparison with levofloxacin and ofloxacin (Fig. **4**) against rifampicin-tolerant bacteria, moxifloxacin is much more effective with better bactericidal and sterilizing activity. Moxifloxacin has also excellent oral bioavailability and long t1/2 and the elimination half-life of the drug in man is about 12 hours in comparison with 1 to 2 hours for isoniazid [2,4]. Because of its good results moxifloxacin is under clinical studies for TB treatment with promising perspectives. For example, by substituting moxifloxacin by ethambutol or isoniazid, and the use against MDR-TB and TB/HIV coinfections, because of this fluoroquinolone has not cross-resistance to others TB drugs [4]. Another promising application is the reduction of the period of time in the TB treatment by using the combination of moxifloxacin and other TB drugs due to its great sterilizing effect [4,10-14].

Table 4: Moxifloxacin compared with other known fluoroquinolones [2].

Drug	Tablet	MIC_{90}	AUC	$t_{1/2}$	Cmax
Moxifloxacin	400 mg	0.25	45-51	12	5
Gatifloxacin	400 mg	0.25	29-40	08	5
Sparfloxacin	400 mg	0.5	41-54	20	1
Levofloxacin	500 mg	1.0	34	07	6

Moxifloxacin Synthesis

Basically, there are two principal strategies for the construction of the quinolin-4-one nucleus of the quinolone antibacterials, boths proceeding *via* enaminones intermediates, the Bayer and the Gould-Jacobs route (Scheme **1**) [5,6]. In the route developed by chemists at Bayer AG, the quinolone nucleus is formed by base-induced cyclisation of 2-(2-halobenzoyl)-3-aminoacrylates. The Gould-Jacobs cyclisation employs a thermal or acid-catalysed of anilinomethylene malonates. This cyclisation is essentially a modification of the classical Conrad-Limpach synthesis of 4-quinolones from anilines and acetoacetic esters [5,6].

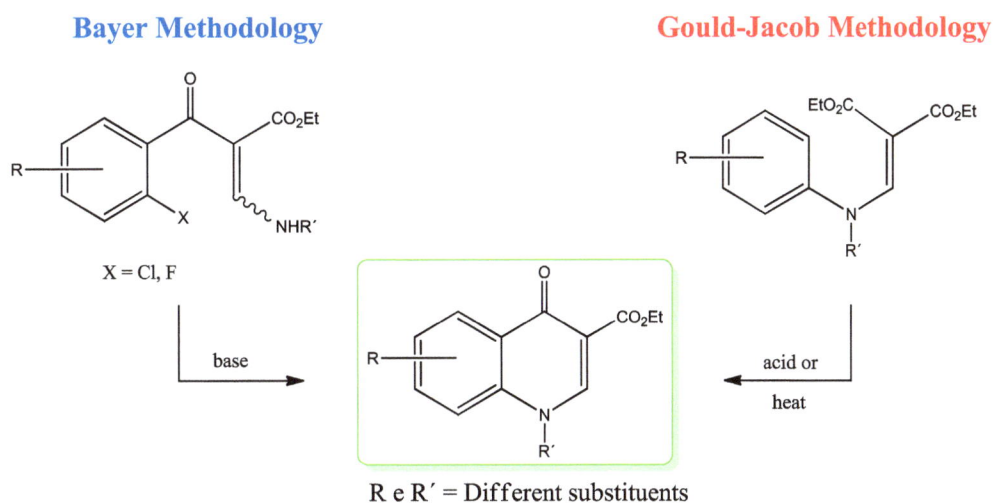

Scheme 1: Principal strategies for the construction of the quinolin-4-one nucleus [5,6].

The synthesis of moxifloxacin (Scheme **2,3**) [2,4] is based on the acid chloride **1** as the starting material, which was transformed into the β-Ketoester **2** and subsequently converted to its ethoxyacrylate derivative **3**. Treatment of this ethoxy acrylate derivative with the cyclopropylamine gave the enamine **4**. Cyclization of the enamine and hydrolysis gave the 4-oxoquinoline-3-carboxylic acid **5**. The substitution of fluorine atom at the C-7 position by byciclo **6**, which was prepared (Scheme **2,3**) using pyridine-2,3-carboxylic acid **7** as starting material gave moxifloxacin [2,4].

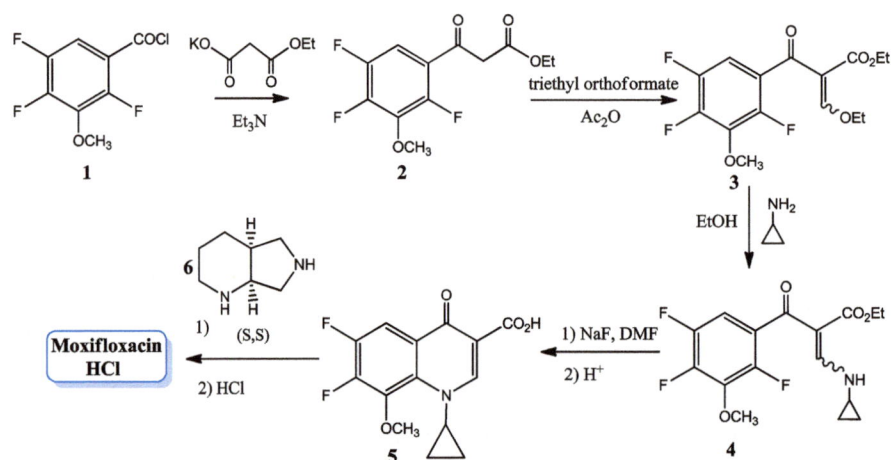

Scheme 2: Synthesis of moxifloxacin.

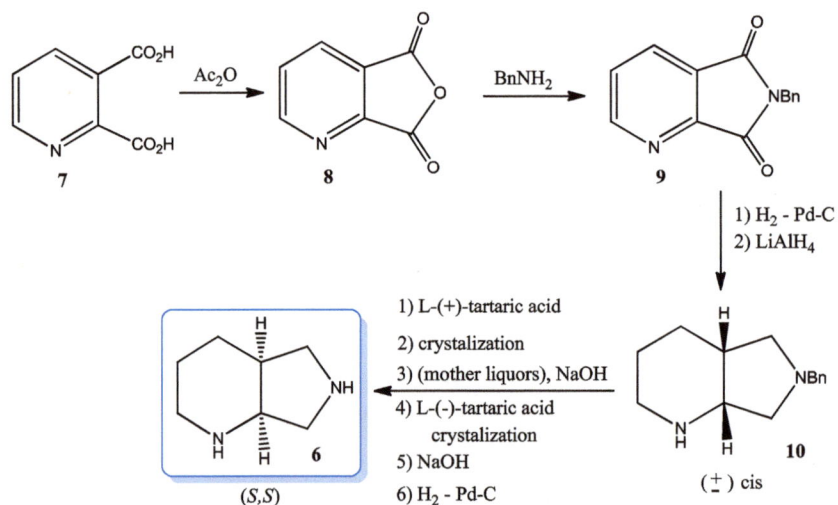

Scheme 3: Synthesis of bicyclo 6 present in moxifloxacin structure.

Gatifloxacin

Gatifloxacin is classified as a fluoroquinolone of third generation and market in the U.S. in 1999 by Bristol-Myers Squibb as Tequin®. This fluoroquinolone possessed a broad-spectrum of a number of bacterial infections and it is available in tablets of 200 and 400mg for oral administration and in injection (gatifloxacin in 5% dextrose) for intravenous administration. The *in vivo* comparison of gatifloxacin with moxifloxacin alone and in combination with anti-tuberculosis drugs were evaluated in mice infected with *Mycobacterium tuberculosis* and the conclusion of Cynamon and co-workers [4,7,15] are that gatifloxacin appears to have sufficient activity alone and in combination to deserve evaluation for treatment of tuberculosis. Different studies also have been demonstrated that gatifloxacin could be useful against MDR-TB and TB/HIV coinfections.

SQ-109

An important work published in 2005 in the field of drug discovered was the study of Protopopova and co-workers [16] in collaboration with Clif Barry (NIH/NIAID), which build a library of 63 238 compounds based on the pharmacophore of ethambutol, 1,2-ethylenediamine by solid-phase synthesis using an acylation-reduction sequence, which is compatible with high-throughput screening [3,4]. These compounds were evaluated against *Mycobacterium tuberculosis* and 26 have demonstrated *in vitro* activity equal to or greater (up to 14 fold) than ethambutol. The compound named SQ-109 (Fig. **6**) was selected for further development due to its potent activity MIC 0.16-0.32 μg/mL an SI of 16.7 and 99% inhibition activity against intracellular bacteria [3,4]. Additionally, it has demonstrated potency *in vivo* and limited toxicity *in vitro* and *in vivo*. Preliminary *in vivo* studies showed that SQ-109 had high activity, mainly in lungs, and it was effective to treat TB infection in mice at 1 mg/kg (ETH at 100 mg/kg) [3,4,17].

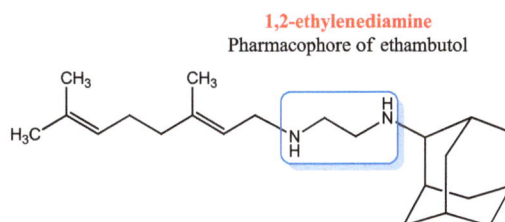

Figure 6: Structure of SQ-109.

Pharmacodynamics and Pharmacokinetics Data

The pharmacodynamics and pharmacokinetics of SQ-109 were studied by Jia and co-workers [4,18]. The results of *in vitro* and *in vivo* indicated that the SQ-109 has antimicrobial activity, potency and efficacy similar to isoniazid and superior to ethambutol. When administrated *in vivo via* oral to the mice for 28 days (0.1–25 mg kg^{-1} day^{-1}), SQ-109 promotes a dose-dependent reductions of mycobacterial load in both spleen and lung comparable to that of ETH administered at 100 mg kg^{-1} day^{-1}, but was less potent than INH at 25 mg kg^{-1} day^{-1}. The study of monitoring of drug levels in mouse tissues demonstrated that lungs and spleen contained the highest concentration of SQ-109, at least 10 times above its MIC [4].

Jia and co-worker [19] also characterized the interspecies absorption, distribution, metabolism and elimination (ADME) profile of SQ-109. They observed that after oral administration of [^{14}C]SQ-109 to rats the highest level of radioactivity was in the liver, followed by the lung, spleen and kidney. After that, they determined the main metabolites in the human liver microsomes as products of oxidation, epoxidation and *N*-dealkylation of SQ109 [4]. Another relevant information is that SQ-109 is predominantly metabolized by CYP2D6 and CYP2C19. These facts evidenced that the rapid liver microsomal metabolism of SQ-109 is the key to the significant observed first-pass effect [4].

Mycobacterial Cell Wall

Before describe the mechanism of action of SQ-109, it is important to be mentioned its target, the mycobacterial cell wall, which is very important as a cellular component surrounding the cell membrane providing additional support and protection. Basically, the mycobacterial cell wall is constituted of three covalently linked substructures: mycolic acids, peptidoglycan and arabinogalactan, which represents over 60% of cell dry weight (Fig. **7**) [20,21].

Mycolic acids are an important class of compounds, basically found in the cell walls of a group of bacteria known as mycolata taxon, exemplified by the most famous bacteria of this group, the *Mycobacterium tuberculosis*, which are very important for the survival of this bacterial. For example, they are able to help to

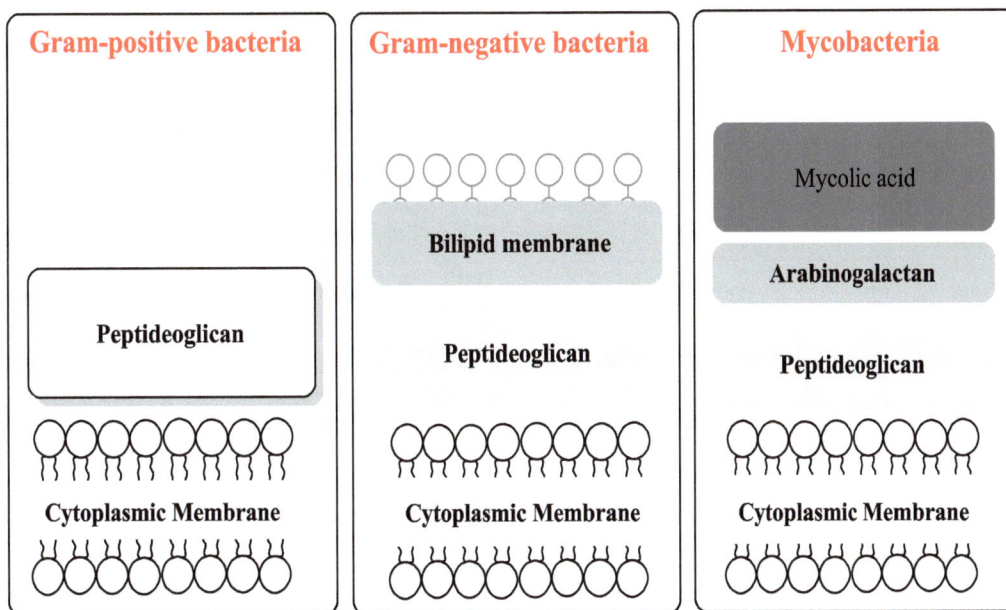

Figure 7: Cell walls of bacterial [20].

fight against hydrophobic drugs and dehydration, and also allow this bacterial to be more effective in the host´s immune system by growing inside macrophages. Structurally, mycolic acids are constituted of long fatty acids containing different functional groups, such as, double bonds, keto, ester, epoxy, methoxy group and cyclopropane ring. They possess a broad family of over 500 species, which are commonly characterized by the numbers of carbons atoms presented in the fatty acids. For example, mycolic acids, which posses 60-90 carbon atoms are commonly isolated from *Mycobacterium* and they are called mycolic or eumycolic acids. In the case of the mycolic acids containing carbon atoms between 22-60 units, they are isolated from other species, such as *Nocardia* and *Corynobacterium,* and they are named nocardomycolic and corynomycolic acids, which contain 44-60 and 22-36 carbon atoms, respectively [20,21]. Fig. **8** shows some of the mycolic acid class. For example, compound **11**, which is a key structural components of the cell envelope of *Mycobacterium tuberculosis*, and other compounds present in different mycobacterial cell wall, such as, α–methyl-trans-cyclopropanes (α-mycolic acids) **12**, α-methyl-β-methoxy groups (methoxymycolates) **13**, α-methyl-β-keto groups (ketomycolates) **14**, α–methyl-trans-epoxy groups **15**.

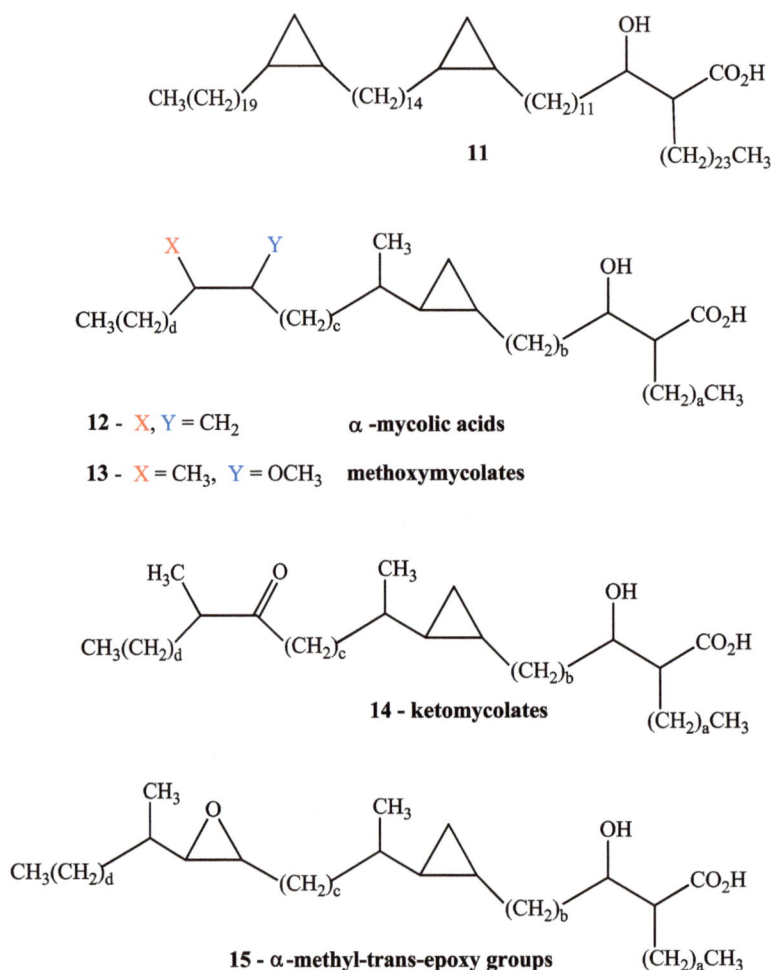

Figure 8: Structure of the mycolic acid class [21].

Peptidoglycan and Arabinogalactan

Peptidoglycan and arabinogalactan are also important polysaccharides in the mycobacterial cell walls, which are linked by covalent attachment to arabiongalactan (AG), a polymer composed primarily of D-galactofuranosyl and D-arabinofuranosyl residues, attached to mycolic acids and is known as coreF the mycolyl-arabinogalactan–peptidoglycan (mAGP) complex (Scheme **4**) [21,22]. The biosynthesis of this complex involves different enzymes, such as, galactopyranosyl mutase and epimerases and arabinosyl and galactofuransyl transferases (Scheme **4**).

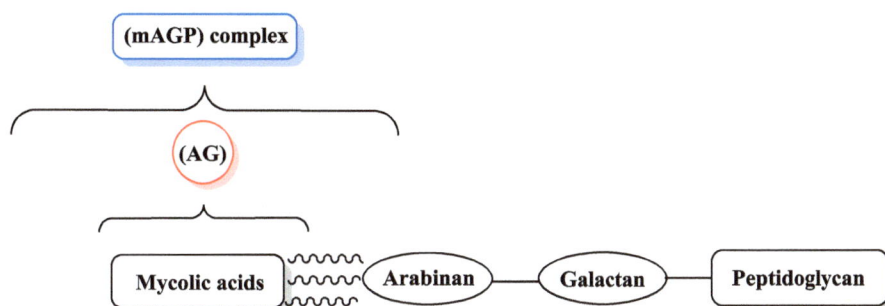

Scheme 4: (mAGP) complex [21].

The mycobacterial cell wall is also constituted of 6,6´-dimycolyltrehalose **16** (Fig. **9**), biosynthesized by three homologous proteins, Ag85, A, B and C, which possess mycolyltransferase. The antigen 85 (Ag 85) complex is a major protein component of the mycobacterial cell wall, composed of three proteins (Ag 85 A, B and C) all of which contribute to cell wall biosynthesis and help maintain its integrity, catalyzing the transfer of mycolic acids into the envelope [21,23].

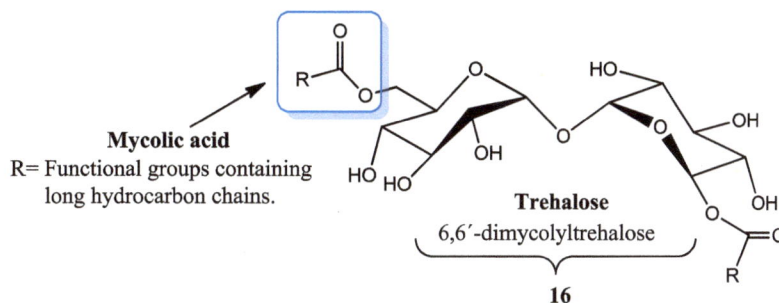

Figure 9: Structure of 6,6´-dimycolyltrehalose [21].

Ethambutol (ETH)

Despite the mycolic acids are an important target in the cell wall of *Mycobacterium tuberculosis*, there are other targets in mycobacterial cell wall. For example, the arabinogalactan (AG), an important polysaccharide which forms mAGP complex of cell wall (Scheme **8**). In this context, it can be mentioned the first-line drug ethambutol (ETH), which is capable of promoting inhibition in the biosynthesis of this constituent (Fig. **10**). It is important to highlight that the (*S,S*)-ethambutol is the isomeric form used, because the (*R,R*)-ethambutol causes blindness [21].

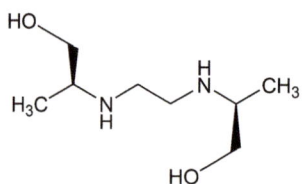

Figure 10: Structure of ethambutol.

AG = Arabiongalactan;

DPA = β-D-arabinofuranosyl-1-monophosphoryldecaprenol

DP = Decaprenol phosphate; *AftA* = Enzyme; *EmbA and EmbB* = Arabinofuranosyl transferases

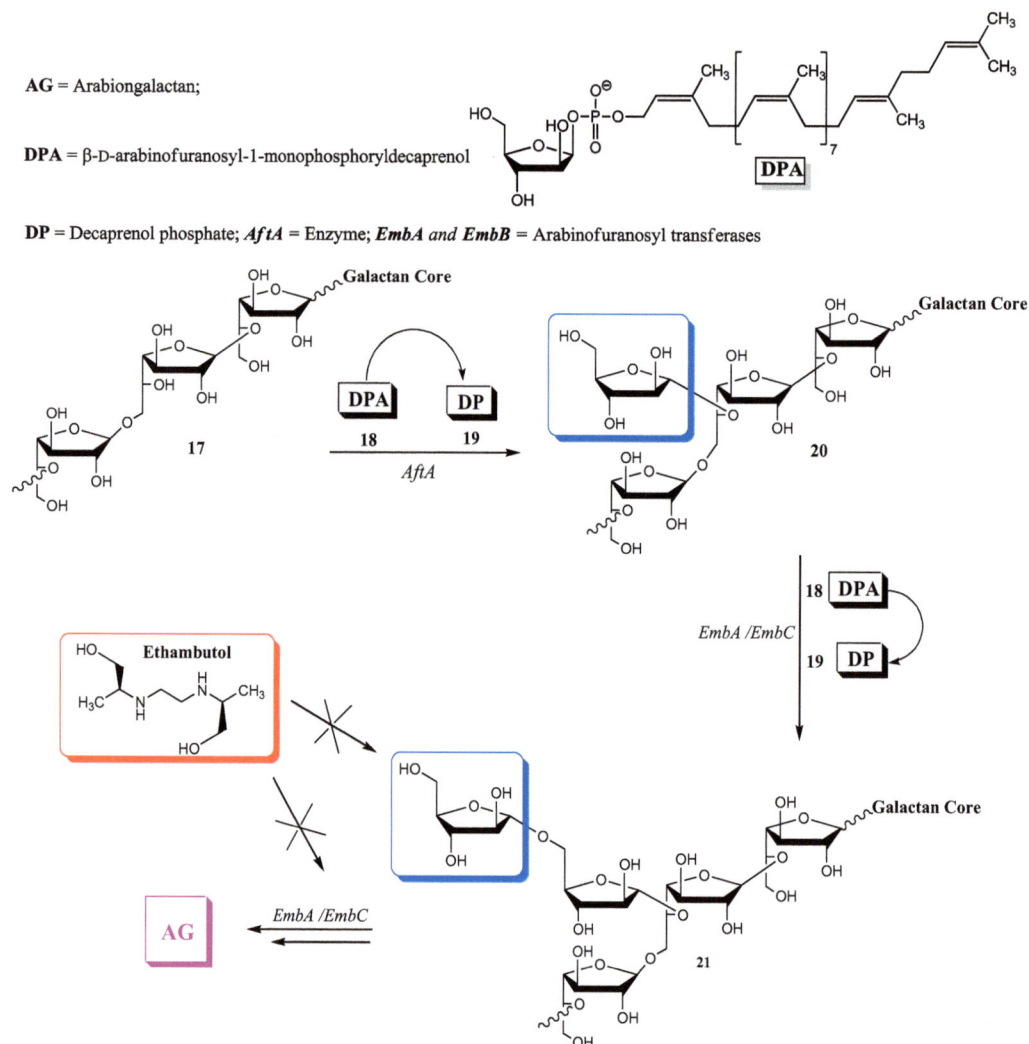

Scheme 5: Proposed action mechanism of ETH, an inhibitor of arabinogalactan biosynthesis [21].

The probable action mechanism of ETH involves the inhibition of the arabinofuranosyl transferases, important enzymes, which promote the polymerization of arabinose into the arabinan domain of AG [21,24,25]. The enzyme named *AftA* catalyzes the addition of the first key arabinofuranosyl residue **19** from the sugar donor β-D-arabinofuranosyl-1-monophosphoryldecaprenol (DPA) **18** to the galactan domain of the cell wall [21,26,27]. Subsequently, additions are promoted by other arabinofuranosyl transferases, called *EmbA* and *EmbB*, which are inhibited by ETH. With the inhibition of AG synthesis, the formation of mAGP complex is interrupted and may lead to increase permeability of the cell wall [21,28,29] (Scheme **10**).

Mechanism of Action of SQ-109

The precise target(s) for SQ-109 activity is not yet known, but it affects the synthesis of *M. tuberculosis* cell walls. Protapopova *et al.* postulated that SQ-109 and ETH have different mechanism of action or activating mechanism, because SQ-109 possess activity against ETH-resistant strains and it shows differences of behavior in genearray studies [17,30]. Another evidence of this difference was reported by Jia and co-workers [31]. Through a proteomic approach comparing the effects of 24-hour drug on *Mycobacterium tuberculosis* H37Rv, they demonstrated that SQ-109 did not affect *EmbA* or *EmbB*, the target of ETH.

PA-824

The history of the bicyclic nitroimidazofurans in the drug development was initially based as anticancer class [32] being the lead compound of this series CGI 17341 (Fig. **11**) [33]. Based on its structure, a structure-activity relationship (SAR) (Fig. **12**) was built and the compound named PA-824 was found and developed by PathoGenesis Inc in 1995 for cancer treatment [34-37]. However, the project was aborted and in 2000 this class showed potent activity against *Mycobacterium tuberculosis*. For example, PA-824 showed potent *in vitro* activity against all tested drug-resistant clinical isolates with MIC of 0.03-0.2 µg/mL [36]. This compound also possesses high activity in mince with no toxicity in rodent models, as well as excellent sterilize activity compared with isoniazid and rifampin. In addition, your novel mechanism of action is responsible for avoiding cross-resistance to current anti-TB drugs [4]. Due to its promising TB activity reported in 2000 and to the decision taken by Chiron, which bought PathoGenesis Inc in 2000, of not to continue the development of PA-824, TB Alliance and

Chiron signed a license agreement that gave TB Alliance rights to develop this compound [2,37,38].

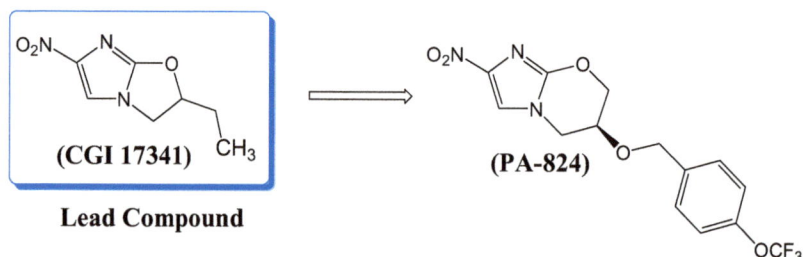

Figure 11: Structures of the nitroimidazoles CGI 17341 and PA-824.

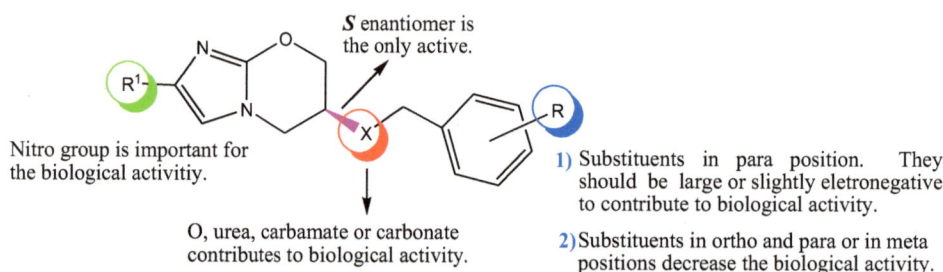

Figure 12: SAR of imidazo[2,1-b]oxazine series [4] (adapted from reference [39]).

Mechanism of Action

The mechanism of action of PA-824 is complex. This prodrug, which requires activation, is due to a flavinoid known as F-420 cofactor, which activates PA-824, which subsequently inhibits the synthesis of protein and cell wall lipids [3]. Therefore, Singh and co-workers [39] have found that PA-824 is converted into three main metabolites by Rv3547, a deazaflavin-dependent nitroreductase (Dnd). The major metabolite is the des-nitroimidazole (des-nitro), which is directly related to the anaerobic killing of *M. tuberculosis* by generation of reactive nitrogen species, such as nitric oxide. These species react with cytochromes and cytochrome C oxidase leading to interference in the electron flow, interruption the coupling of respiration to reduction of oxygen and, consequently, the cell killing [4,38,39].

In vitro, *in vivo* and Phase I of PA-824

The *in vitro* evaluation against a variety of resistant strains demonstrated that PA-824 was highly active (MIC < 1µg/mL) against all strains tested being also assessed against *M. tuberculosis* isolates grown under conditions of transient oxygen depletion and PA-824 showed a strong activity against these persistent bacteria in a dose-dependent manner [4,40]. This compound when compared to GAT and MXF was slightly less, however it was very similar to that of metronidazole (MET) (Fig. **13**), which is an antibiotic that possess activity against *M. tuberculosis* isolates that survive under anaerobic conditions [4,41]. The experiments were formulated in cyclodextrin/lecitin (CM2) due to the poor solubility of PA-824 in aqueous solution.

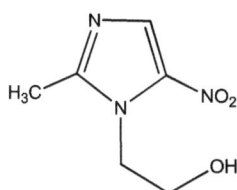

Figure 13: Structure of metronidazole.

The MIC of PA-824 in murine model was (0.125 µg/mL), and the minimal effective dose (MED) and the minimal bacterial dose (MBD) were 12.5 and 100 mg/Kg of body weight/day, respectively. Tyagi and co-workers [4,42] also characterize the bactericidal activity of PA-824 during the initial phase of therapy.

In 2009, Ginsberg and co-workers [43] reported the phase I study of PA-824 where they evaluated the safety, tolerability and pharmacokinetics of this substance. This study was divided in two stages: a single-dose and a multiple-dose (up to 7 days of daily dosing). In both cases, PA-824 was readily absorbed, bioavailable and well tolerated. The pharmacokinetics parameters indicated oral bioavailability and a half-life consistent with a once-per-day dose–regimen. Furthermore, no significant or serious adverse events were observed in the 58 subjects dosed with up to 1.000 mg PA-824 for up to 7 days (the multidosing was halted at 5 days at 1.000 mg due to increases in serum creatinine). Furthermore, serum creatinine elevation has been shown to be unrelated to human safety when directly examined in a renal effects study.

The phase I study of PA-824 started in 2009 by Ginsberg and co-workers [43], which evaluated the safety, tolerability and pharmacokinetics of this substance. This study was divided in two stages: a single-dose and a multiple-dose (up to 7 days of daily dosing). In both cases, PA-824 was readily absorbed, bioavailable and well tolerated. The pharmacokinetics parameters indicated oral bioavailability and a half-life consistent with a once-per-day dose–regimen. Furthermore, no significant or serious adverse events were observed in the 58 subjects dosed with up to 1.000 mg PA-824 for up to 7 days (the multidosing was halted at 5 days at 1.000 mg due to increases in serum creatinine). Furthermore, serum creatinine elevation has been shown to be unrelated to human safety when directly examined in a renal effects study [4,43].

OPC-67683

Sasaki and co-workers [44,45] at Otsuka Pharmaceutical Development & Commercialization, Inc. (OPDC) synthesized a series of 6-nitro-2,3-dihydroimidazo[2,1-*b*]oxazoles (CGI 17341 core), which produce the lead compound named OPC-67683 being the structure-activity relationship (SAR) of this class summarized in Fig. **14**.

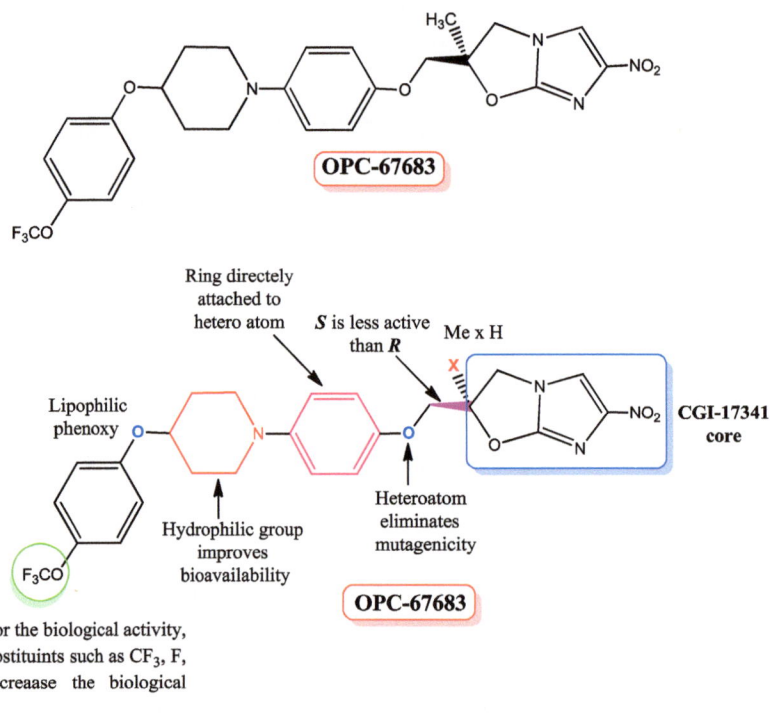

Figure 14: Structure of OPC-67683 and SAR of 6-nitro-2,3-dihydroimidazo[2,1-*b*]oxazoles series [4].

Synthesis

The synthesis of OPC-64683 was based on the key intermediate (*R*)-form of epoxide **26** with a specific phenol **30**, by ring formation in basic conditions being this key intermediate synthesized in four steps. The first step was the coupling between the nitroimidazole **21** and the epoxide **22**, which furnished the compound **23**. After that, the diol **24** was produced by using MeOH and K_2CO_3 followed by reaction with MsCl in pyridine to furnish the mesylate **25**, which was converted into the epoxide **26** by using DBU in AcOEt. The other intermediate, the phenol **30** was prepared by using Buchwald palladium catalyzed amination methodology between 2-(4-bromophenoxy) tetrahydropyran **27** and 4-phenoxypiperidine **28**, followed by deprotection in acid conditions (Scheme **5**) [45].

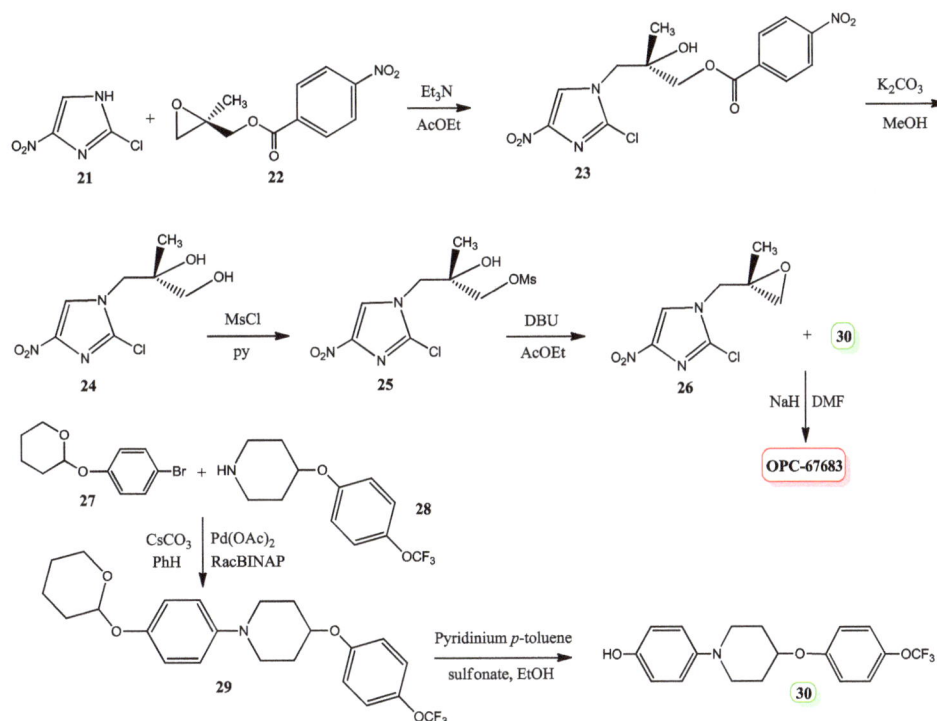

Scheme 5: Synthetic route to preparation of OPC-67683 [4].

In vitro, in vivo and Phase II of OPC-67683

This compound when evaluated *in vitro* showed potent activity in a wide variety of sensitive and resistant strains with MIC ranging from 0.006 to 0.012 µg/mL, being most potent than streptomicyn, INH, RIF, ETH, CGI-17341 and PA-824. Other important information about this compound made by Matsumoto and co-workers is that no cross-resistance to any currently used anti-TB drug was observed [4,46]. This authors also evaluated evaluated the inhibitory activity against mycolic acid biosynthesis and the results showed that OPC-67683 inhibits the synthesis of methoxy and keto-mycolic acids, but not the synthesis of α–mycolic acids while INH inhibits all mycolic acid subclasses. Another study indicated that the major metabolite of OPC-67683 was identified as a non-active desnitro-imidazooxazole. This information suggests that Rv3547 has a reduction potency of the nitro group and that an intermediate between OPC-67683 and desnitro-imidazooxazole could be the active form [4].

Similarly to PA-824, OPC-67683 also needs metabolic activation by *M.tuberculosis* to produce its anti-TB activity. Through the isolation of OPC-67683-resistant strains, they observed that these strains did not metabolize the compound. Thus, they confirmed a mutation in the Rv3547 gene among these strains, which shows that Rv3574 is the key enzyme involved in the activation of OPC-68673. Furthermore, in an experiment with radioactive OPC-67683, they found that in standard strains, 20% of the radioactive substances were not recovered at the end of the exposure while in OPC-67683-resistant strains 100% of radioactivity was recovered. This data suggests that a radical intermediate that appears as the intermediate for the metabolism of a nitro residue covalently binds to the target molecule. This hypothesis could explain the strong post-antibiotic effect observed with OPC-67683 against intracellular mycobacterium, which was demonstrated in an experiment that examined the killing activity intracellular TB in macrophages. This study is an important information about the capacity of this drug to be effective against latent TB [4,46].

In this model, OPC-67683 exhibited the most potent anti-tubercular activity in comparison with the standard anti-TB drugs. The viable bacterial counts in the lung were clearly reduced dose-dependently this substance at 0.313 mg/kg and higher. Moreover, OPC-67683 was so effective in a TB model established using immunodeficient mice than using standard mice. These data are an important evidence that this substance could be helpful in the treatment of TB patients co-infected with HIV/AIDS [4,46].

The evaluation of the safety, efficacy and pharmacokinetics proprieties of OPC-67683 were made in phase II trial. This study was based on four oral doses of this compound in patients with uncomplicated, smear-positive, pulmonary tuberculosis being successfully completed in 2007. Currently, OPC-67683 is in phase III.

LINEZOLID

Oxazolidinones represent the first new class of antibacterial drugs in the last 35 years [2,47,48]. The history of oxazolidinones as drugs started in 1978, when a patent of El DuPont de Nemours & Co., Inc. reported a series of 5-(halomethyl)-3-aryl-2-oxazolidinones with biological activity against a certain plant pathogen [2,49]. After this discovery, (5*R*)-(hydroxymethyl)-3-aryl-2-oxazolidinone, S-6123 (Fig. **15**) was reported to have weak *in vitro* activity against human pathogens. The optimization of this compound in 1987 lead to the discovery of two compounds DuP 721 and DuP 105 (Fig. **15**), which possessed both parental and oral activity [2,49]. However, due to their toxicity, the development of these compounds was aborted. In spite of these problems, Upjohn Laboratories (latterly Pharmacia Corporation, Peapack, NJ) and Pfizer continued to study this class of compounds and in 1996 two non toxic derivatives U-100592 and U-100766 (Fig. **15**) were reported [49]. They were named eperezolid and linezolid, respectively. Linezolid was developed by Pharmacia Corporation, Peapack, NJ with the brand name Zyvox as oral and intravenous dosage forms [2,50]. This compound, approved by FDA in 2000 is used to treat infections caused by Gram-positive strains, which are resistant to different antibacterial drugs, such as vancomycin and penicillin. However it has limited activity against Gram-negative bacteria. This class possesses new mechanisms of action based on block protein synthesis by stopping translation at the initiation step, which involves the binding of *N*-formylmethionyl-tRNA to the 70S ribosome [2,50]. Oxazolidinones possess promising activity against *M. tuberculosis* especially for the treatment of multi-drug resistant strains with *in vitro* MIC_{90} from 0.5 to 2.0 mg/l and inhibition of growth in murine model. In 2003, Hadjiangelis and co-workers reported the effectiveness of linezolid in humans with MDR-TB [2,51]. A recent study done by Lippe and co-workers showed the efficacy and safety of linezolid in patients with MDR-TB in ten patients treated with this drug in combination with others TB drugs [2,51].

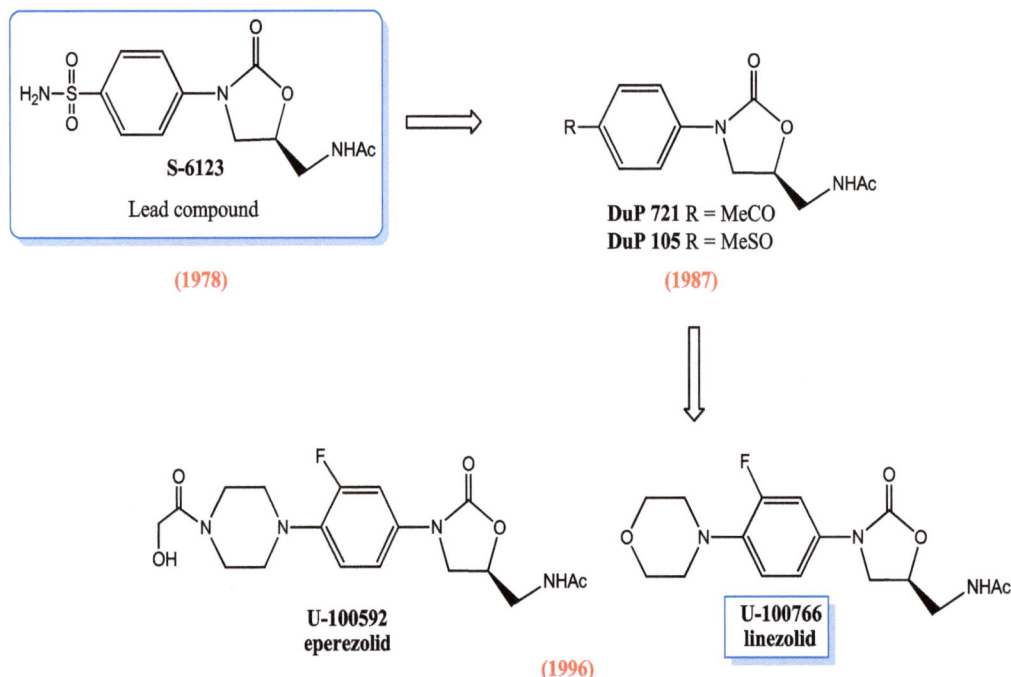

Figure 15: Structures of some important linezolids.

The synthesis of linezolid (Scheme **6**) [47] was firstly described in nine steps being the first step responsible for the formation of the intermediate **33**, due to the reaction between morpholine **31** and 3,4-difluoronitrobenzene **32**. The second and third steps were respectively, the reduction and attachment of a carbobenzoxy (Cbz) activating group, which produced the intermediate **35**. The key intermediate (5*R*)-(hydroxymethyl)-2-oxazolidinone **36** was synthesized by using compound **35** in presence of *n*-BuLi followed by the addition of (*R*)-glycidyl butyrate. The yield of this key step was 85% with a high enantiomeric excess >99.7% ee. The final steps were mesilation, introduction of the azide group, its reduction and acetylation of the amino group, which furnished the drug linezolide.

Due to the importance of this drug several analogues have been synthesized with important information for the SAR indicating the critical positions (Scheme **7**) [52].

In this context it could be mention the Subezolid and AZD-5847, which are currently in phase II (Fig. **16**) [52,53].

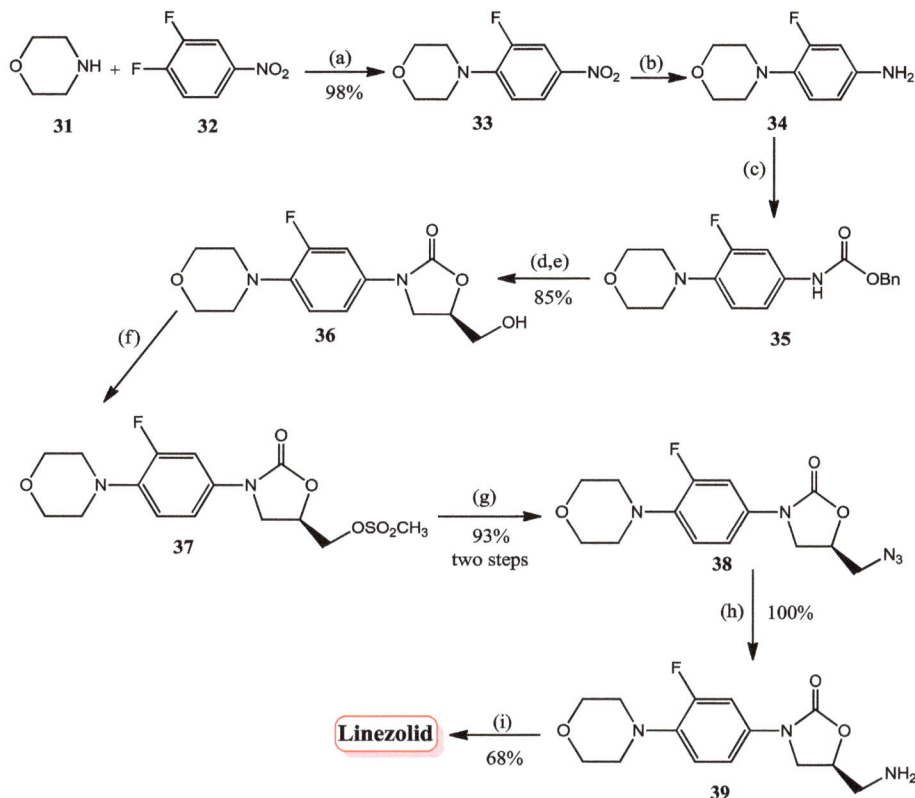

(a) (i-Pr)$_2$EtN, EtOAc; (b) HCO$_2$NH$_4$, 10% Pd-C, THF-MeOH; (c) CBzCl, NaHCO$_3$ or NaCO$_3$, acetone-H$_2$O; (d) *n*-BuLi, THF, 78°C; (e) (*R*)-glycidyl butyrate; (f) MsCl, Et$_3$N, CH$_2$Cl$_2$; (g) NaN$_3$, DMF, 75°C; (h) 10% Pd-C, H$_2$, EtOAc; (i) Ac$_2$O, py.

Scheme 6: Synthesis of linezolid [2].

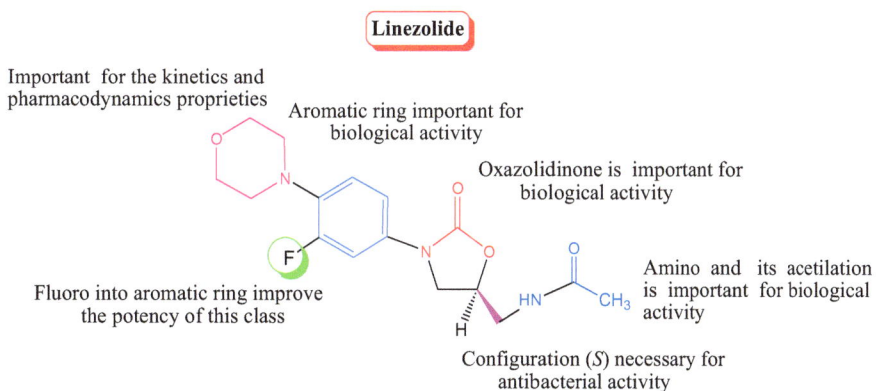

Scheme 7: SAR of linezolid.

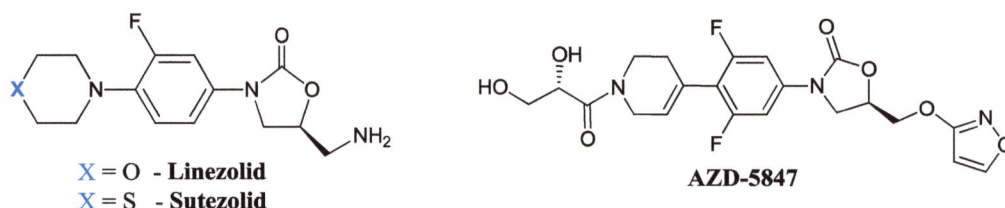

X = O - **Linezolid**
X = S - **Sutezolid**

AZD-5847

Figure 16: Structures of sutezolid and AZD-5847.

DIARYLQUINOLINE BEDAQUILINE (TMC207) AN APPROVED DRUG BY FDA IN DECEMBER, 2012

The company Johnson & Johnson Pharmaceutical Research & Development synthesized and evaluated several compounds of the diarylquinolines class, and some of them displayed potent anti-TB activity (MIC below 0.5 µg/mL). The most active compound was R207910 (after called TMC207 and now bedaquiline) (Fig. **17**), exhibiting promising *in vitro* activities with MIC values ranging from 0.03 to 0.12 µg/mL [54-60]. Recently, due to its excellent results bedaquiline was approved by FDA for multidrug-resistant tuberculosis in December, 2012. Unfortunately, it is important to mention that we were almost half a century without a new drug against tuberculosis being bedaquiline the first one to be developed since rifampicin (1966-1970). This new TB drug is also the first anti-bacterial with a new mechanism of action in 40 years being its mechanism of action based on the inhibition of the enzyme ATP synthase, which is essential for this proton transport (the proton pump). It also important to mention that this enzyme could be an attractive target for the treatment of latent TB infections being bedaquiline a excellent candidate, as well as a good start point for the development of new drugs with this purpose [57].

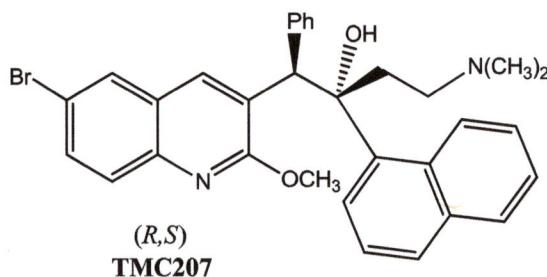

(*R,S*)
TMC207

Figure 17: Structure of bedaquiline (TMC207).

Synthesis

The synthesis of TMC207, which has two stereogenic centers (configuration *R,S*) was made in four steps. It is important to mention that in one of these steps there are the formations of four isomers that need to be separated by chiral HPLC. The first step was based on the amide formation between 4-bromo aniline **40** and 3-phenylpropionyl chloride **41** in the presence of triethylamine and methylene chloride producing the intermediate **42**. After that, a Vilsmeier-Haack formylation, cyclization using $POCl_3$ in DMF and introduction of methoxy group furnished the quinoline **44**. The coupling reaction between **44** and **45** was made by using diisopropylamine lithium (LDA), which led the compound **46** (TMC207) as a mixture of 4 diastereoisomers, which were separated by column chromatography, obtaining two pure fractions of the diastereoisomers (*R,R* and *S,S*) and (*R,S* and *S,R*), being isolated by chiral HPLC (Scheme **8**) [4].

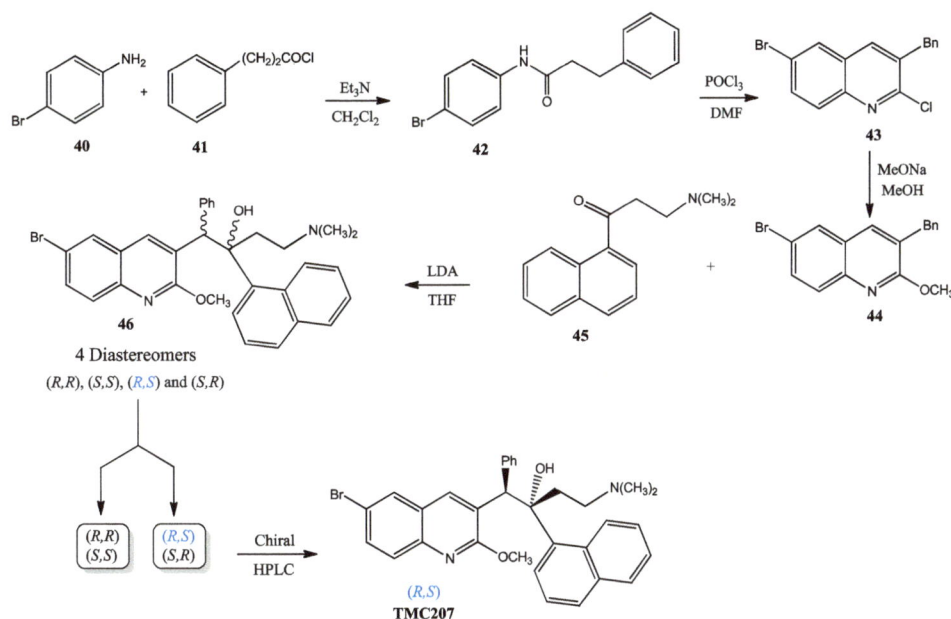

Scheme 8: Synthetic route for the preparation of the diarylquinoline Bedaquiline (TMC207) [4].

COMPARATIVE EFFICACIES OF NEW TB DRUG COMBINATIONS

Drug combinations (DCs) have been used successfully in different kinds of diseases such as cancer, AIDS, malaria, infectious diseases, asthma, diarrhea, hypertension, neurological disorders and others. In this context, one important concept in drug discovery is fixed-dose combination (FDC), which can be defined as a formulation of two or more substances biologically active, combined in a single drug, available in certain fixed doses [61]. Nowadays, this strategy has been used successfully in different kinds of diseases, such as cancer, AIDS, malaria, infectious diseases, asthma, diarrhea, hypertension, neurological disorders and others [61-63]. This strategy is usually used with only one disease; however it can also be used to treat more than one. For example, the drug named Caduet or Exforge, which contains artovastatin and amlodipine is used to treat hypercholesterolemia and hypertension, respectively. Several advantages can be mentioned in favor of FDC such as reduced risk of emergence of drug resistant strains, better patient compliance, reduced cost of treatment, fewer risks of medication errors, dosages adjustment according to patient's needs and simplified drug supply management, shipping and distribution. Despite the vital importance of FDCs in the treatment of several diseases, there are also some disadvantages and problems to be solved such as drug interactions, instability of the formulation and adverse drug reactions. It is also important to mention that FDCs can be protected by patents, even if the drugs included into the formulation are off-patent. In this context, FDCs are an important strategy, which can be used by pharmaceutical companies as an alternative to extend the life time of their drugs [61,64].

The Importance of DCs in the Modern Tuberculosis Treatment

Due to the resurgence of TB, new drugs and DCs are necessary or a tragedy might happen. However, the pharmaceutical development of FDCs is complex and there are many variants and problems to be considered. In this context, cost, excipients, methods of manufacture, bioavailability, bioequivalence, stability, polymorphic forms, bulk density, solubility, pKa, impurities and drug interactions can be mentioned. A known example of problems of FDCs in TB [65] is the bioavailability of rifapetine [66,67], which can decrease in the stomach, due to the chemical reaction with isoniazid catalyzed by ethambutol and pyrazinamide [68]. Considering the importance of the DCs for the modern treatment of tuberculosis nowadays, the next section will present some new DCs focus on MDR and XDR-TB. These combinations were based on between the drugs used against tuberculosis and the compounds in advanced clinical trials, as well as the new drug bedaquiline and they are summarized in the tables (Tables **5-9**).

Moxifloxacin

Table 5: Moxifloxacin combined with other anti-TB drugs [4].

Tests	Drugs	Results
In vitro	MXF + INH	Improvement in the activity of both drugs [69-71].
	MXF + RIF	Low concentrations of RIF increase MXF activity. High concentrations of RIF decrease MXF activity [69-71].
	MXF + ETH	Decrease in MXF activity [69].
	MXF + Cm	More active than each drug separately [69].
	MXF + Cs	Little effect in MXF activity [69].
In mice	MXF + RIF + PYZ	Treatment time reduction [13,14]
In humans	MXF + INH	Keeps the activity unchanged [72].
	MXF + INH + RIF + PYZ	Higher rate of culture negativity in the first month than the standard regimen but similar effect after 2 months [73].
	MXF + ETH + RIF + PYZ	The activity was similar to the standard regimen [74].

Gatifloxacin

Table 6: Gatifloxacin combined with other anti-TB drugs [4].

Tests	Drugs	Results
In vitro	GTX + ETH	Decreased GTX activity [69].
In mice	GTX + ETH	Kept the activity unchanged [75].
	RIF + GTX	Improved the activity of GTX. Similar activity to that of INH + RIF [75].
	INH + GTX + RIF	Improved the activity of GTX. Similar activity to that of INH + RIF [75].
	GTX + Eti	Improved the activity of GAT [76].
	GTX + Eti + PZA	Similar activity to that of GTX + ETA [76].
	GTX + Eti + PZA + ETH	Similar activity to that of GTX + Eti [76].
In humans	GTX + INH + PZA + RIF	Significant acceleration of bacillary elimination during the late phase [77,78].

SQ-109

Table 7: SQ-109 combined with other anti-TB drugs [4].

Tests	Drugs	Results
In vitro	SQ-109 + PYZ or ETH	No additive or synergistic effect [79].
	SQ-109 + STM	Additive effect [79].
	SQ-109 + INH + RIF	Synergistic effect [79].
In mice	SQ109 + INH + RIF + PYZ	Intensive phase treatment regimen having a better and faster rate of mycobacterial killing than the therapeutic regimen INH-RIF-ETH-PYZ [80]

PA-824 and OPC-67683

Table 8: *In vivo* studies with PA-824 and OPC-67683 combined with other anti-TB drugs [4].

Drugs	Results
PA-824 + INH	Prevented the selection of INH-resistant mutants [81,82].
PA-824 + 2 months with INH, RIF and PYZ	Demonstrated activity in persistent bacilli that, survived after the intensive initial phase [83].
PA-824 + 6 months with INH, RIF and PYZ	It was not able to improve its sterilizing activity and, consequently, to decrease the period of treatment [83].
PA-824 + 6 months with RIF and PYZ	No difference in the proportion of mice relapsing after completing 6 months of therapy [83].
PA-824 + RIF-PYZ	Led to all mice culture negative, after 2 months of treatment and free of relapse, after 4 months of treatment [84].
PA-824 + PYZ	Exhibited synergistic activity that was equivalent to that combination of first-line drugs [84].
PA-824 + RIF-MXF-PYZ	Incorporation of PA-824 to the experimental 4-month RIF-MXF-PYZ regimen did not allow the shortening of the treatment duration to 3 months [84].
PA-824 + MXF-PYZ	Regimen cured mice more quickly than the first-line regimen (RIF, INH and PYZ) [82].
OPC-67683 + RIF and PYZ (2 months) + RIF for more two months	produced a rapid reduction in bacterial load over the first 3 months [46].

Table 9: *In vivo* studies with TMC207 combined with other anti-TB drugs [4].

Drugs	Results
TCM+RIF-INH-PYZ	Promoted a greater decrease in bacterial load in the lungs [59].
TMC207+INH-RIF, TMC207+INH-PYZ and TMC207+RIF-PYZ	The lungs of all animals were culture-negative. However, the differences among the bactericidal activities of the combinations were not significant [59].

Table 9: contd....

TMC207-INH-PYZ and TMC207-RIF-PYZ	Comparable to the combinations RIF-INH-PYZ after 2 months of therapy [59].
TMC207 + PYZ	Important synergistic interaction between murine models [85].
TMC207-PYZ + RIF, INH or MXF	Regimen could not increase the activity after 2 months of treatment [85].
TMC207 + RIF	The interaction of TMC207 with RIF in the standard treatment (RIF-INH-PYZ) [86].
TMC207 + Am, PYZ, MXF or Eti	All TMC207-containing regimens were significantly more active than the non-TMC207-containing regimens after 1 month of therapy [87].

ACKNOWLEDGEMENT

None Declare.

CONFLICT OF INTEREST

The author(s) confirm that this chapter content has no conflict of interest.

REFERENCES

[1]   Spigelman M and Ginsbrg AM. Challenges in tuberculosis drug research and development. *Nature Medicine* 2007;**13**:290-294.

[2]   Souza, MVN. Promising drugs against tuberculosis. *Rec Pat Anti-Infect Drug Discov* 2006;**1**:33-45.

[3]   De Souza MVN. *New Strategies Combating Bacterial Infection*. Iqbal A and Farrukh A. Ed.;Wiley-VCH Verlag GmbH and Co. KGaA:Weinheim **2008**;vol *3*, p. 71-87.

[4]   De Souza MVN, Gonçalves RSB, Ferreira ML. *Frontiers in Anti-Infective Drug Discovery*. Atta-ur-Rahman FRS & Iqbal CM. Ed.;Bentham **2009**;vol *9*, p. 176-201.

[5]   De Souza MVN, De Almeida MV, Da Silva AD, Couri MRC. Biological activity and synthetic metodologies for the preparation of fluoroquinolones, a class of potent antibacterial agents. *Curr Med Chem* 2003;**10**:21-39.

[6]   De Souza MVN. New Fluoroquinolones:A Class of Potent Antibiotics. *Mini-Review in Medicinal Chemistry* 2005;**5**:1009-1018.

[7]   De Souza MV, Vasconcelos TR, de Almeida MV, Cardoso SH. Fluoroquinolones:an important class of antibiotics against tuberculosis. *Curr Med Chem* 2006;**13**:455-63.

[8]   Tsukamura M. *In vitro* antituberculosis activity of a new antibacterial substance ofloxacin (DL8280). *Am Rev Resp Dis* 1985;**131**:348-51.

[9]   Kohno S, Koga H, Kaku M. Prospective comparative study of ofloxacin or ethambutol for the treatment of pulmonary tuberculosis *Chest.* 1992;**102**:1815-8.

[10]   Drusano GL, Sgambati N, Eichas A, Brown D, Kulawy R, Louie A. Effect of Administration of Moxifloxacin plus Rifampin against *Mycobacterium tuberculosis* for 7 of 7 Days *vs.* 5 of 7 Days in an *In Vitro* Pharmacodynamic System. *MBio* 2011;**2**:e00108-11.

[11] Miyazaki E, Miyazaki M, Chen JM, Chaisson RE, Bishai WR. Moxifloxacin (BAY12-8039), a New 8-Methoxyquinolone, Is Active in a Mouse Model of Tuberculosis. *Antimicrob Agents Chemother* 1999;**43**:85-89.

[12] Yoshimatsu T, Nuermberger E, Tyagi S, Chaisson R, Bishai W, Grosset J. Bactericidal Activity of Increasing Daily and Weekly Doses of Moxifloxacin in Murine Tuberculosis. *Antimicrob Agents Chemother* 2002;**46**:1875-1879.

[13] Nuermberger EL, Yoshimatsu T, Tyagi S, *et al.* Moxifloxacin-containing regimen greatly reduces time to culture conversion in murine tuberculosis. *Am J Respir Crit Care Med* 2004;**169**:421-426.

[14] Nuermberger EL, Yoshimatsu T, Tyagi S, *et al.* Moxifloxacin-containing regimens of reduced duration produce a stable cure in murine tuberculosis. *Am J Respir Crit Care Med* 2004;**170**:1131-1134.

[15] Freites EJA, Carter, JL, Cynamon MH. *In Vitro* and *In Vivo* Activities of Gatifloxacin against *Mycobacterium tuberculosis Antimicrob Agents Chemother* 2002;**46**:1022-25.

[16] Lee RE, Protopopova M, Crooks E, Slayden RA, Terrot M, Barry CE. Combinatorial lead optimization of [1,2]-diamines based on ethambutol as potential antituberculosis preclinical candidates. *J Comb Chem* 2003;**5**:172-187.

[17] Protopopova M, Hanrahan C, Nikonenko B, *et al.* Identification of a new antitubercular drug candidate, SQ109, from a combinatorial library of 1,2-ethylenediamines. *J Antimicrob Chem* 2005;**56**:968-974.

[18] Jia L, Tomaszewski JE, Hanrahan C, *et al.* Pharmacodynamics and pharmacokinetics of SQ109, a new diamine-based antitubercular drug. *Brit J Pharmacol* 2005;**144**:80–87.

[19] Jia L, Noker PE, Coward L, Gorman GS, Protopopova M, Tomaszewski JE. Interspecies pharmacokinetics and *in vitro* metabolism of SQ109. *Brit J Pharmacol* 2006;**147**:476–485.

[20] De Souza MVN, Facchinetti V, Cardinot D. Natural Products with Translocase I inhibitory activity, as new lead compounds against tuberculosis. *Boletín Latinoamericano y del Caribe de Plantas Medicinales y Aromáticas* 2010;**9**:1-12.

[21] De Souza MVN, Ferreira ML, Pinheiro AC, Saraiva MF, Almeida MV, Valle MS. Synthesis and Biological Aspects of Mycolic Acids:An Important Target Against *Mycobacterium tuberculosis. The Scientific World Journal* 2008;**8**:720-751.

[22] Crick DC, Mahapatra S, and Brennan PJ. Biosynthesis of the arabinogalactan-peptidoglycan complex of *Mycobacterium tuberculosis. Glycobiology* 2001;**11**:107R–118R.

[23] Content J, Cuvellerie A, Wit L, Vicent-Levy-Frebault V, Ooms J, Bruyn J. The genes coding for the antigen 85 complexes of *Mycobacterium tuberculosis* and Mycobacterium bovis BCG are members of a gene family:cloning, sequence determination, and genomic organization of the gene coding for antigen 85-C of M. tuberculosis. *Infect Immun* 1991;**59**:3205–3212.

[24] Deng L, Mikusova K, Robuck KG, Scherman M, Brennan PJ, McNeil MR. Recognition of multiple effects of ethambutol on metabolism of mycobacterial cell envelope. *Antimicrob Agents Chemother* 1995;**39**;694-701.

[25] Takayama K, Kilburn JO. Inhibition of synthesis of arabinogalactan by ethambutol in Mycobacterium smegmatis. *Antimicrob. Agents Chemother* 1989;**33**:1493-99.

[26] Alderwick LJ, Seidel M, Sahm H, Besra GS, Eggeling L. Identification of a novel arabinofuranosyltransferase (AftA) involved in cell wall arabinan biosynthesis in *Mycobacterium tuberculosis. J. Biol. Chem* 2006;**281**:15653-15661.

[27] Mikuová K, Huang H, Yagi T, Holsters M, Vereecke D, D'Haeze W, Scherman MS, Brennan PJ, McNeil MR, Crick DC. Decaprenylphosphoryl arabinofuranose, the donor of the D-arabinofuranosyl residues of mycobacterial arabinan, is formed *via* a two-step epimerization of decaprenylphosphoryl ribose. *J Bacteriol* 2005;**187**:8020-25.

[28] Belanger AE, Besra GS, Ford ME, Mikušová K, Belisle JT, Brennan PJ, Inamine JM. The embAB genes of Mycobacterium avium encode an arabinosyl transferase involved in cell wall arabinan biosynthesis that is the target for the antimycobacterial drug ethambutol. *Proc Natl Acad Sci USA* 1996;**93**:11919-24.

[29] Escuyer VE, Lety M, Torrelles JB, Khoo K, Tang J, Rithner, CD, Frehel C, McNeil MR, Brennan PJ, Chatterjee D. The role of the embA and embB gene products in the biosynthesis of the terminal hexaarabinofuranosyl motif of *Mycobacterium smegmatis* arabinogalactan. *J Biol Chem* 2001:**276**;48854-62.

[30] Nikonenko BV, Protopopova M, Samala R, Einck L, Nacy AC. Drug Therapy of Experimental Tuberculosis (TB):Improved Outcome by Combining SQ109, a New Diamine Antibiotic, with Existing TB Drugs. *Antimicrob Agents Chemother* 2007;**51**:1563-1565.

[31] Jia L, Coward L, Gorman GS, Noker PE, Tomaszewski JE. Pharmacoproteomic Effects of Isoniazid, Ethambutol, and *N*-Geranyl-*N'*-(2-adamantyl)ethane-1,2-diamine (SQ109) on *Mycobacterium tuberculosis* H37Rv. *J Pharmacol Exp Ther* 2005;**315**:905-911.

[32] Agrawal KC, Bears KB, Sehgal RK, Brown JN, Rist PE, Rupp WD. Potential radiosensitizing agents. Dinitroimidazoles. *J Med Chem* 1979;**22**:583-586.

[33] Ashtekar DR, Costa-Perira R, Nagrajan K, Vishvanathan N, Bhatt AD, Rittel W. *In vitro* and *in vivo* activities of the nitroimidazole CGI 17341 against *Mycobacterium tuberculosis*. *Antimicrob Agents Chemother* 1993;**37**:183-186.

[34] Baker, W.R, *et al.* US5668127 (**1997**).

[35] Baker W.R, *et al.* US6087358 (**2000**).

[36] Stover CK, Warrener P, Van Devanter DR, Sherman DR, Arain TM, Langhorne MH, Anderson SW, Towell JA, Yuan Y, McMurray DN, Kreiswirth BN, Barry CE, Baker WR. A small-molecule nitroimidazopyran drug candidate for the treatment of tuberculosis. *Nature* 2000;**405**:962-966.

[37] http://www.tballiance.org/home/home.php (date of access:09-20-2010)

[38] Barry, Clifton E, Boshoff HIM, Dowd CS. Prospects for Clinical Introduction of Nitroimidazole Antibiotics for the Treatment of Tuberculosis. *Current Pharmaceutical Design* 2004;**10**:3239-3262.

[39] Singh R, Manjunatha U, Boshoff HIM, Ha YH, Niyomrattanakit P, Ledwidge R, Dowd CS, Lee IY, Kim P, Zhang L, Kang S, Keller TH, Jiricek J, Barry CE. PA-824 Kills Nonreplicating *Mycobacterium tuberculosis* by Intracellular NO Release. *Science* 2008;**28**:1392-1395.

[40] Lenaerts AJ, Gruppo V, Marietta KS, Johnson CM, Driscoll DK, Tompkins NM, Rose JD, Reynolds RC, Orme IM. Preclinical Testing of the Nitroimidazopyran PA-824 for Activity against *Mycobacterium tuberculosis* in a Series of *In Vitro* and *In Vivo* Models. *Antimicrob Agents Chemother* 2005;**49**:2294-2301.

[41] Wayne LG, Hayes LG. An *in vitro* model for sequential study of shiftdown of *Mycobacterium tuberculosis* through two stages of nonreplicating persistence. *Infect Immun* 1996;**64**:2062–2069.

[42]   Tyagi S, Nuermberger E, Yoshimatsu T, Williams K, Rosenthal I, Lounis N, Bishai W, Grosset J. Bactericidal Activity of the Nitroimidazopyran PA-824 in a Murine Model of Tuberculosis. *Antimicrob Agents Chemother* 2005;**49**:2289-2293.

[43]   Ginsberg AM, Laurenzi MH, Rouse DJ, Whitney KD, Spigelman MK. Safety, Tolerability, and Pharmacokinetics of PA-824 in Healthy Subjects. *Antimicrob Agents Chemother* 2009;**53**:3720-3725.

[44]   Rivers EC, Mancera RL. New anti-tuberculosis drugs in clinical trials with novel mechanisms of action. *Drug Dis Today* 2008,**13**:1090-1098.

[45]   Sasaki H, Haraguchi Y, Itotani M, Kuroda H, *Hashizume* H, Tomishige T, Kawasaki M, Matsumoto M, Komatsu M, Tsubouchi H. Synthesis and Antituberculosis Activity of a Novel Series of Optically Active 6-Nitro-2,3-dihydroimidazo[2,1-*b*]oxazoles. *J Med Chem* 2006;**49**:7854-7860.

[46]   Matsumoto M, Hashizume H, Tomishige T, Kawasaki M, Tsubouchi H, Sasaki H, Shimokawa Y, Komatsu M. OPC-67683, a Nitro-Dihydro-Imidazooxazole derivative with promising action against tuberculosis *in vitro* and in mice. *PloS Medicine* 2006;**3**:2131-2144.

[47]   Zurenko GE, Gibson JK, Shinabarger DL, Aristoff PA, FordCW, Tarpley WG. Oxazolidinones:a new class of antibacterials. *Int J Antimicrob Agents* 2004;**23**:113-9.

[48]   Brickner SJ, Hutchinson, DK, Barbachym, MR, *et al.* Synthesis and antibacterial activity of U-100592 and U-100766, two oxazolidinone antibacterial agents for the potential treatment of multidrug-resistant Gram-positive bacterial infections. *J Med Chem* 1996;**39**:673-9.

[49]   Ross JE, Anderegg TR, Sader HS, Fritsche TR, Jones RN. Trends in linezolid susceptibility patterns in 2002:Reports fromthe worldwide Zyvox annual appraisal of potency and spectrumprogram. *Diag Microbiol Infect Dis* 2005;**52**:53-8.

[50]   Hadjiangelis NO, Leibert E, Harkin TJ. Linezolid:a promising new agent for multidrug resistant tuberculosis treatment. *Am J Respir Crit Care Med* 2003;**167**:A868.

[51]   Lippe B, Sandven P, Brubakk O. Efficacy and safety of linezolidin multidrug resistant tuberculosis (MDR-TB) – a report of tencases. *J Infections* 2005;1-5.

[52]   Barbachyn MR, Ford CW. Oxazolidinone structure-activity relationships leading to linezolid. *Angew Chem Internat Ed* 2003;**42**:2010-2023.

[53]   Shaw KJ, Barbachyn MR. The oxazolidinones:past, present, and future. *Ann NY Acad Sci.* 2011;**1241**:48-70.

[54]   Cole ST, Alzari PM. Enhanced:TB A New Target, a New Drug. *Science* 2005;**14**:214-5.

[55]   Andries K, *et al.* A diarylquinoline drug active on the ATP Synthase of *Mycobacterium tuberculosis*. *Science* 2006;**307**:223-7.

[56]   Haagsma AC, Abdillahi-Ibrahim R, Wagner MJ, Klaas Krab K, Vergauwen K, Guillemont J, Andries K, Lill H, Koul A, Bald D. Selectivity of TMC207 towards Mycobacterial ATP Synthase Compared with That towards the Eukaryotic Homologue. *Antimicrob Agents Chemother* 2009;**53**:1290-2.

[57]   Koul A, Vranckx L, Dendouga N, Balemans W, Van den Wyngaert I, Vergauwen K, Göhlmann HWH, Willebrords R, Poncelet A, Guillemont J, Bald D, Andries K. Diarylquinolines Are Bactericidal for Dormant Mycobacteria as a Result of Disturbed ATP Homeostasis. *J Biol Chem* 2008;**283**:25273-25280.

[58]   Huitric E, Verhasselt P, Andries K, Hoffner SE. *In Vitro* Antimycobacterial Spectrum of a Diarylquinoline ATP Synthase Inhibitor. *Antimicrob Agents Chemother* 2007;**51**:4202-4204.

[59]   Rustomjee R, Diacon AH, Allen J, Venter A, Reddy C, Patientia RF, Mthiyane TCP, De Marez T, Van Heeswijk R, Kerstens R, Koul A, De Beule K, Donald PR, McNeeley DF. Early Bactericidal Activity and Pharmacokinetics of the Diarylquinoline TMC207 in Treatment of Pulmonary Tuberculosis. *Antimicrob Agents Chemother* 2008;**52**:2831-2835.

[60]   Diacon AH, Pym A, Grobusch M, Patientia R, Rustomjee R, Page-Shipp L, Pistorius C, Krause R, Bogoshi M, Churchyard G, Venter A, Allen J, Palomino JC, De Marez T, van Heeswijk RPG, Lounis N, Meyvisch P, Verbeeck J, Parys W, de Beule K, Andries K, Mc Neeley DF. The Diarylquinoline TMC207 for Multidrug-Resistant Tuberculosis. *N Engl J Med* 2009;**360**:2397-2405.

[61]   Pinheiro AC, De Souza MVN. The Relevance of New Drug Combinations for Modern Tuberculosis Treatment – A Patent Perspective. *Rec Pat Anti-Infect Drug Discov* 2013;**8**:130-138.

[62]   Herrick TM, Million RP, 2006. Tapping the potential of fixed-dose combinations. *Nature* 2006;**6**:513-14.

[63]   Zumla A, Nahid P, Cole ST. Advances in the development of new tuberculosis drugs and treatment regimens. *Nature Reviews Drug Discovery* 2013;**12**:308-404.

[64]   http://cdsco.nic.in/FDC%20Guidelines%20_%20Revised1.pdf

[65]   Singh S, Bhutani H, Mariappan TT, 2006. Quality problems of anti-tuberculosis fixed-dose combinations (FDCs):A way forward. Indian *J Tuberc* 2006;**53**:201-205.

[66]   Prasad B, Bhutani H, Singh S. Study of the interaction between rifapentine and isoniazid under acid conditions. *J Pharm Biomed Anal* 2006;**41**:1438-1441.

[67]   Panchagnula R, Agrawal S. Biopharmaceutic and pharmacokinetic aspects of variable bioavailability of rifampicin. *Int J Pharmac* 2004;**271**:1–4.

[68]   Bhutani H, Singh S, Jindal KC, Chakraborti AK, 2005. Mechanistic explanation to the catalysis by pyrazinamide and ethambutol of reaction between rifampicin and isoniazid in anti-TB FDCs. *J Pharm Biomed Anal* 2005;**39**:892-899.

[69]   Lu T, Drlica K. *In vitro* activity of C-8-methoxy fluoroquinolones against mycobacteria when combined with anti-tuberculosis agents. *J Antimicrob Chemother* 2003;**52**:1025-1028.

[70]   Pletz MWR, De Roux A, Roth A, Neumann KH, Mauch H, Lode H. Early Bactericidal Activity of Moxifloxacin in Treatment of Pulmonary Tuberculosis:a Prospective, Randomized Study. *Antimicrob Agents Chemother* 2004;**48**:780-782.

[71]   Gosling RD, Uiso LO, Sam NE, *et al*. 2003. The Bactericidal Activity of Moxifloxacin in Patients with Pulmonary Tuberculosis. *Am J Respir Crit Care Med* 2003;**168**:1342-5.

[72]   Gillespie SH, Gosling RD, Uiso L, Sam NE, Kanduma EG, McHugh TD. Early bactericidal activity of a moxifloxacin and isoniazid combination in smear-positive pulmonary tuberculosis. *J Antimicrob Chemother* 2005;**56**:1169-1171.

[73]   Burman WJ, Goldberg S, Johnson JL, *et al*. Moxifloxacin *vs.* ethambutol in the first 2 months of treatment for pulmonary tuberculosis. *Am J Respir Crit Care Med* 2006;**174**:331-8.

[74]   Dorman SE, Johnson JL, Goldberg S, *et al*. 2009. Substitution of moxifloxacin for isoniazid during intensive phase treatment of pulmonary tuberculosis. *Am J Respir Crit Care Med* 2009;**180**:273-280.

[75]   Alvirez-Freites EJ, Carter JL, Cynamon MH. *In Vitro* and *In Vivo* Activities of Gatifloxacin against *Mycobacterium tuberculosis*. *Antimicrob Agents Chemother* 2002;**46**:1022-5.

[76]   Cynamon MH, Sklaney M. Gatifloxacin and Ethionamide as the Foundation for Therapy of Tuberculosis. *Antimicrob Agents Chemother* 2003;**47**:2442-4.

[77]   Rustomjee R, Lienhardt C, Kanyok T, *et al*. A Phase II study of the sterilising activities of ofloxacin, gatifloxacin and moxifloxacin in pulmonary tuberculosis. *Int J Tuberc Lung Dis* 2008;**12**:128-138.

[78]   Van den Boogaard J, Kibiki GS, Kisanga ER, Boeree MJ, Aarnoutse RE. New Drugs against Tuberculosis:Problems, Progress, and Evaluation of Agents in Clinical Development. *Antimicrob Agents Chemother* 2009;**53**:849-862.

[79]   Chen P, Gearhart J, Protopopova M, Einck L, Nacy CA. Synergistic interactions of SQ109, a new ethylene diamine, with front-line antitubercular drugs *in vitro*. *Antimicrob Chem* 2006;**58**:332-7.

[80]   Nikonenko B.V., Protopopova M., Samala R., Einck L., Nacy A.C., 2007. Drug Therapy of Experimental Tuberculosis (TB):Improved Outcome by Combining SQ109, a New Diamine Antibiotic, with Existing TB Drugs. *Antimicrob. Antimicrob Agents Chemother* 2007;**51**:1563-1565.

[81]   Tyagi S, Nuermberger E, Yoshimatsu T, *et al*. 2005. Bactericidal Activity of the Nitroimidazopyran PA-824 in a Murine Model of Tuberculosis. *Antimicrob Agents Chemother* 2005;**49**:2289-2293.

[82]   Nuermberger E., Rosenthal I., Tyagi S., *et al*. Combination Chemotherapy with the Nitroimidazopyran PA-824 and First-Line Drugs in a Murine Model of Tuberculosis. *Antimicrob Agents Chemother* 2006;**50**:2621-5.

[83]   Tasneen R, Tyagi S, Williams K, Grosset J, Nuermberger E. Enhanced Bactericidal Activity of Rifampin and/or Pyrazinamide When Combined with PA-824 in a Murine Model of Tuberculosis. *Antimicrob Agents Chemother* 2008;**52**:3664-3668.

[84]   Nuermberger E, Tyagi S, Tasneen R, *et al*. 2008. Powerful Bactericidal and Sterilizing Activity of a Regimen Containing PA-824, Moxifloxacin, and Pyrazinamide in a Murine Model of Tuberculosis. *Antimicrob Agents Chemother* 2008;**52**:1522-1524.

[85]   Ibrahim M., Andries K., Lounis N., *et al*. Synergistic Activity of R207910 Combined with Pyrazinamide against Murine Tuberculosis. *Antimicrob Agents Chemother* 2007;**51**:1011-5.

[86]   Lounis N., Gevers T., Van Den Berg J., Andries K., 2008. Impact of the Interaction of R207910 with Rifampin on the Treatment of Tuberculosis Studied in the Mouse Model. *Antimicrob Agents Chemother* 2008;**52**:3568-3572.

[87]   Lounis N, Veziris N, Chauffour A, Truffot-Pernot C, Andries K, Jarlier V. Combinations of R207910 with Drugs Used To Treat Multidrug-Resistant Tuberculosis Have the Potential To Shorten Treatment Duration. *Antimicrob Agents Chemother* 2006;**50**:3543-7.

CHAPTER 3

Known Drugs Against Different Targets or Diseases Evaluated Against Tuberculosis

Marcus V.N. de Souza[*]

Instituto de Tecnologia em Fármacos – Farmanguinhos, FioCruz – Fundação Oswaldo Cruz, R. Sizenando Nabuco, 100, Manguinhos, 21041-250, Rio de Janeiro, RJ, Brazil

Abstract: Nowadays, the evaluation of known drugs against different targets or diseases has become a new strategy in drug discovery. Many of known drugs have exhibited very good efficacy against TB and this methodology is very fruitful because PK-PD (Pharmacokinetic-pharmacodynamic), toxicity and preclinical studies are known for such drugs, which can be useful for conducting clinical trials directly. Fluoroquinolones are the best example, where moxifloxacin and, gatifloxacin used as antiinfective drugs are in advanced clinical trials against TB (Chapter **2**). Known drugs exhibiting anti TB activity can also be used as a start point for chemical modifications in the search of new TB lead compounds. In this context several known drugs, such as antimalarial drugs, isoxyl, thiosemicarbazone, clofazimine, diclofenac, macrolide and thioridazine will be highlight in this chapter.

Keywords: Tuberculosis, *Mycobacterium tuberculosis*, known drugs, drug development, treatment, clinical trials, multi-drug-resistant tuberculosis (MDR TB), extensive-drug-resistant tuberculosis (XDR TB), AIDS, target, mechanism of action, synthesis.

INTRODUCTION

Evaluation of drugs indicated for other disease areas has currently become an important strategy in TB research. A few examples in this context, there are the antibacterial agents, fluoroquinolones, moxifloxacin and gatifloxacin which are in advanced clinical trials against TB (Chapter **2**). This strategy is also an important starting point for chemical modifications in the search for new lead compounds, which will also be highlighted in this chapter.

*Adress correspondence to Marcus V.N. de Souza: Instituto de Tecnologia em Fármacos – Farmanguinhos, FioCruz – Fundação Oswaldo Cruz, R. Sizenando Nabuco, 100, Manguinhos, 21041-250, Rio de Janeiro, RJ, Brazil; E-mail: marcos_souza@far.fiocruz.br

ANTIMALARIAL DRUGS

The quinoline derivatives are known to be particularly important in antimalarial drug research. Quinine (Fig. **1**), an alkaloid first isolated from the bark of cinchona tree in Peru, was the first effective treatment for malaria. The medicinal properties of cinchona tree (antipyretic, analgesic, antimalarial and anti-inflamatory activities) were originally discovered by the Indians of Peru. However, during the colonization period of the Americas (17th century), the Jesuits were the first to bring cinchona to Europe. Despite its toxicity, bitter taste and adverse effects, such as nausea, tinnitus and deafness), quinine remained the antimalarial drug of choice until the 1940s, when other drugs with better pharmacological profile were developed [1].

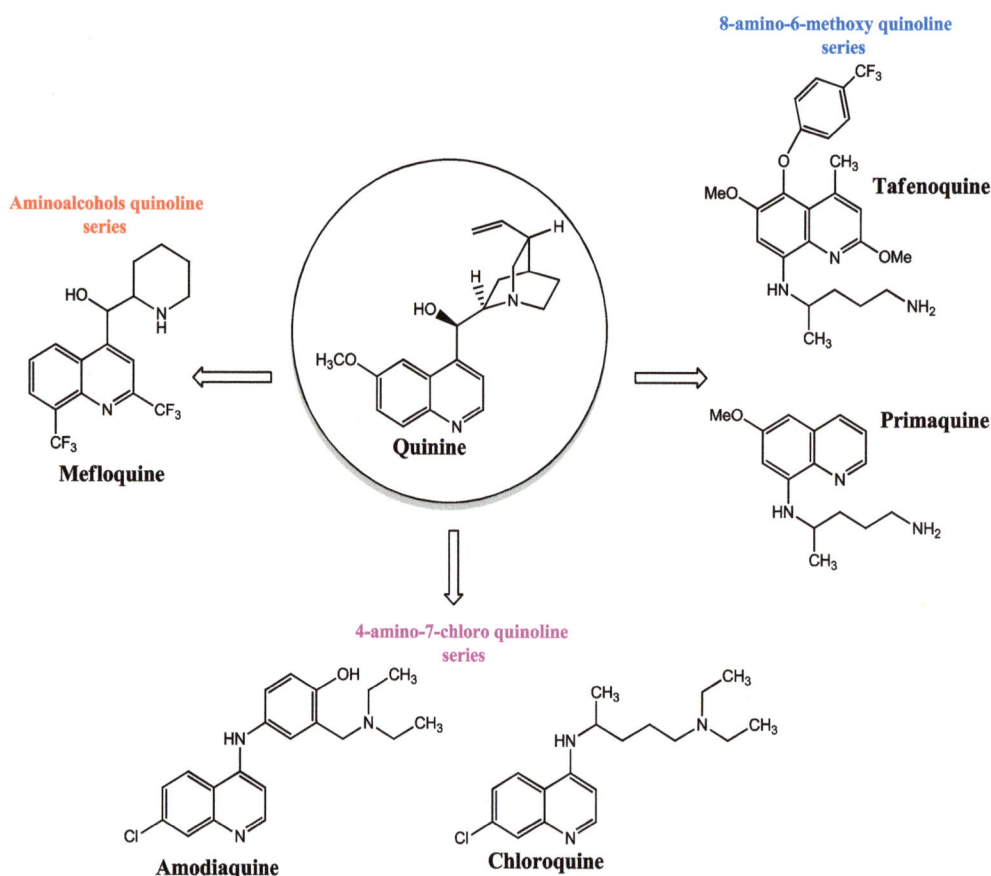

Figure 1: Quinoline antimalarial drugs derived from Quinine.

Nevertheless, quinine served as a starting point to design new antimalarial drugs, such as the 4-amino-quinoline series (chloroquine and amodiaquine), the aminoalcohols quinoline (mefloquine) and the 8-amino-6-methoxy quinoline series (primaquine and tafenoquine) (Fig. **1**). The mechanisms of action of these quinoline anti-malarial drugs have not been fully resolved, but the most widely accepted hypothesis is based on the inhibition of the hemozoinbiocristallization, which facilitates the aggregation of cytotoxic heme. Toxic free heme accumulates in the parasites, leading to their death [2].

In addition to their antimalarial activity, these quinoline drugs showed promising perspectives when they were assayed against TB using the microplate alamar blue assay (MABA). These results indicate that quinoline antimalarial drugs such as quinine, chloroquine, mefloquine, primaquine, and amodiaquine are good starting points for the development of new anti-TB drugs (Table **1**) [3].

Table 1: Minimal inhibitory concentration (MIC) in μg/mL of quinoline antimalarial drugs.

Drugs	MIC (μg/mL)
Amodiaquine	100
Chloroquine	Res
Mefloquine	25
Primaquine	50
Quinine	100

Mefloquine Analogues

Mefloquine (Fig. **1**) is a renowned drug used to prevent malaria (prophylaxis) and also in the treatment of chloroquine-resistant falciparum malaria. Despite its well-known side-effects, such as dizziness, headache, insomnia and vivid dreams [4], this drug and several analogues have been studied as possible antibacterial agents [5-8]. Kozikowski´s research group has developed a relevant study about the potential of mefloquine-based compounds as anti-TB agents [9-13]. In their first report [9], they performed different biological assays on the (+) and (-) forms of the *erythro* and *threo*isomers of mefloquine in replicating (R-TB) and nonreplicating persistant (NRP-TB) phenotypes (Table **2**), which included MABA (microplate Alamar Blue assay), GFP (green fluorescent protein microplate assay), LORA (low oxygen recovery assay – luciferase readout) and MBC [minimal bactericidal concentration, which was determined by quantification of colony forming units (CFU)]. These results showed that erythro isomers were more active against *M. tuberculosis*, as expected through findings made in the malaria field and the (+)-erythro isomer appeared to be less cytotoxic than the (-)-erythro isomer. In this test, the mefloquine MIC and MBC values are in the same range as those rifampin and PA-824, compounds that previously have demonstrated activity against NRP-TB. Because of these observations, they have chosen the (+)-*erythro*isomer of mefloquine as the lead candidate.

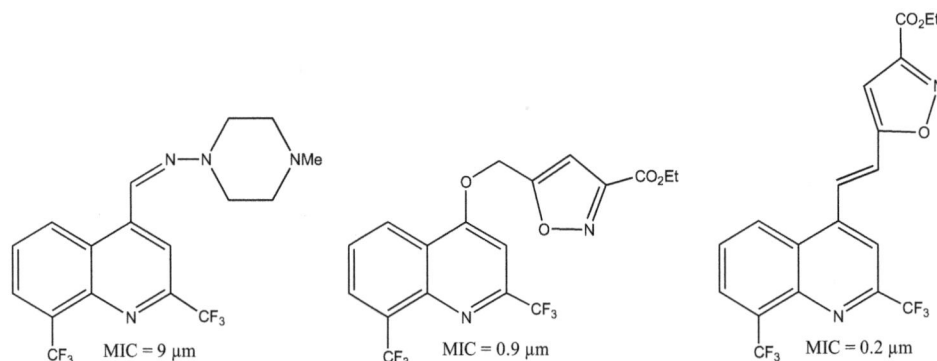

Figure 2: Lead compounds found by SAR information about mefloquine analogues made by Kozikowski's research group [9-13].

Table 2: Anti-TB activity of mefloquine isomers [9].

Compound	MIC (µM)			MBC (µM)	IC$_{50}$	Selectivity Index SI = IC$_{50}$/ MIC		
	MABA	GFP	LORA	CFU	Vero	MABA	GFP	LORA
(+)-*threo*-Mefloquine.HCl	21.3	14.4	19.2	32	25.1	1.2	1.7	1.3
(-)-*threo*-Mefloquine.HCl	12.8	11.7	17.3	32	30.1	2.3	2.6	1.7
(+)-*erythro*-Mefloquine.HCl	7.8	11.2	7.2	8	17.2	2.2	1.5	2.4
(-)-*erythro*-Mefloquine.HCl	6.7	3.8	7.3	4	38.1	5.6	9.9	5.2
Moxifloxacin			42.3	2				
PA-824			7.6	4				
Rifampicin	0.08	0.04	6.5	2	99.7	1246.6	2492.8	15.4

Due to this work, Kozikowski´s research group proposed the synthesis of several mefloquine analogues furnishing important SAR information for this class (Fig. **2**) [9-13].

Mefloquine-Oxazolidine Derivatives

Our group evaluated the introduction of a conformational restriction in the rotation of the piperidinyl ring of mefloquine, by the construction of an oxazolidine ring and the subsequent evaluation of the role of different aryl substituent bounded to the oxazolidine nucleus (Fig. **3** and Scheme **1**). Conformational restriction of flexible drugs has proved to be a very useful strategy in medicinal chemistry, helping to determine the drug receptor steric requirements and in the identification of new structures with greater efficacy and selectivity [14,15].

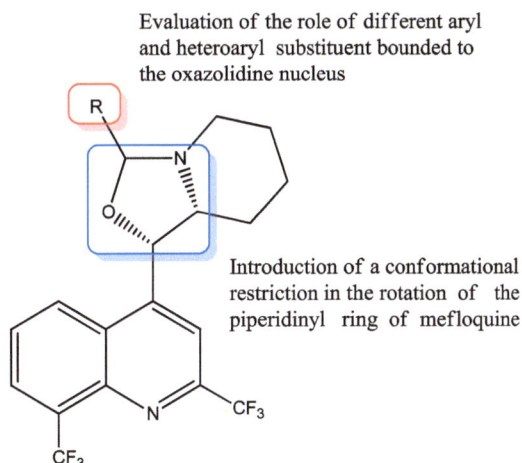

Evaluation of the role of different aryl and heteroaryl substituent bounded to the oxazolidine nucleus

Introduction of a conformational restriction in the rotation of the piperidinyl ring of mefloquine

Figure 3: Design of mefloquine-oxazolidine derivatives.

A series of mefloquine-oxazolidine derivatives, containing phenyl and heteroaryl substituents on the oxazolidine nucleus, has been synthesized and tested against *M. tuberculosis* by our group [14,15]. Among them, two compounds displayed very good antimicobacterial activities in the *in vitro* microplate Alamar Blue assay (Fig. **4**). The compounds **1** and **2** (MICs = 11.9 and 12.1 µM respectively) were around 2.7 times more active than mefloquine and close to the first line tuberculostatic agent ethambutol (MIC = 15.9). The compounds were evaluated against a MDR-TB strain and the same MICs were observed. The resistant strain T113 was isolated from a clinical case of pulmonary tuberculosis in the city of Rio de Janeiro and belonged to the collection of the Bacteriology and Bioassay Laboratory – Instituto de Pesquisa Clínica Evandro Chagas – IPEC – FIOCRUZ. This strain is resistant to the drugs isoniazid, rifampicin, ethambutol and ofloxacin. The cell viability assay also displayed that the compounds were not cytotoxic to Murine Macrophages Cells in a concentration near the MIC being less cytotoxic than mefloquine. These results show that the introduction of the oxazolidine nucleus in mefloquine structure can improve the activity against *M. tuberculosis*.

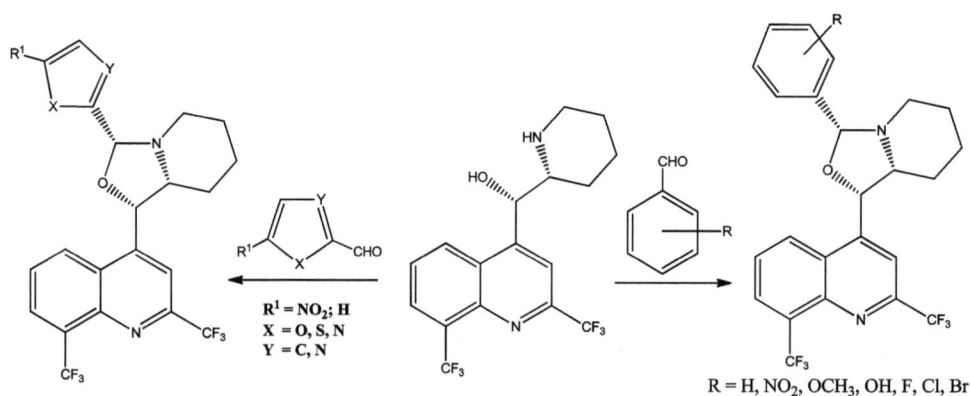

Scheme 1: Synthesis of mefloquine-oxazolidine derivatives.

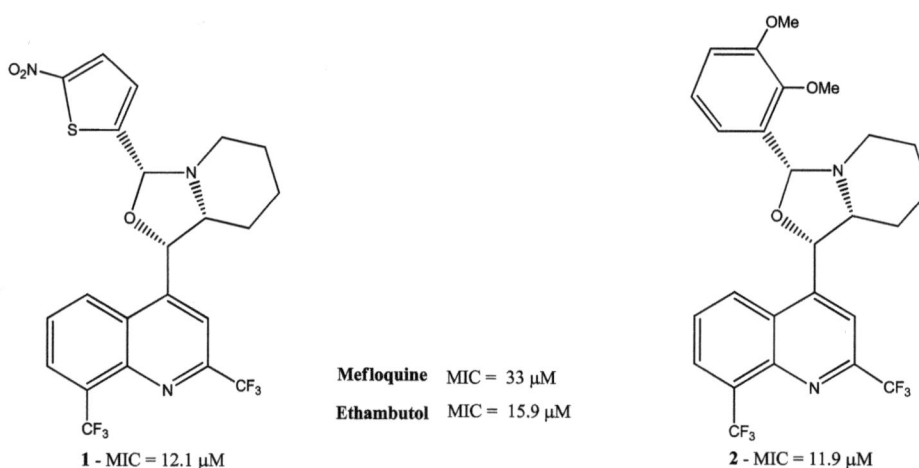

Mefloquine   MIC = 33 μM
Ethambutol   MIC = 15.9 μM

1 - MIC = 12.1 μM

2 - MIC = 11.9 μM

Same MIC for H37Rv (ATCC 27294) and MDR-TB strain T113
(resistant to isoniazid, rifampicin, ethambutol and ofloxacin)

Figure 4: Lead compounds of mefloquine-oxazolidine derivatives.

7-Chloro-Quinoline Derivatives

De Souza and co-workers [3,16,17] have reported the synthesis of several 7-chloro-quinoline derivatives. Their interest in this class of compounds appeared with the evaluation of antimalarial drugs, such as quinine, chloroquine, mefloquine, primaquine, and amodiaquine against TB (Table **1**), using the microplate Alamar Blue Assay (MABA). Despite the lack of activity of chloroquine, the increase in activity of amodiaquine indicates that the biological activity of 7-chloro quinoline derivatives can be modulated by different substitutions at the C4 position. Considering that the design concept of quinoline derivatives attempts to introduce the ethambutol pharmacophore, a first line TB drug, into the core structure of the starting material 4,7-dichloroquinoline, in the expectation to improve its activity, possible by the incorporation of a different mode of action through a different target. Based on this design concept, they proposed the synthesis of 7-chloroquinoline C4-functionalized derivatives (Scheme **2**).

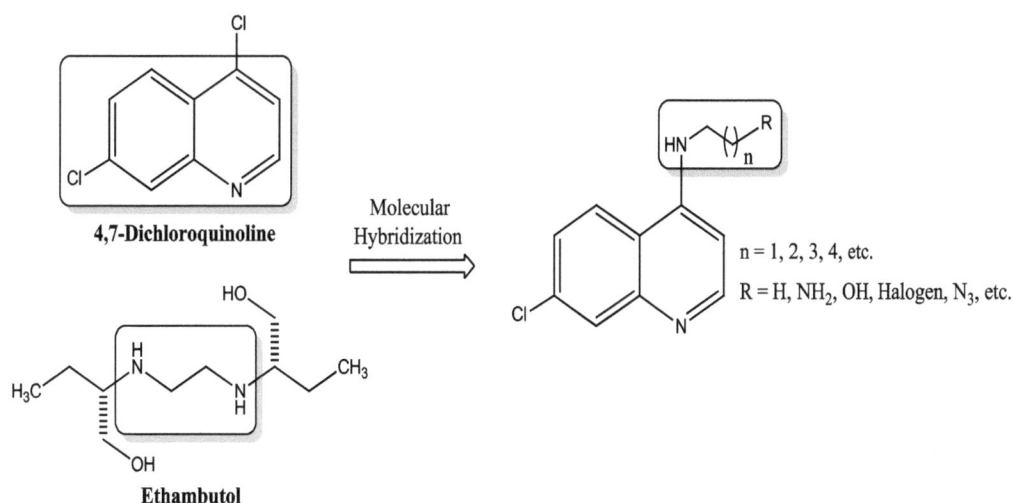

Scheme 2: Design concept of quinoline derivatives prepared by De Souza and co-workers [3].

The synthesis of 7-chloroquinoline C4-functionalized derivatives is described in the Scheme **3**. All the synthesized compounds were assessed against *M. tuberculosis ATTC 27294* using MABA and the best results obtained are described in the Fig. **5**.

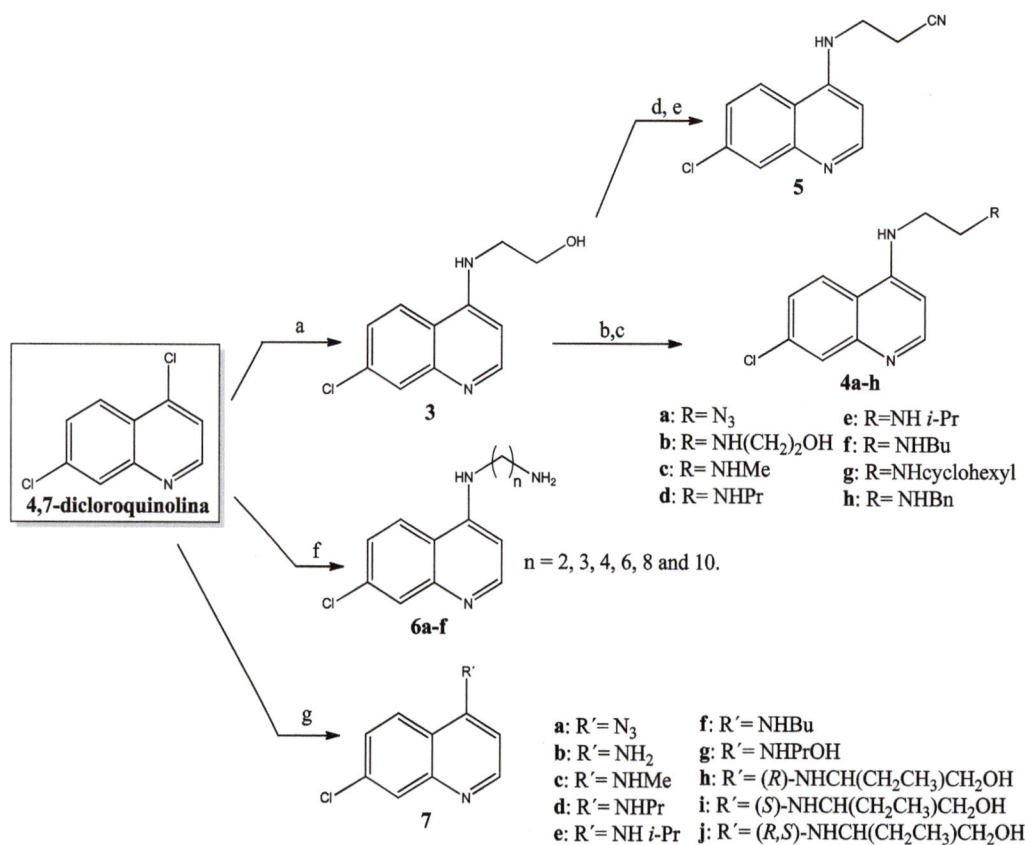

Scheme 3: *Reagents and conditions:* (a) 1-Ethanolamine, Et$_3$N, 120°C, 2h, 94%; (b) SOCl$_2$, DMF, 24h, 94%; (c) Compound 4a: NaN$_3$; DMF; 4h; 46%; Compunds 4b-h corresponding amine, Et$_3$N; 1 -24h, 80-120°C, 72-95%; (d) TsCl, Py, 50°C, 4h; (e) KCN, DMF, 100°C, 1h, 35% in two steps; (f) corresponding diamine, 80-135°C, 4h, 51-94%; (g) Compound 7a: NaN$_3$, DMF, 100°C, 3h, 70%; Compound 7b: phenol, NH$_3$(g), 170°C, 2h, 82%; Compounds 11c-j: corresponding amine or aminoalcohol, Et$_3$N, 60-120°C, 2-24h, 66-96%.

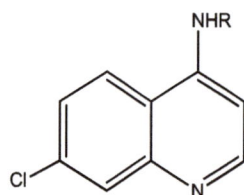

6d: R= (CH$_2$)$_6$NH$_2$ (MIC = 25µg/mL)

6e: R= (CH$_2$)$_8$NH$_2$ (MIC = 6.25µg/mL)

6f: R= (CH$_2$)$_{10}$NH$_2$ (MIC = 3.12µg/mL)

7f: R=Bu (MIC=12.5µg/mL)

Figure 5: The most active derivatives synthesized by De Souza *et al.* [3].

This study furnished some important information about SAR (structure-activity relationship) of 7-chloro-quinoline derivatives based on the activity against *M. tuberculosis*. For example, the presence of a chlorine atom in position 7 and the size of alkyl chain contribute towards the increase of anti-TB activity in this series of compounds. Alkyl groups with large chains lead to more active derivatives, indicating that lipophilicity is an important parameter for the biological activity. Moreover, the group attached in the terminal nitrogen is also a relevant factor that influences the antitubercular activity. In conclusion, some information about SAR of these quinoline derivatives are summarized in Fig. **6**.

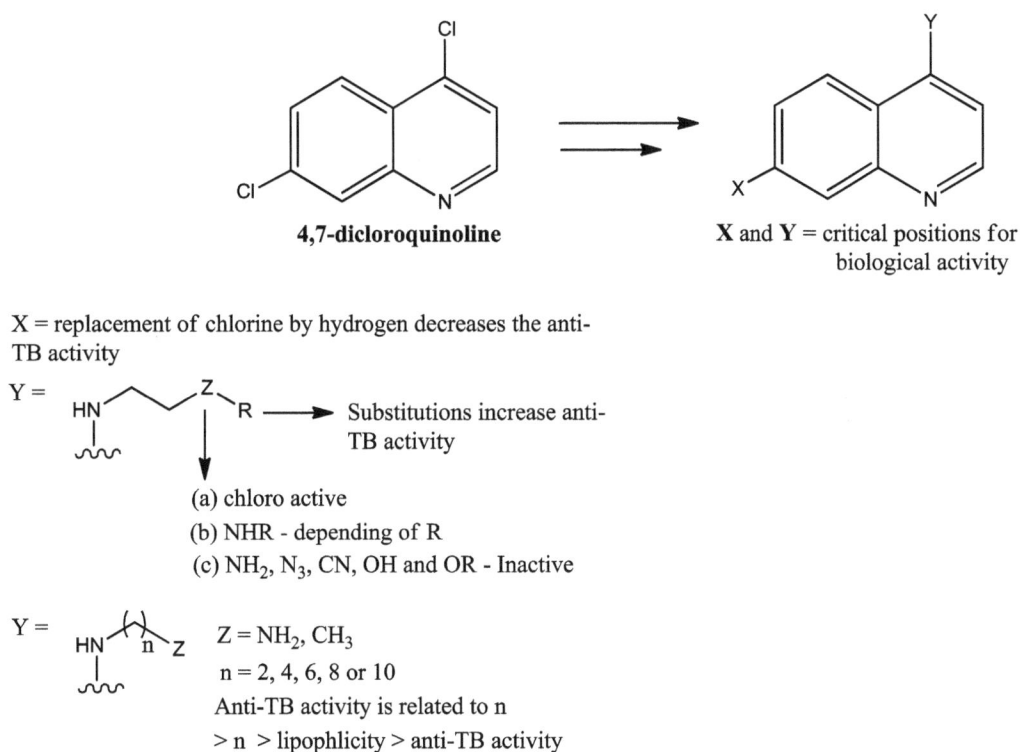

4,7-dicloroquinoline

X and **Y** = critical positions for biological activity

X = replacement of chlorine by hydrogen decreases the anti-TB activity

Y = $\longrightarrow$ Substitutions increase anti-TB activity

(a) chloro active
(b) NHR - depending of R
(c) NH_2, N_3, CN, OH and OR - Inactive

Y = $Z = NH_2$, CH_3
n = 2, 4, 6, 8 or 10
Anti-TB activity is related to n
> n > lipophlicity > anti-TB activity

Figure 6: Important remarks about SAR of quinoline derivatives prepared by De Souza and co-workers [3].

In their continuous efforts in the search for new candidates to antitubercular agents, De Souza and co-workers proposed the synthesis of some hydrazones, containing the 7-chloro-quinoline moiety that was designed by molecular hybridization [16,17]. Due to its synthetic and biological versatility, hydrazones are attractive target compounds for new drug development. In the literature, many pharmacological activities have been associated to hydrazones, such as antidepressant, anticonvulsant, anti-inflammatory, antimicrobial and antitubercular activities. In conclusion, some information about SAR of these quinoline derivatives are summarized in Fig. **7** [16,17].

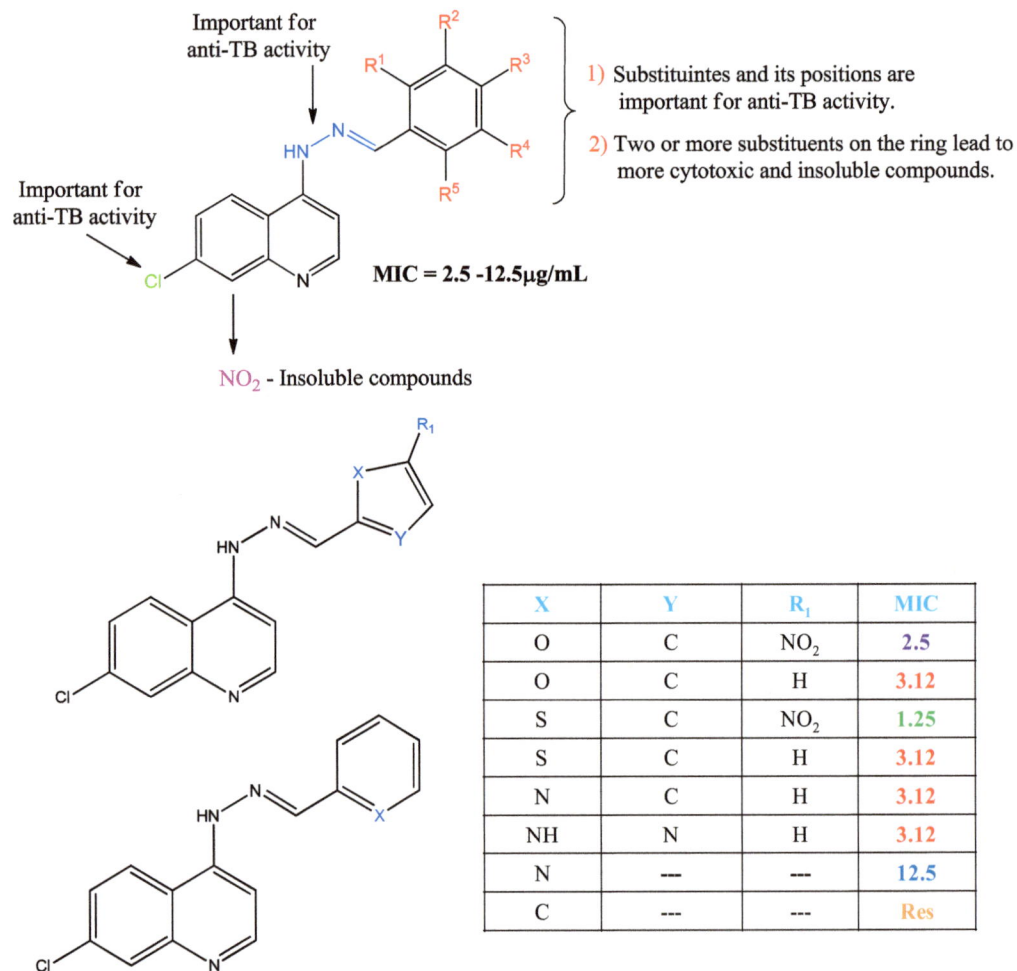

X	Y	R₁	MIC
O	C	NO_2	2.5
O	C	H	3.12
S	C	NO_2	1.25
S	C	H	3.12
N	C	H	3.12
NH	N	H	3.12
N	---	---	12.5
C	---	---	Res

Figure 7: Important remarks about SAR of quinolinehydrazones prepared by De Souza and co-workers [16,17].

Anti-TB Quinolines Made by Other Research Groups

Because of the importance of the quinoline nucleus in the development of new drugs and their potential in TB field, other research groups have synthesized and evaluated various compounds containing this core. The Fig. **8** shows some promising anti-TB compounds of this class.

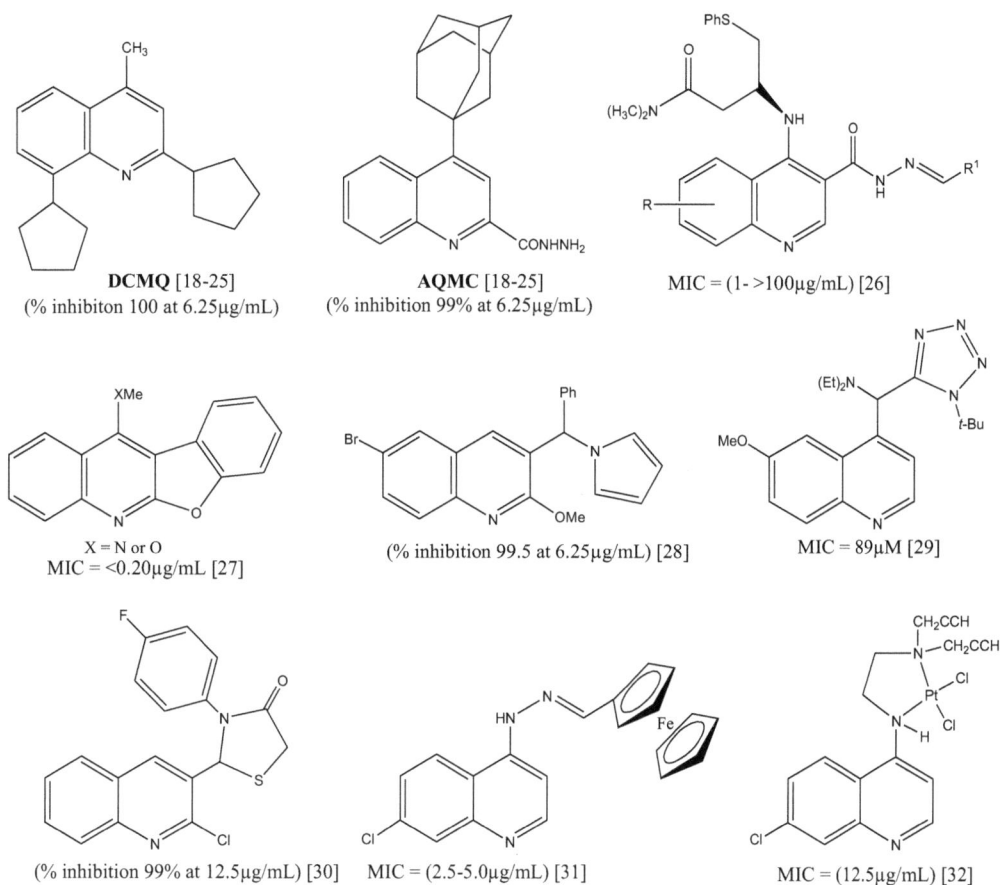

DCMQ [18-25]
(% inhibiton 100 at 6.25μg/mL)

AQMC [18-25]
(% inhibition 99% at 6.25μg/mL)

MIC = (1- >100μg/mL) [26]

X = N or O
MIC = <0.20μg/mL [27]

(% inhibition 99.5 at 6.25μg/mL) [28]

MIC = 89μM [29]

(% inhibition 99% at 12.5μg/mL) [30]   MIC = (2.5-5.0μg/mL) [31]

MIC = (12.5μg/mL) [32]

Figure 8: Anti-TB compounds based on quinoline nucleus.

ISOXYL

The thiourea known as thiocarlide (isoxyl; 4,4′-diisoamyloxythiocarbanilide) (Fig. **9**) was used in the 1960s to treat tuberculosis, whose mechanism of action is similar to INH and ETH *i.e.*, the strong inhibition of mycolic acid synthesis. However, today this drug has regained special attention, owing to its promising *in vitro* antimycobacterial activity (between 1-10 μg/mL), against different clinical multidrug-resistant strains (MDR). Brennan and co-workers made important contributions to this class of compounds by studying its mechanism of action and evaluated several symmetrical and unsymmetrical isoxyl analogues, of which several of them were more potent against *M. tuberculosis* and other *Mycobacterium* species than isoxyl (Table **3**) [33-36].

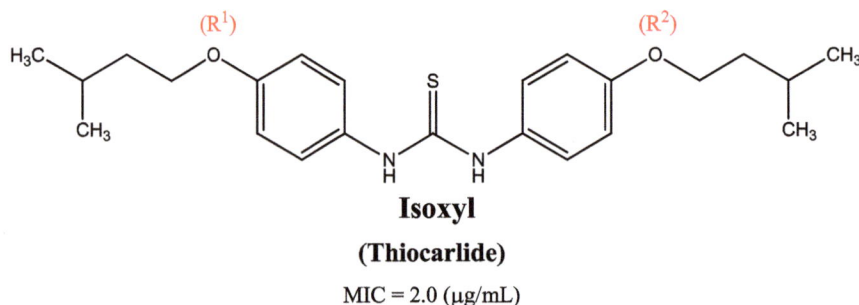

Isoxyl

(Thiocarlide)

MIC = 2.0 (μg/mL)

Figure 9: Structure of isoxyl.

Table 3: Symmetrical and unsymmetrical isoxyl analogues made by Brennan and co-workers.

Number	R^1	R^2	MIC (μg/mL)
8	$OCH_2C(CH_3)_2$	$OCH_2C(CH_3)_2$	1.0
9	$OCH_2CH_2CH_2CH_3$	$OCH_2CH_2CH_2CH_3$	0.1-0.5
10	$OCH_2CH_2CH_3$	$OCH_2CH_2CH_3$	0.1-0.5
11	OCH_3	OCH_3	1.0
12	$SCH_2CH_2CH_2CH_3$	$SCH_2CH_2CH_2CH_3$	2.5
13	$SCH_2CH_2CH_3$	$SCH_2CH_2CH_3$	<0.1
14	SCH_3	SCH_3	0.5
15	$C(CH_3)_3$	$C(CH_3)_3$	>20
16	$CH_2CH_2CH_2CH_3$	$CH_2CH_2CH_2CH_3$	0.1-0.5
17	$OCH_2CH_2C(CH_3)_2$	$SCH_2CH_2CH_3$	2.5-5.0
18	$CH_2CH_2CH_2CH_3$	$OCH_2CH_2C(CH_3)_2$	0.5
19	$CH_2CH_2CH_2CH_3$	OCH_3	0.5
20	$CH_2CH_2CH_2CH_3$	$SCH_2CH_2CH_3$	0.5

In the search for potent isoxyl analogues Besra and co-workers have synthesized different symmetrical and unsymmetrical analogues of isoxyl by two methodologies (Scheme **4**), which were evaluated against *Mycobacterium tuberculosis* H37Rv and *Mycobacterium bovis* BCG with promising results (Fig. **9**) [36]. Compounds 1-(*p-n*-butylphenyl)-3-(4-propoxy-phenyl) thiourea **30** and 1-(*p-n*-butylphenyl)-3-(4-*n*-butoxy-phenyl) thiourea **31**, when compared to isoxyl

(Table **4**), have demonstrated a nearly a 10-fold increase *in vitro* activity in the inhibition of mycolic acid biosynthesis in *M. bovis* BCG. Another important information provided by these compounds was that their poor inhibition of oleate production indicated that the modifications made in the aromatic ring have an influence in the biologic activity [36].

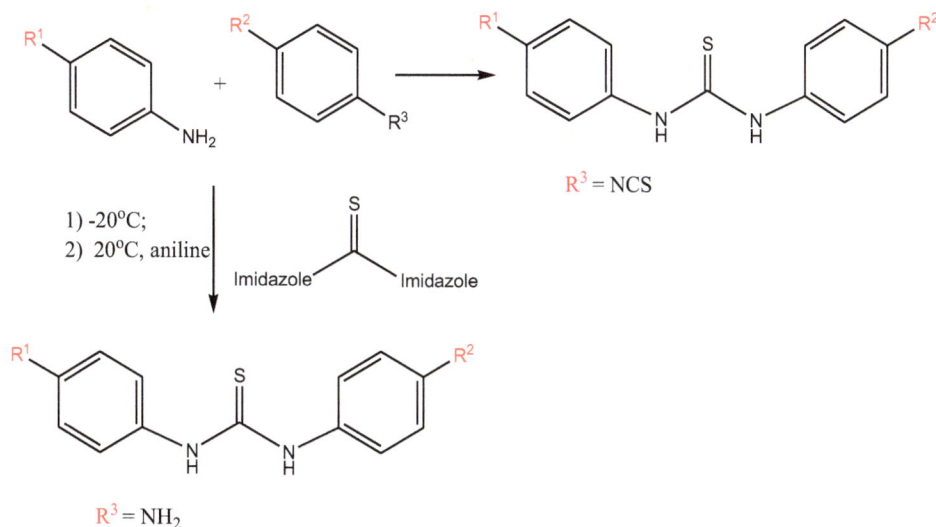

Scheme 4: Synthesis of symmetrical and unsymmetrical analogues of isoxyl.

Table 4: Symmetrical and unsymmetrical isoxyl analogues made by Besra and co-workers.

Number	R^1	R^2	MIC$_{99}$ (µg/mL)
21	$OCH_2CH_2C(CH_3)_2$	$OCH_2CH_2C(CH_3)_2$	2.0
22	$OCH_2CH(CH_3)_2$	$OCH_2CH(CH_3)_2$	ND
23	$OCH_2CH(CH_3)_2$	$OCH_2CH_2CH(CH_3)_2$	0.39
24	$OCH_2CH(CH_3)_2$	$OCH_2CH_2CH_2CH_3$	0.1
25	$OCH_2CH_2CH_3$	$OCH_2CH_2CH_3$	0.2
26	$OCH_2CH_2CH_2CH_3$	$OCH_2CH_2CH_2CH_3$	ND
27	$OCH_2CH_2CH_2CH_3$	$OCH_2CH_2CH(CH_3)_2$	<0.1
28	$CH_2CH_2CH_2CH_3$	$CH_2CH_2CH_2CH_3$	ND
29	$CH_2CH_2CH_2CH_3$	$OCH_2CH_2CH(CH_3)_2$	ND
30	$CH_2CH_2CH_2CH_3$	$OCH_2CH_2CH_3$	<0.1
31	$CH_2CH_2CH_2CH_3$	$OCH_2CH_2CH_2CH_3$	<0.1
32	$SCH_2CH(CH_3)_2$	$SCH_2CH(CH_3)_2$	0.78
33	$SCH_2CH_2CH_3$	$OCH_2CH_2CH_2CH_3$	0.2

34	$SCH_2CH_2CH_3$	$OCH_2CH_2CH_2CH_3$	0.2
35	$SCH_2CH_2CH_3$	$OCH_2CH_2CH(CH_3)_2$	ND
36	$PhCH_2Ph$	$OCH_2CH_2CH(CH_3)_2$	0.2
37	$PhCH_2Ph$	$OCH_2CH_2CH_2CH_3$	0.39
38	$PhCH_2Ph$	$SCH_2CH_2CH_3$	1.56

Other research groups have synthesized and evaluated the anti-TB activity of different thioureas in different scaffolds [37-43] (Fig. **10**).

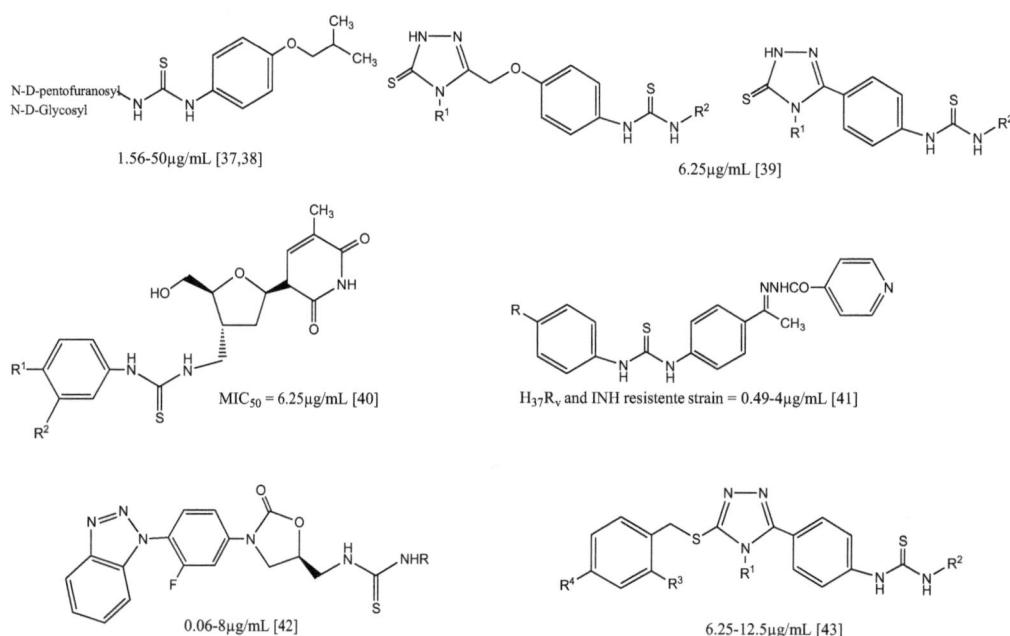

Figure 10: Structure of isoxyl analogues.

THIOSEMICARBAZONE

Semicarbazide, semicarbazone, and thiosemicarbazone are organic functions closely related with hydrazones, and the last one has a wide range of biological activity, especially, antitumor and antiviral activities by acting as a ligand in the complexation of iron and copper from the cell. A special thiosemicarbazone in TB field is thiacetazone, discovered by Gerhard Domagk (1895-1964) in 1946, which showed promising perspectives (Fig. **11**). However, due to problems with clinical trials and toxicity this compound was only introduced in the market in 1962. This drug regained attention due to MDR advent and several analogues have been synthesized and evaluated by different research groups. For example, Kremer and co-workers made outstanding contributions in the synthesis and evaluation of new thiacetazone analogues, as well as by studying the mechanism of action of thiacetazone (Fig. **12**) [44]. Similarly Karali and co-workers, synthesized and evaluated 5-methyl/trifluoromethoxy-1H-indole-2,3-dione3-thiosemicarbazone derivatives (Fig. **13**) [45].

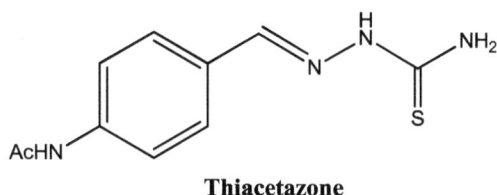

Thiacetazone

Figure 11: Structure of the anti-TB drug thiacetazone.

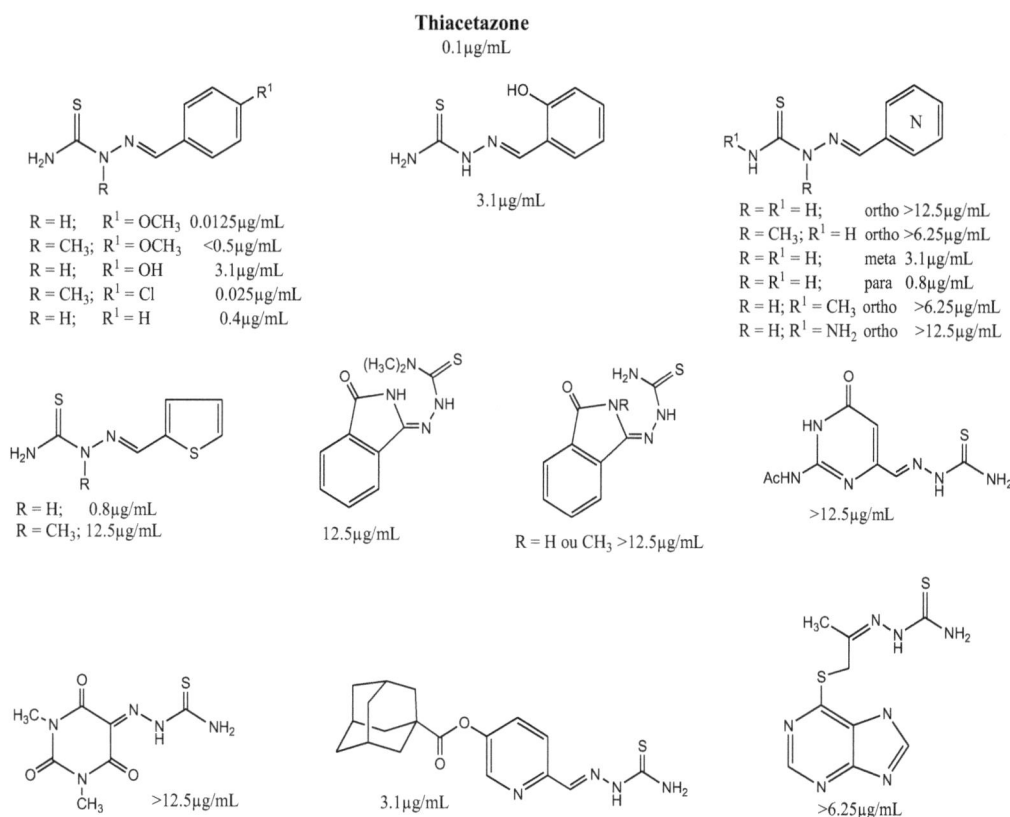

Figure 12: Structure of thiacetazone analogues in different scaffolds.

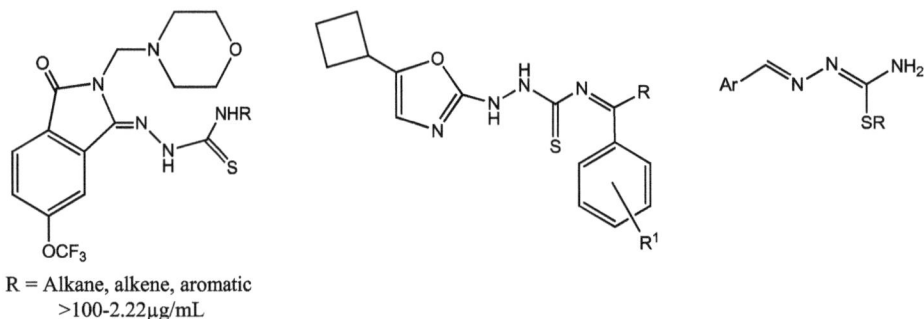

R = Alkane, alkene, aromatic
>100-2.22µg/mL

Figure 13: Structures of 5-methyl/trifluoromethoxy-1H-indole-2,3-dione 3-thiosemicarbazone derivatives.

CLOFAZIMINE

Clofazimine (CFM) is a soluble riminophenazine dye used in the therapy of leprosy in combination with rifampin and dapsone. There are also studies with this drug in combination with other antimycobacterial drugs to treat AIDS patients with *Mycobacterium avium* infections (MAC) (Fig. **14**). It is important to mention that this drug was initially developed to be used in tuberculosis treatment by Barry and co-workers (MIC = 0.12 µg/mL, H37Rv) [46]. However, despite good activity in hamster and mouse models, CFM had problems in monkeys and guinea pigs, suggesting absorptions problems due to the decreased levels of the drug in serum of these animals. Due to the advent of AIDS and MDR-TB, this drug was evaluated alone and as combination against several TB resistant strains with good results, however few analogues of this class have been synthesized and evaluated [47]. The mechanism of action of this class against TB is not well established. However, there are some theories such as, the generation of intracellular hydrogen peroxide, CFM binding to the guanine base of DNA and its stimulation of phospholipase A_2 (PLA_2) activity, responsible for the accumulation of lypophospholipids [47].

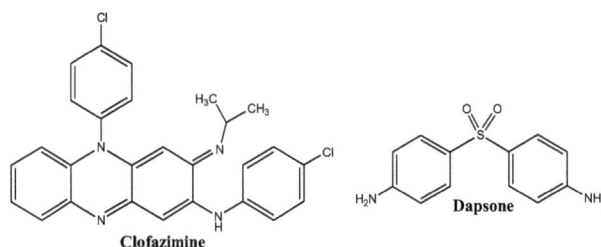

Figure 14: Structure of clofazimine and dapsone.

DICLOFENAC

The drug diclofenac (Fig. **15**) is a non steroidal anti-inflamatory, which has a broad antibacterial activity spectrum against both drug sensitive and resistant clinical isolates of several class of bacterial such as, *Staphylococcus aureus*, *Listeria monocytogenes*, *Escherichia coli*, and *Mycobacterium* spp. In the case of *Mycobacterium tuberculosis*, this drug is also able to inhibit MDR-TB and also possessing synergism *in vitro* and *in vivo* when combined with the anti-TB drug streptomycin, which augments its potency [48].

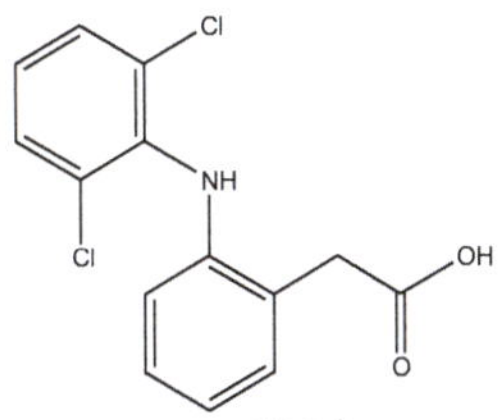

Diclofenac
MIC = 20 µM

Figure 15: Structure of diclofenac.

Sriramsome synthesized and evaluated some diclofenac derivatives by changing the acid function by hydrazone and amides (Fig. **16**) [49]. Among the derivates evaluated compound **39** furnished the best result MIC = 0.36µM being more active than the fluoroquinolones ciprofloxacin (MIC = 9.41µM) and gatifloxacin (MIC = 2.07µM). The coupling reaction between diclofenac and the respective fluoroquinolones lead the compound **40** as the best derivative of this series (MIC = 0.0383 µM), being more potent than first line antitubercular drug isoniazid (MIC= 0.1822 µM).

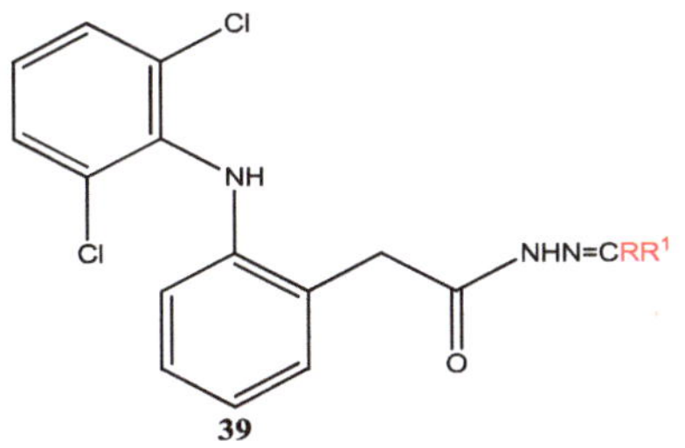

39
R = Ph and **R**^{1} = *p*-PhBr
MIC = 0.3614 µM

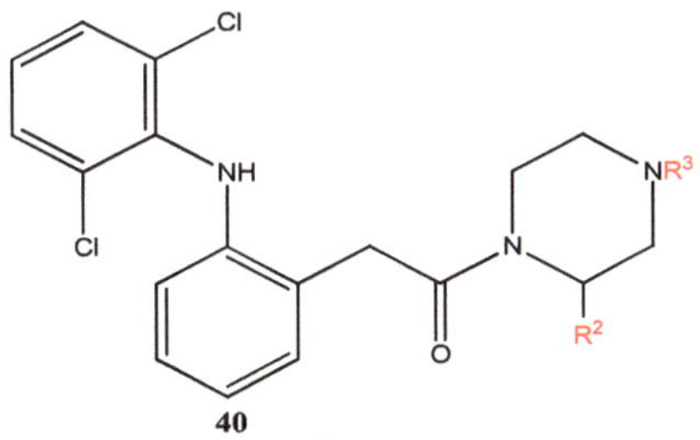

40
R^2 = CH$_3$ and **R**^{3} = Gatifloxacin
MIC = 0.0383 µM

Figure 16: Structure of diclofenac analogues.

It is important to be considered that there are two compounds used in the market that have some similarities with diclofenac, triclosan and hexachlorophene, which also possesses biological activity against *Mycobacterium tuberculosis* (Fig. **17**). Triclosan was first discovered and employed as herbicide, being later identified as an antibacterial agent with a broad spectrum of activity. Nowadays, this compound has several applications such as, antiseptic proprieties being used in laboratories, hospitals and medical surgeries. Due to their safe profile, triclosan has been used in many products used daily by such as, mouthwashes, hand soaps, cutting boards, deodorants and toothpastes. In this context, hexachlorophene also known as Nabac is structurally analogous to triclosan having similar applications. It is also being used in agriculture as acaricide, plant bactericide and soil fungicide. This compound like triclosan also possesses biological activity against *Mycobacterium tuberculosis*.

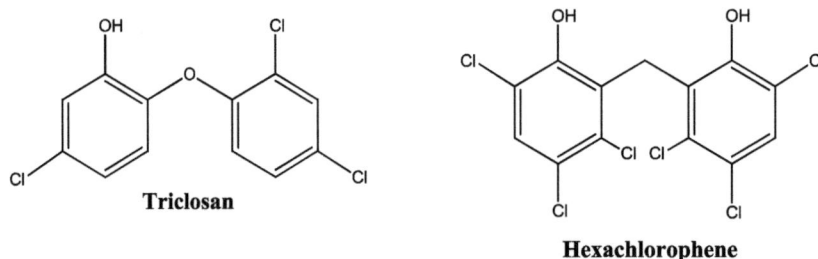

Figure 17: Structure of triclosan and hexachlorophene.

MACROLIDE

The class of drugs known as macrolide belongs to the poliketide class of natural products and possess in its structure a macrocyclic lactone, usually 14-16-member ring, with one or more deoxy sugars, basically cladinose and an amino sugar desosamine. Macrolides are used to treat *Haemophilus influenza*, *Streptococcus pneumonia*, Gram positive bacteria andpenicillin-allergic patients, its mechanism of action being the inhibition of bacterial protein biosynthesis. The first macrolide identified was erythromycin, an antibiotic produced from a strain of the actinomycete *Saccharopolysporaerythraea* discovered in 1949 by the company Eli Lilly [50]. Erythromycin is usually used to treat penicillin-allergic patients, being also effective against species of *Chlamydia*, *Legionella* and *Myoplasma*, however this drug have some side effects, such as gastrointestinal problems, nausea, vomiting and diarrhea, as well as a short serum half-life. Due to this problem, several modifications have been made in the structure of erythromycin with the goal to improve pharmacodynamic proprieties, the spectrum of activity, increase the half life and reduce side effects. In this context, clarithromycin and azitromycin were approved by US Food and Drug Administration (FDA) in 1990's being used against respiratory tract infections, *Helicobacter* and STD (Sexually Transmitted Disease). Another class of macrolides recently discovery was the ketolides, which are erythromycin analogues possessing in its structure a keto-group in the place of cladinose sugar and a cyclic carbamate function in the macrolide. The first ketolide to be approved in clinical use was telithromycin [51] used in respiratory tract infections including erythromycin-resistant bacteria.

Franzblau and co-workers made outstanding contributions in the search for new macrolides and ketolides to be used against *M. tuberculosis* (Fig. **18**) [52,53]. It is important to mention that this scientist made several contributions in TB-drug discovery based on natural, semisynthetic, and synthetic products being an expert in this field. In this study [52] Franzblau's team evaluated several macrolides and ketolides against *M. tuberculosis* selecting three of them for further studies, one macrolide RU60887 MIC = 0.125 µg/mL and two ketolideos RU69874 MIC = 0.38 µg/mL and RU66252 MIC = 0.25 µg/mL having potent anti-TB activity against resistant clinical isolates (MIC = 0.125-4.0 µg/mL) (Fig. **18**). The ketolide RU66252 showed the best results *in vivo* suggesting that modifications in the macrolides and ketolides structures could further lead to improvement toward new lead anti-TB drugs demonstrating that these classes of compounds could be useful against MDR and XDR-TB.

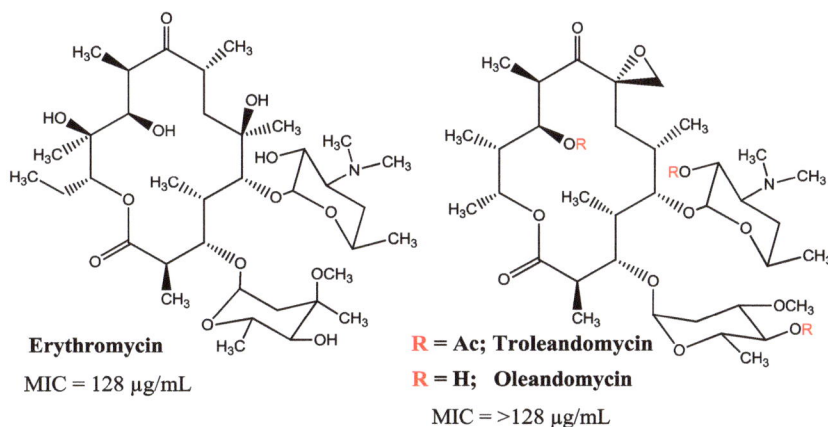

Erythromycin
MIC = 128 µg/mL

R = Ac; Troleandomycin
R = H; Oleandomycin
MIC = >128 µg/mL

Tylosin
MIC = 64 μg/mL

Spiramycin
MIC = >128 μg/mL

Rosamycin
MIC = >128 μg/mL

Midecamycin
MIC = >128 μg/mL

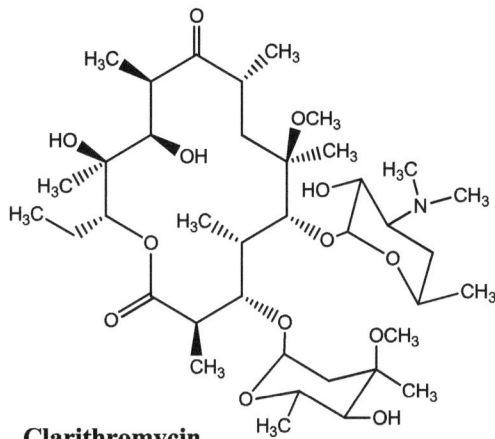

Clarithromycin
MIC = 8 μg/mL

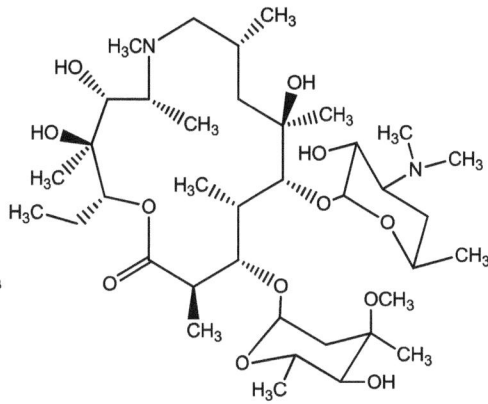

Azithromycin
MIC = 128 μg/mL

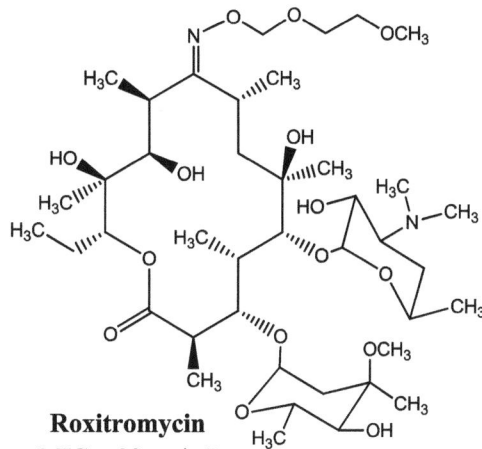

Roxitromycin
MIC = 32 μg/mL

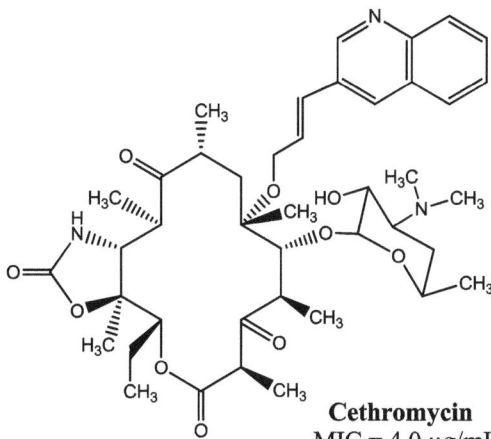

Cethromycin
MIC = 4.0 μg/mL

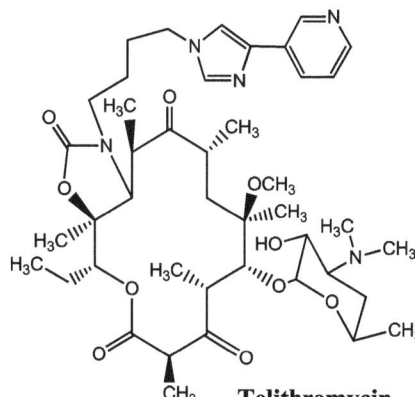

Telithromycin
MIC = 128 μg/mL

RU60887

MIC = 0.125 µg/mL

RU69874

MIC = 0.38 µg/mL

RU66252

MIC = 0.25 µg/mL

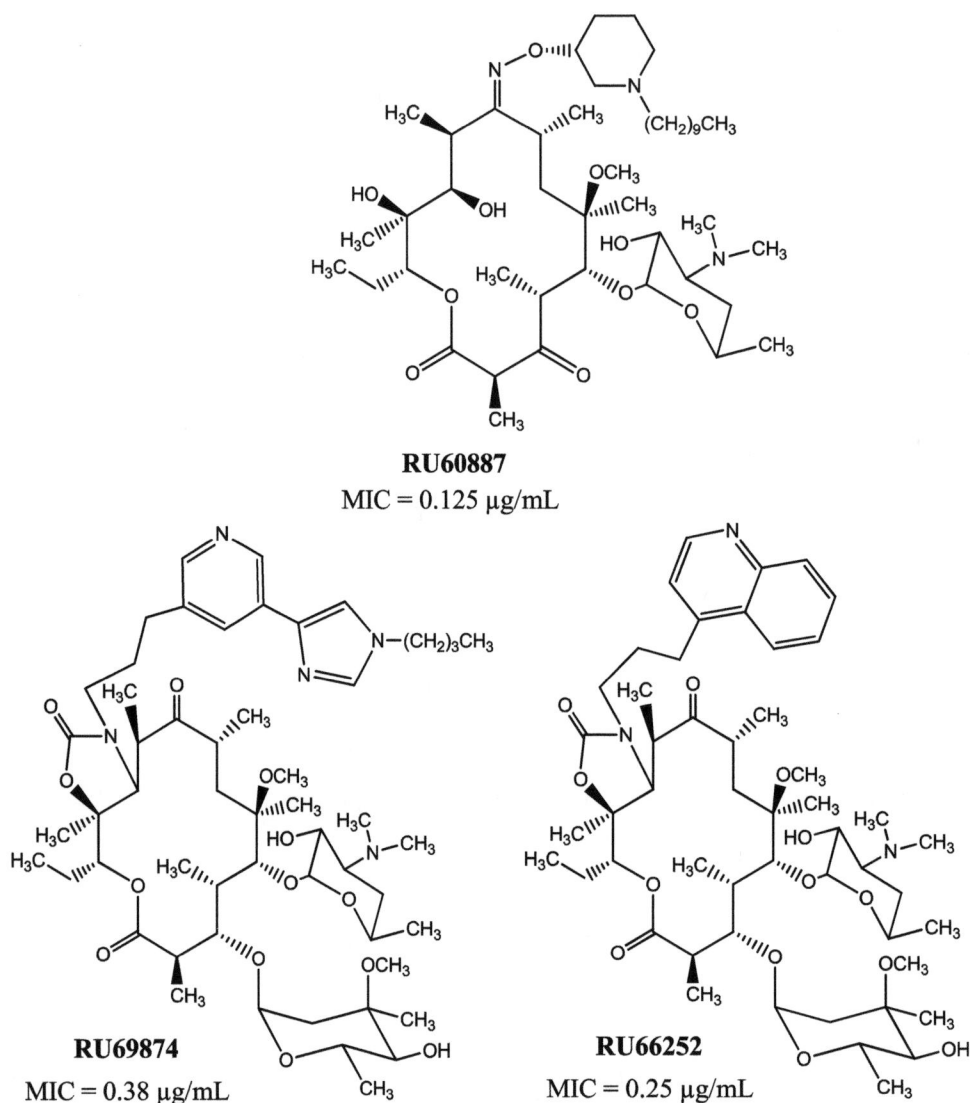

Figure 18: Structure of several macrolides evaluated against *Mycobacterium tuberculosis*.

THIORIDAZINE

This drug is used as an antipsychotic to treat schizophrenia and psychosis, however it has been used with promising perspectives against MDR and XDR-TB. For example, thioridazine was used to cure 10 of 12 XDR-TB patients in Buenos Aires, Argentina being also used in terminal XDR-TB patients in Mumbai, India [54] (Fig. **19**).

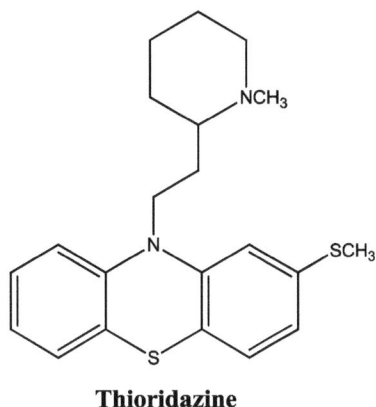

Thioridazine

Figure 19: Structure of thioridazine.

ACKNOWLEDGEMENT

None Declare.

CONFLICT OF INTEREST

The author(s) confirm that this chapter content has no conflict of interest.

REFERENCES

[1]   Foley M, Tilley L. Quinoline antimalarials: mechanisms of action and resistance and prospects for new agents. *PharmacolTher* 1998;**79**:55-87.

[2]   Muraleedharan KM, Avery MA. *Comprehensive Medicinal Chemistry II*. Taylor, JB and Triggle, DJ: Elsevier Science: Amsterdã, **2006**, vol. *8*, p.765-814.

[3]   De Souza MVN, Pais KC, Kaiser CR, Peralta MA, Ferreira ML, Lourenço MCS. Synthesis and *in vitro* antitubercular activity of a series of quinoline derivatives. *Bioorg Med Chem* 2009;**17**:1474-1480.

[4]   Murai Z, Baran B, Tolna J, Szily E, Gazdag G. Neuropsychiatric symptoms caused by mefloquine (report of several cases). *OrvHetil* 2005;**146**:133-136.

[5]   Kunin CM, Ellis WY. Antimicrobial activities of mefloquine and a series of related compounds. *Antimicrob Agents Chemother* 2000;**44**:848-852.

[6]   Bermudez LE, Kolonoski P, Wu M, Aralar PA, Inderlied CB, Young LS. Mefloquine is active *in vitro* and *in vivo* against *Mycobacterium avium* complex. *Antimicrob Agents Chemother* 1999;**43**:1870-1874.

[7]   Bermudez LE, Kolonoski P, Seitz LE, Petrofsky M,Reynolds R, Wu M, Young LS. SRI-286, a thiosemicarbazole, in combination with mefloquine and moxifloxacin for treatment of murine *Mycobacterium avium* complex disease. *Antimicrob Agents Chemother* 2004;**48**:3556-3558.

[8]   Bermudez LE, Kolonoski P, Petrofsky M, Wu M, Inderlied, CB, Young JLS.Mefloquine, moxifloxacin, and ethambutol are a triple-drug alternative to macrolide-containing regimens for treatment of *Mycobacterium avium* disease. *Infect Dis* 2003;**187**:1977-1980.

[9]   Jayaprakash S, Iso Y, Wan B, Franzblau SG, Kozikowski, AP. Design, synthesis, and SAR studies of mefloquine-based ligands as potential antituberculosis agents. *ChemMed Chem* 2006;**1**:593-597.

[10]   Mao J, Wan B, Wang Y, Franzblau SG, Kozikowski AP. HTS, chemical hybridization, and drug design identify a chemically unique antituberculosis agent-coupling serendipity and rational approaches to drug discovery. *ChemMedChem* 2007;**2**:811-813.

[11]   Mao J, Yuan H, Wang Y, Wan B, Pieroni M, Huang Q, *et al.* From serendipity to rational antituberculosis drug discovery of mefloquine-isoxazole carboxylic acid esters *J Med Chem* 2009;**52**:6966-6978.

[12]   Lilienkampf A, Jialin M, Baojie W, Yuehong W, Franzblau SG, Kozikowski AP. Structure-activity relationships for a series of quinoline-based compounds active against replicating and nonreplicating mycobacterium tuberculosis. *J Med Chem* 2009;**52**:2109-2118.

[13]   Lilienkampf A, Pieroni, M, Franzblau, SG, Bishai, WR, Kozikowski, AP. Derivatives of 3-Isoxazolecarboxylic Acid Esters - A Potent and Selective Compound Class against Replicating and Nonreplicating *Mycobacterium tuberculosis*. *Curr Top Med Chem* 2012;**12**:729-734.

[14]   Gonçalves, RSB, Kaiser CR, Lourenço MCS, Bezerra, Flavio AFM, De Souza MVN, Wardell JL, Wardell SMSV, Henriques MGMO, Henriques, Costa, Thadeu. Mefloquine oxazolidine derivatives, derived from mefloquine and arenecarbaldehydes: *In vitro* activity including against the multidrug-resistant tuberculosis strain T113. *Bioorganic & Medicinal Chemistry* 2012;**20**:243-248.

[15]   Gonçalves RSB, Kaiser CR, Lourenço MCS, De Souza MVN, Wardell JL, Wardell SMSV, Da Silva AD. Synthesis and antitubercular activity of new mefloquine-oxazolidine derivatives. *Eur J Med Chem* 2010;**45**:6095-6100.

[16]   Candéa ALP, Ferreira ML, Pais KC, Cardoso LNF, Kaiser CR, Henriques, MGMO, *et al.* Synthesis and antitubercular activity of 7-chloro-4-quinolinylhydrazones derivatives. *Bioorg Med Chem Lett* 2009;**19**:6272-6274.

[17]   Ferreira ML, Goncalves, RSB, Cardoso, LNF, Kaiser CR, Candea ALP, Henrique MGMO, Lourenco MC, Bezerra AFM, De Souza MVN. Synthesis and Antitubercular Activity of Heteroaromatic Isonicotinoyl and 7-Chloro-4-Quinolinyl Hydrazone Derivatives. *The Scientific World Journal* 2010;**10**:1347-1355.

[18]   Jain, R.; Vaitilingam, B.; Nayyar, A.; Palde, P.B. Substituted 4-methylquinolines as a new class of anti-tuberculosis agents. *Bioorg Med Chem Lett* 200;**13**:1051-1054.

[19]   Vangapandu, S.; Jain, M.; Jain, R.; Kaur, S.; Singh, P.P. Ring-substituted quinolines as potential anti-tuberculosis agents. *Bioorg Med Chem* 2004;**12**:2501-2508.

[20]   Vaitilingam B, Nayyar A, Palde PB, Monga V, Jain R, Kaur S, *et al.* Synthesis and antimycobacterial activities of ring-substituted quinolinecarboxylic acid/ester analogues. part 1. *Bioorg Med Chem* 2004;**12**:4179-4188.

[21]   Monga V, Nayyar A, Vaitilingam B, Palde PB, Singh Jhamb S, Kaur S, *et al.* Ring-substituted quinolines. part 2: Synthesis and antimycobacterial activities of ring-substituted quinolinecarbohydrazide and ring-substituted quinolinecarboxamide analogues. *Bioorg Med Chem* 2004;**12**:6465-6472.

[22]   Nayyar A, Malde A, Jain R, Coutinho E. 3D-QSAR study of ring-substituted quinoline class of anti-tuberculosis agents. *Bioorg Med Chem* 2006;**14**:847-856.

[23]   Nayyar A, Malde A, Coutinho E, Jain R. Synthesis, anti-tuberculosis activity, and 3D-QSAR study of ring-substituted-2/4-quinolinecarbaldehyde derivatives. *Bioorg Med Chem* 2006;**14**:7302-7310.

[24]   Nayyar A, Monga V, Malde A, Coutinho E, Jain R. Synthesis, anti tuberculosis activity, and 3D-QSAR study of 4-(adamantan-1-yl)-2-substituted quinolines. *Bioorg Med Chem* 2007;**15**:626-640.

[25]   Nayyar A, Patel SR. Shaikh M, Coutinho E, Jain R. Synthesis, anti-tuberculosis activity and 3D-QSAR study of amino acid conjugates of 4-(adamantan-1-yl) group containing quinolines. *Eur J Med Chem* 2009;**44**:2017-2029.

[26]   Eswaran S, Adhikari AV, Pal NK, Chowdhury IH. Design and synthesis of some new quinoline-3 carbohydrazone derivatives as potential antimycobacterial agents. *Bioorg Med Chem Lett* 2010;**20**:1040-4.

[27]   Yang CL, Tseng CH, Chen YL, Lu CM, Kao CL, Wu MH, Tzeng CC. Identification of benzofuro[2,3-b]quinoline derivatives as a new class of antituberculosis agents. *Eur J Med Chem* 2010;**45**:602-7.

[28]   Upadhayaya RS, Vandavasi JK, Vasireddy NR, Sharma V, Dixit SS, Chattopadhyaya J. Design, synthesis, biological evaluation and molecular modelling studies of novel quinoline derivatives against *Mycobacterium tuberculosis*. *Bioorg Med Chem* 2009;**17**:2830-41.

[29]   Tukulula M; Little S, Gut J, Rosenthal PJ, Wan B, Franzblau SG, Chibale K. The design, synthesis, *in silico* ADME profiling, antiplasmodial and antimycobacterial evaluation of new arylamino quinoline derivatives. *Eur J Med Chem* 2012;**57**:259-67.

[30]   Bhupendra MM, Smita J. Quinoline-based azetidinone and thiazolidinone analogues as antimicrobial and antituberculosis agents. *Med Chem Res* 2013;**22**:647–658.

[31]   Mahajan A, Kremer L, Louw S, Guéradel Y, Chibale K, Biot, C. Synthesis and *in vitro* antitubercular activity of ferrocene-based hydrazones. *Bioorg & Med Chem Lett* 2011; **21**:2866–2868.

[32]   Carmo AML, Silva FMC, Machado PA, Fontes, APS, Pavan FR, Leite CQF, Leite SRA, Coimbra, ES, Da Silva, AD. Synthesis of 4-aminoquinoline analogues and their platinum(II) complexes as new antileishmanial and antitubercular agents. *Biomedicine & Pharmacotherapy* 2011;**65**:204-209.

[33]   Phetsuksiri B, Baulard AR, Cooper AM, Minnikin DE, Douglas JD, Besra GSBrennan PJ.Antimycobacterial Activities of Isoxyl and New Derivatives through the Inhibition of Mycolic Acid Synthesis. *Antimicrob Agents Chemother* 1999;**43**:1042-51.

[34]   Phetsuksiri B, Jackson M, Scherman H, McNeil M, Besra GS, Baulard AR, Slayden RA, Debarber AE, Barry CE, Baird MS, CrickDC, Brennan PJ. Unique mechanism of action of the thiourea drug isoxyl on Mycobacterium tuberculosis. *J Biol Chem* 2003;**278**:53123-30.

[35]   Kordulakova J, Janin YL, Liav A, Barilone N, Dos VUltos T, Rauzier J, Brennan PJ, Gicquel B, Jackson M. Isoxyl Activation Is Required for Bacteriostatic Activity against *Mycobacterium tuberculosis*. *Antimicrob Agents Chemother* 2007;**51**:3824-3829.

[36]   Bhowruth V, Brown AK, Reynolds RC, Coxon GD, Mackay SP, Minnikin DE, Besra GS. Symmetrical and unsymmetrical analogues of isoxyl; active agents against *Mycobacterium tuberculosis*. *Bioorg Med Chem Lett* 2006;**16**:4743-47.

[37]   Liav A, Angala SK, Brennan PJ. *N*-Glycosyl-*N'*-[*p*-(isoamyloxy)phenyl]-thiourea Derivatives: Potential Anti-TB Therapeutic Agents. *Synth Comm* 2008;**38**:1176–1183.

[38]   Liav A, Angala SK, Brennan PJ Jackson M. *N*-D-Aldopentofuranosyl-*N′*-[*p*-(isoamyloxy)phenyl]-thiourea derivatives: Potential anti-TB therapeutic agents. *Bioorg & Med Chem Lett* 2008;**18:**2649–2651.

[39]   Kucukguzel I, Tatar E, GunizKucukguzel S, Rollas S, De Clercq E. Synthesis of some novel thiourea derivatives obtained from 5-[(4-aminophenoxy)methyl]-4 alkyl/aryl-2,4-dihydro-3H-1,2,4-triazole-3-thiones and evaluation as antiviral/anti-HIV and anti-tuberculosis agents. *Eur J Med Chem* 2008;**43:**381-392.

[40]   Rational Design of 5′-Thiourea-Substituted α-Thymidine Analogues as Thymidine Monophosphate Kinase Inhibitors Capable of Inhibiting Mycobacterial Growth. Daele IV, Lehmann, HM, Froeyen M, Balzarini J, Calenbergh SV. *J. Med. Chem.* 2007;**50:**5281-5292.

[41]   Synthesis and in vitro antitubercular activity of some 1-[(4-sub)phenyl]-3-(4-{1-[(pyridine-4-carbonyl) hydrazono]ethyl}phenyl)thiourea. Sriram D, Yogeeswari P, Madhu, K *Bioorg & Med Chem Lett* 2006;**16:**876–878.

[42]   Dixit PP, Patil VJ, Nair PS, Jain S, Neelima Sinha, Arora SK. Synthesis of 1-[3-(4-benzotriazol-1/2-yl-3-fluorophenyl)-2-oxo-oxazolidin-5-ylmethyl]-3-substituted-thiourea derivatives as antituberculosis agents. *Eur J Med Chem* 2006;**41:**423–428.

[43]   Kucukguzel I, GunizKucukguzel S, Rollasa S, Kirazb M. Some 3-Thioxo/Alkylthio-1,2,4-triazoles with a Substituted Thiourea Moiety as Possible Antimycobacterials. *Bioorg & Med Chem Lett* 2001;**11:**1703–1707.

[44]   Thiacetazone, an Antitubercular Drug that Inhibits Cyclopropanation of Cell Wall Mycolic Acids in Mycobacteria. Alahari A, Trivelli X, Guerardel Y, Dover LG, Besra GS, Sacchettini JC, Reynolds RC, Coxon GD, Kremer L, *PLoS ONE* 2007;**12:**e1343 1-12.

[45]   Synthesis and antituberculosis activity of 5-methyl/trifluoromethoxy-1H-indole-2,3-dione 3-thiosemicarbazone derivatives. Güzel O, Karalı N, Salman A. *Bioorg & Med Chem* 2008;**16:**8976–8987.

[46]   Barry VC, Belton JG, Conalty ML, Twomey D. Antitubercular activity of oxidations products of substituted o-phenylene diamines. *Nature* 1948;**162:**622-3.

[47]   Reddy VM, Sullivan JFO, Gangadharam PRJ. Antimycobacterial activities of riminophenazines *Antimicrobial Chemotherapy* 1999;**43:**615-623.

[48]   Dutta NK, Mazumdar K, Dastidar SG, Park JH. Activity of diclofenac used alone and in combination with streptomycin *against Mycobacterium tuberculosis* in mice. *Int J Antimicrob Agents* 2007;**30:**336-40.

[49]   Sriram D, Yogeeswari P, Vandana RD. Synthesis, *in vitro* and *in vivo* antimycobacterial activities of diclofenac acid hydrazones and amides. *Bioorg Med Chem* 2006;**14:**3113-18.

[50]   Kirst HA, Sides GD New directions for macrolide antibiotics: structural modifications and in vitro activity. *Antimicrob Agents Chemother* 1989;**33:**1413-18.

[51]   Speirs KM, Zervos M. Telithromycin. *J Expert Review of Anti-Infective Therapy* 2004;**2:**685-93.

[52]   Zhu ZJ, Krasnykh O, Pan D, Petukhova V, Yu G, Liu Y, Liu H, Hong S, Wang Y, Wan B, Liang W, Franzblau SG. Structure-activity relationships of macrolides against *Mycobacterium tuberculosis. Tuberculosis* 2008;**88:**S49-S63.

[53]   Falzari K, Zhu Z, Pan D, Liu H, Hongmanee P, Franzblau, SG. *In Vitro* and *In Vivo* Activities of Macrolide Derivatives against *Mycobacterium tuberculosis. Antimicrob Agents Chemother* 2005;**49:**1447-54.

[54]   Amarala L, Boereeb MJ, Gillespie SH, Udwadiad ZF, Soolingene DV. Thioridazine cures extensively drug-resistant tuberculosis (XDR-TB) and the need for global trials is now! *Int J Antimicro Ag* 2010;**35:**524–526.

CHAPTER 4

Synthetic Anti-TB Compounds

Marcus V.N. de Souza[*]

Instituto de Tecnologia em Fármacos – Farmanguinhos, FioCruz – Fundação Oswaldo Cruz, R. Sizenando Nabuco, 100, Manguinhos, 21041-250, Rio de Janeiro, RJ, Brazil

Abstract: TB became again an important infectious disease worldwide in the mid-1980's, and several factors are responsible for this, such as AIDS epidemic, the advent of multidrug resistant strains (MDR), poor socioeconomic condition and immigration. Unfortunately, due to the disadvantages of the first and second line drugs, and the increase of MDR strains worldwide, nowadays we urgent need new drugs to improve the TB treatment or a tragedy can happen. Considering this problem, several actions have been made, and in 2000 it was established the Global Alliance for TB Drug Development (GATB; www.tballiance.org). In this context, GATB have been working in partnership with different kinds of organizations, such as academic institutions, government research laboratories, non-governmental organizations, pharmaceutical industries and contract research houses. Due to its important work, GATB have changed the perspective of TB drug discovery. Considering that, this chapter aims to highlight synthetic compounds from different chemical classes, which were evaluated against *M. tuberculosis* in the last fifteen years.

Keywords: Tuberculosis, *Mycobacterium tuberculosis*, chemistry, synthetic compound, synthesis, drug development, treatment, multi-drug-resistant tuberculosis (MDR TB), extensive-drug-resistant tuberculosis (XDR TB), target, mechanism of action, biological evaluation.

INTRODUCTION

After the discovery of the natural product streptomycin in 1944 and, the period known as the gold era of TB research (1940-70), which was responsible for the introduction of synthetic drugs, as well as semisynthetic and other natural

---

*Adress correspondence to Marcus V.N. de Souza: Instituto de Tecnologia em Fármacos – Farmanguinhos, FioCruz – Fundação Oswaldo Cruz, R. Sizenando Nabuco, 100, Manguinhos, 21041-250, Rio de Janeiro, RJ, Brazil; E-mail: marcos_souza@far.fiocruz.br

products, the scientific community believed that this disease would be finally eradicated. However, in 1981, a new disease, known as AIDS was identified, being one of the major causes of the resurgence of TB, which was declared by WHO as a global health emergency in 1993. After that, TB research was again regained attention, with important discoveries made by several scientists aiming to solve two new TB problems: MDR and XDR-TB. In this context, known and unknown compounds have been evaluated against *Mycobacterium tuberculosis*, as well as natural products and drugs used against other diseases [1-6]. Considering that, this chapter aims to highlight synthetic compounds from different chemical classes, which were evaluated against *M. tuberculosis* in the last fifteen years.

HYDRAZINE DERIVATIVES AND RELATED COMPOUNDS

Hidrazine, hidrazone, *N*-acylhydrazone and guanylhydrazone are important classes of compounds, which possessed a wide range of pharmacological activities, such as antiviral, antimalarial, antitumoral, antiinflammatory, analgesic, antimicrobial, vasodilator, antischistosomiasis, anticonvulsant, antiplatelet, and antidepressant activities [7]. Due to the versatile biological applications of these classes of compound different research groups have investigated its anti-TB proprieties in different scaffolds [8-15] being described in the Fig. **1**.

Our group has synthesized and evaluated several hidrazone and acyl hidrozone compounds, such as isoniazid, pyrazinamide, thiadiazole, quinoline, coumarine, serine and oxazolidinones derivatives. Some of them demonstrated potent activity, including against isoniazid resistant strains with MIC in the range 0.31 and 3.12 µg/mL (Fig. **2**) [16-22].

In addition we evaluated 48 common aldehydes used to prepare hydrazones (Fig. **3**) [23]. Benzaldehydes are an important class of reagents used for different purposes. For example, in medicinal chemistry they are used in the formation of Schiff bases, amines, hydrazones and *N*-acylhydrazones. These groups are present in several compounds with application in many diseases. However, in despite of commercial aldehydes have been largely used for many research groups, this class was not tested before against *Mycobacterium tuberculosis* [23]. The biological

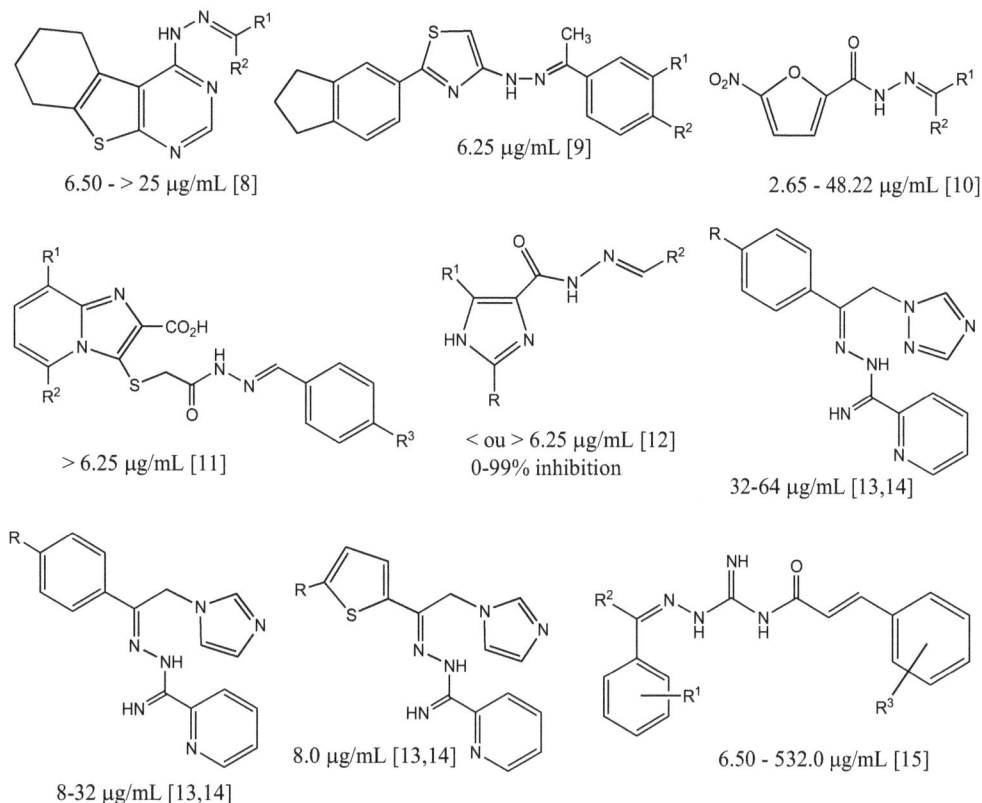

6.50 - > 25 μg/mL [8]

6.25 μg/mL [9]

2.65 - 48.22 μg/mL [10]

> 6.25 μg/mL [11]

< ou > 6.25 μg/mL [12]
0-99% inhibition

32-64 μg/mL [13,14]

8-32 μg/mL [13,14]

8.0 μg/mL [13,14]

6.50 - 532.0 μg/mL [15]

Figure 1: Synthesis and anti-TB evaluation of hidrazine, hidrazone, *N*-acylhydrazone and guanylhydrazone in different scaffolds.

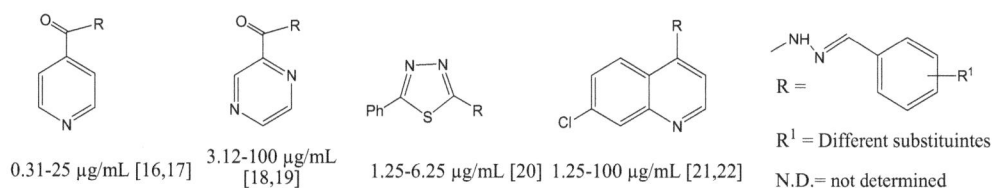

0.31-25 μg/mL [16,17]

3.12-100 μg/mL [18,19]

1.25-6.25 μg/mL [20]   1.25-100 μg/mL [21,22]

R^1 = Different substituintes

N.D.= not determined

Figure 2: Hidrazone and *N*-acylhydrazone compounds synthesized by our group.

evaluation of benzaldehydes suggests that the number and position of substituents are important for the activity against *Mycobaterium tuberculosis*. For example, in the case of cyano group, the position in the ring is important for the biological activity (*orto*-100; *metha*-25 and *para*-12.5 μg/mL). In the case of the group nitro substituent the better positions are in *ortho* and *para* (3.25 μg/mL), but the presence of this group in *meta* position decreases the biological activity. In conclusion, we can observe that when electron withdrawing groups, such as NO_2

and CN are in *para* position, they increase the biological activity of these aldehydes. Another important fact observed is that the position and the number of hydroxyl groups in the ring are critical for the biological activity. The Fig. **3** also summarizes the structure-activity relationship for this class of compounds.

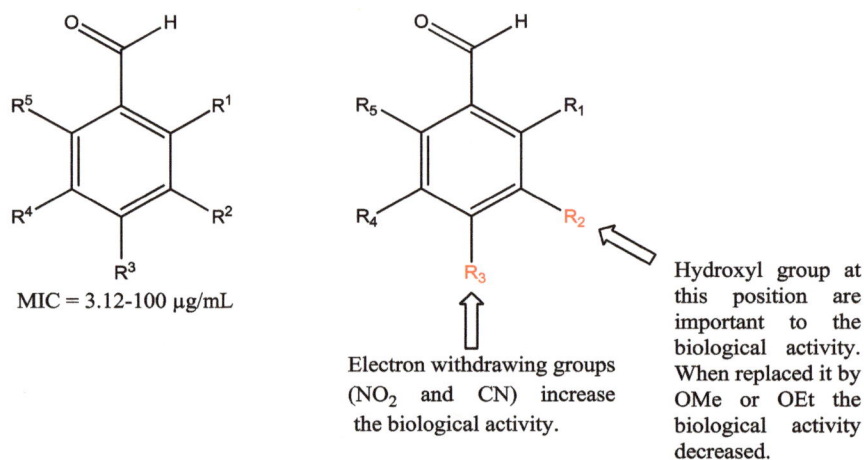

MIC = 3.12-100 µg/mL

Electron withdrawing groups (NO$_2$ and CN) increase the biological activity.

Hydroxyl group at this position are important to the biological activity. When replaced it by OMe or OEt the biological activity decreased.

Figure 3: Anti-TB evaluation of commercial benzaldehydes and SAR of the benzaldehydes series tested against *M. tuberculosis*.

TRIAZOLES

Triazole is a heterocyclic five-membered ring containing three nitrogen atoms with two isomeric chemical compounds, 1,2,3 and 1,2,4 triazole. This class of compounds possesses potent antifungal and fungicides proprieties, with several drugs into the market, such as fluconazole and voriconazole used as antifungal drugs and tebuconazole used in agricultural as fungicide (Fig. **4**). Several researchers have been studied the potential of this class of compounds as anti-TB drug with 1,2,3 and 1,2,4 triazoles substituted in different positions and with a wide range of substituents. In Fig. **5** is described some series of triazoles with its respective anti-TB activities (MIC).

IMIDAZOLE

Imidazole (1,3-diazole), like triazole is a heterocyclic five-membered ring containing two nitrogen atoms into its structure displaying also potent antifungal

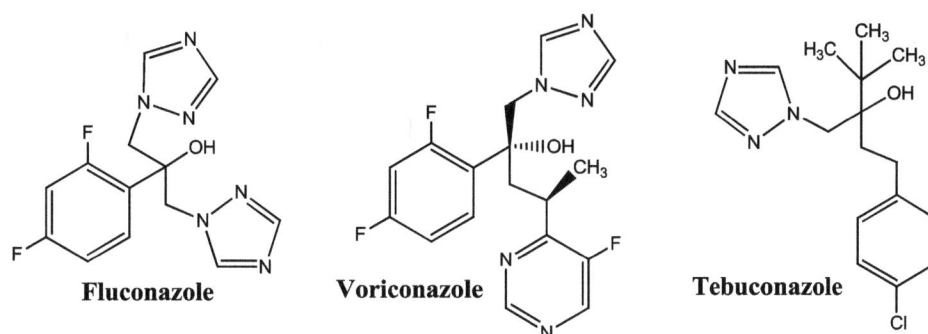

Figure 4: Structure of fluconazole, voriconazole and tebuconazole.

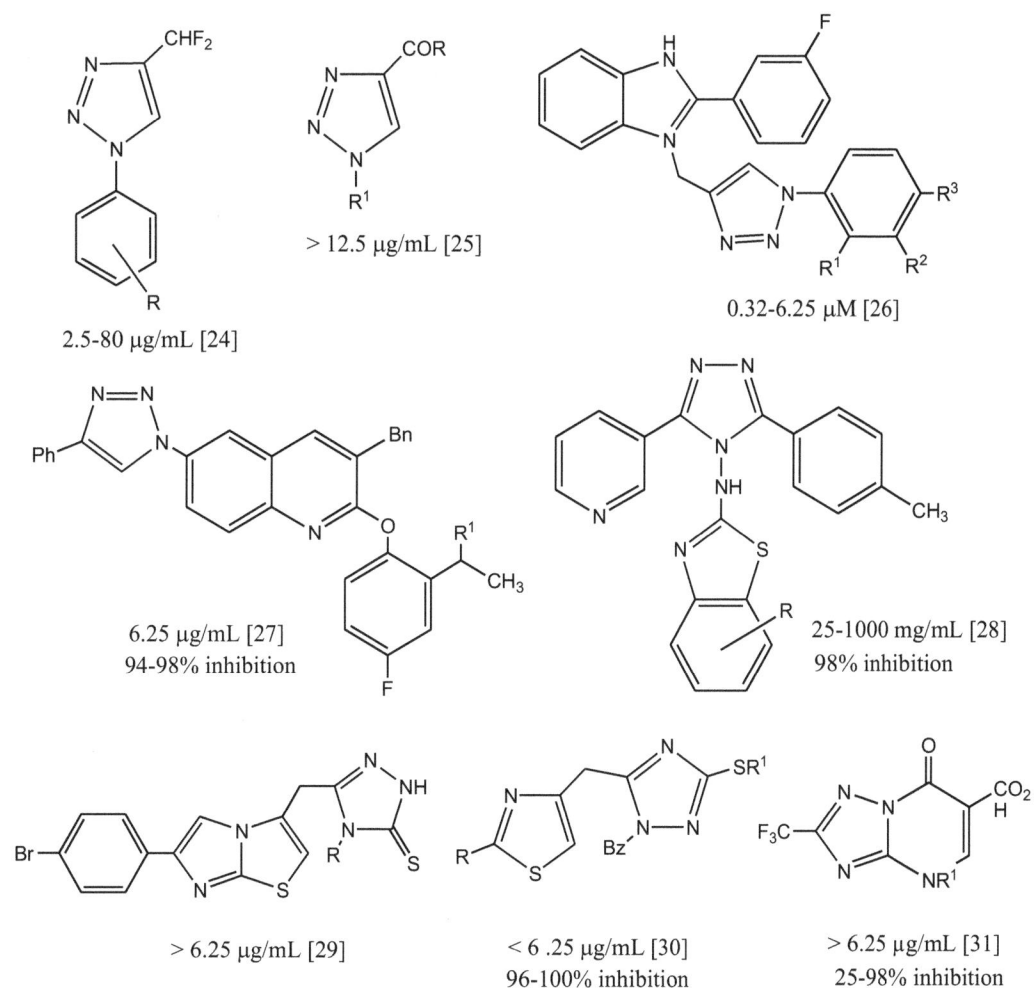

2.5-80 µg/mL [24]

> 12.5 µg/mL [25]

0.32-6.25 µM [26]

6.25 µg/mL [27]
94-98% inhibition

25-1000 mg/mL [28]
98% inhibition

> 6.25 µg/mL [29]

< 6 .25 µg/mL [30]
96-100% inhibition

> 6.25 µg/mL [31]
25-98% inhibition

Figure 5: Synthesis and anti-TB evaluation of imidazole in different scaffolds.

proprieties being clotrimazole, miconazole and ketoconazole drugs used for systemic fungal infections (Fig. **6**). This class of compound showed also other pharmacological activities being incorporated in many anticancer, antihypertensive, fungicides, and antiprotozoal drugs. In this context, several researchers have been studied the potential of this class of compounds as anti-TB drug with imidazole substituted in different positions and with a wide range of substituents. In Fig. **7** is described some series of imidazoles derivatives with its respective anti-TB activities (MIC).

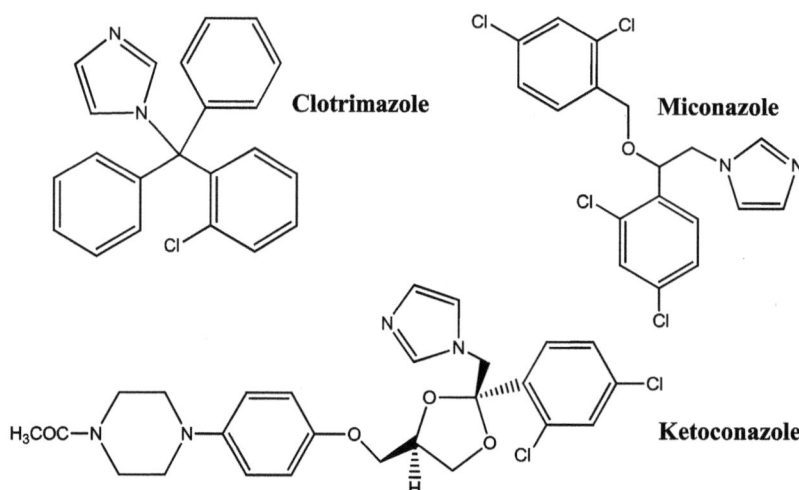

Figure 6: Structure of clotrimazole, miconazole and ketoconazole.

TRIAZINES

Chauhan and co-workers synthesized a series of new 2,4,6-trisubstituted-1,3,5-triazines, which demonstrated potent activity against *Mycobacterium tuberculosis* with MIC in the range of 1.56 to 3.12 µg/mL for the fifteen most active compounds with no citotoxic profile (Scheme **1**) [35]. Another point to be considered is that the inclusion of isoniazid increased the potency of 1,3,5- triazines.

ISATINES

The 1H-indoline-2,3-dione (isatin) is a versatile intermediate used to prepare different class of compounds, being also found in plants, and in the mammalian

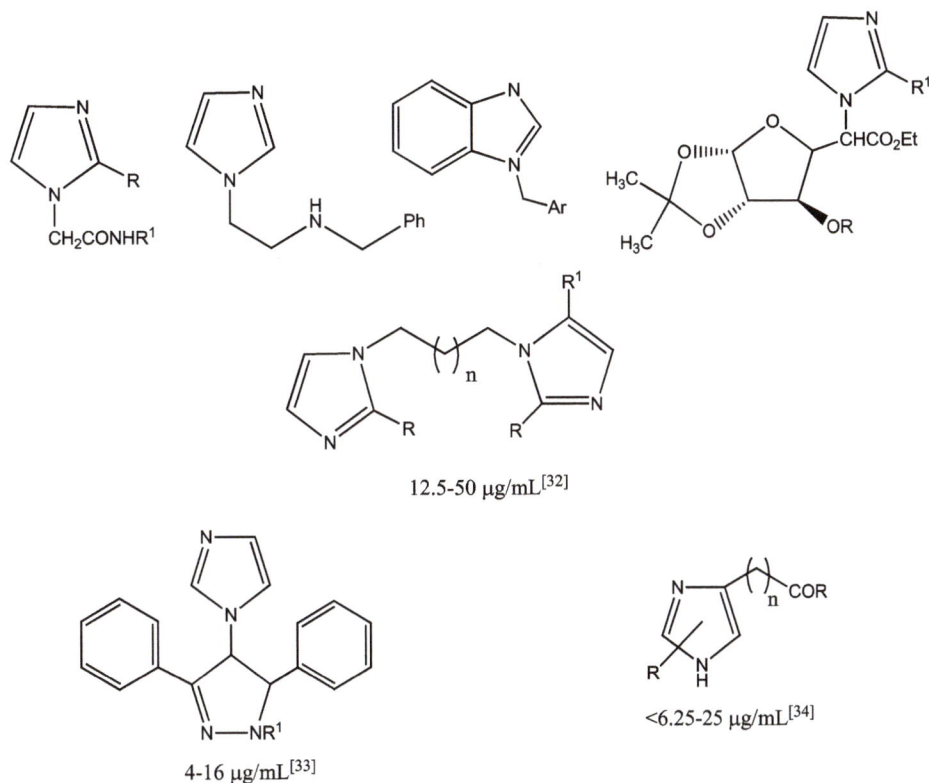

12.5-50 µg/mL[32]

4-16 µg/mL[33]

<6.25-25 µg/mL[34]

Figure 7: Synthesis and anti-TB evaluation of imidazole in different scaffolds.

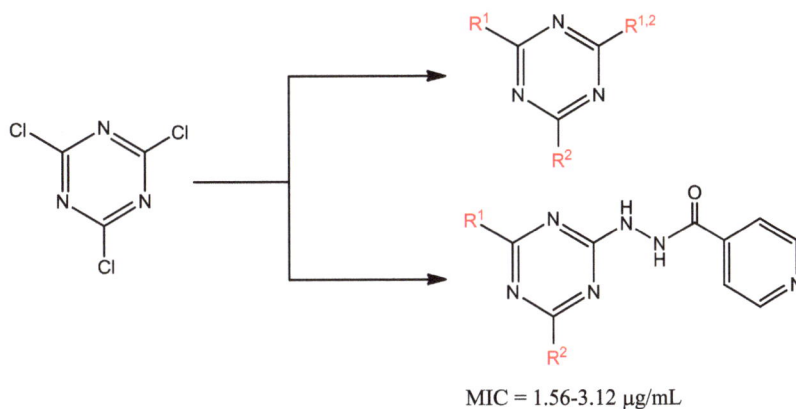

MIC = 1.56-3.12 µg/mL

Scheme 1: New 2,4,6-trisubstituted-1,3,5-triazines.

brain, peripheral tissues, and body fluids. Isatin and its derivatives exhibit a wide range spectrum of biological activities, including anti-TB. In this context, several isatin derivatives have been synthesized and tested against this disease with MIC in the range of 0.0125 to 6.25µg/mL (Fig. **8**). A very good review about this subject was made by Fadl and Jubair [36], which described several isatin derivatives and its anti-TB activity.

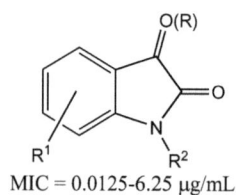

MIC = 0.0125-6.25 µg/mL

Figure 8: General structure of isatine with different substituents.

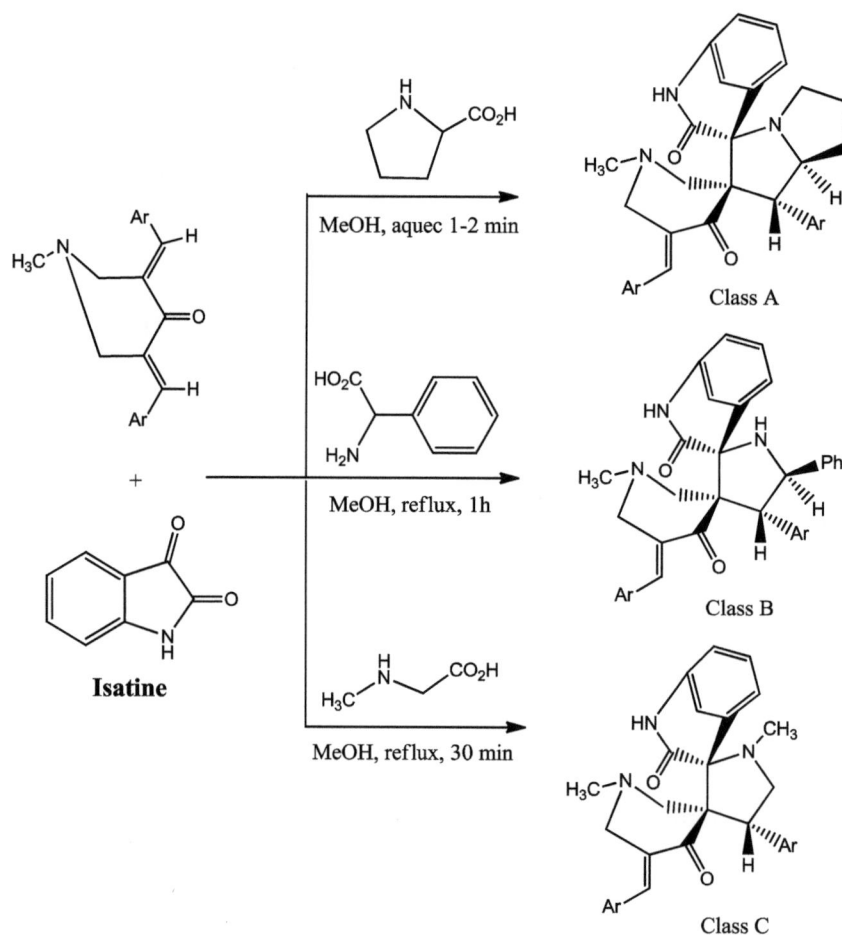

Scheme 2: Stereoselective synthesis of spiro-piperidin-4-ones.

Another example of the versatility of isatine in drug discovery is in the stereoselective synthesis of spiro-piperidin-4-ones made by Perumal and co-workers [37], which through 1,3-dipolar cycloaddition of azomethine ylides generated *in situ* from isatin and (*R*)-amino acids a series of stereoselective spiro-piperidin-4-ones with an atom economic (Scheme **2**). These series were evaluated *in vitro* and *in vivo* against *Mycobacterium tuberculosis* H37Rv and MDR-TB being the compound (Ar = 4-fluorophenyl, class B) one the most potent *in vitro* (MIC = 0.07μM). These values are much lower when compared for example with the first line drugs used against TB. The *in vivo* evaluation of this compound shows promising perspectives in reducing bacterial count in lung and spleen tissues. However, when compared to isoniazid at the same dose level, the compound was found to be less active.

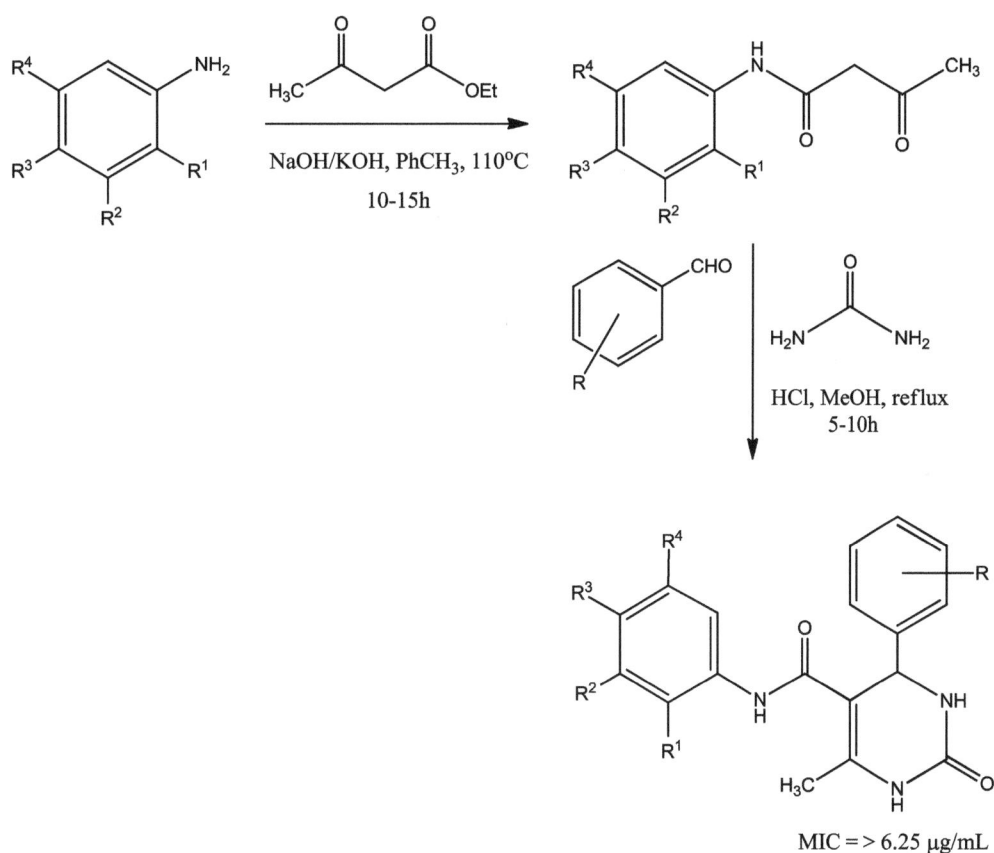

MIC = > 6.25 μg/mL

Scheme 3: Synthesis, evaluation and 3D-QSAR studies of substituted tetrahydro-pyrimidine-5-carboxamides.

TETRAHYDRO-PYRIMIDINE-5-CARBOXAMIDES

Coutinho and co-workers have synthesized, evaluated and made a 3D-QSAR studies of substituted tetrahydro-pyrimidine-5-carboxamides in the search of new TB drugs [38]. This synthesis was based on the reaction between anilines and ethyl acetoacetate leading the respective acetoacetanilides, which reacted with aldehydes and urea to furnish the respective *N*-phenyl-6-methyl-2-oxo-4-phenyl-1,2,3,4-tetrahydro-pyrimidine-5-carboxamides. This class was evaluated against *Mycobacterium tuberculosis* extending from 2 to 63% inhibition (Scheme **3**). These results suggested that methyl groups on phenyl ring of C5 side chain with *meta* substituted 4-phenyl ring displayed good potency being supported by 3D-QSAR models, which also gave information for the improvement of biological activity.

NITROFURAN CLASS

Nitrofuran is a known subunit with potent antibiotic and antimicrobial properties. In this context, it can be mentioned nifuratel used as topic antiprotozoal and antifungal agent in gynecology, nifurtoinol used in bacterial urinary tract infections, nifuroxazide used in the treatment of diarrhea and colitis and nifurtimox to treat Chagas disease and also African trypanosomiasis known as sleeping sickness disease (Fig. **9**). However, this class of compounds was not well studied for TB until 2004 when Lee and co-workers [39] synthesized and evaluated a series of nitrofuranylamides with promising anti-TB perspectives *in vitro* and in mouse model. Due to the good results Lee and co-workers have synthesized and evaluated new generations of nitrofuranyl compounds and also used 3-Dimensional Quantitative Structure-Activity Relationship (3D-QSAR) techniques to correlate the biological activity [40-44]. In Fig. **10** is described some important nitrofuranyl derivatives developed by this group with potent anti-TB activity. For more information about this class its recommend the review wrote by Lee and co-workers [45].

PEPTIDE DEFORMYLASE INHIBITORS

Mukherjee and co-workers synthesized and evaluated promising anti-TB compounds able to act on peptide deformylase (PDF) [46]. This enzyme catalyzes

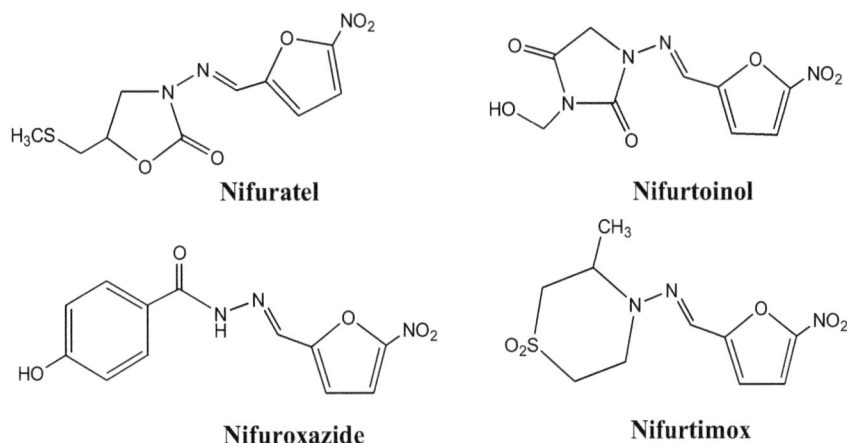

Nifuratel   **Nifurtoinol**

Nifuroxazide   **Nifurtimox**

Figure 9: Structure of nitrofuran drugs.

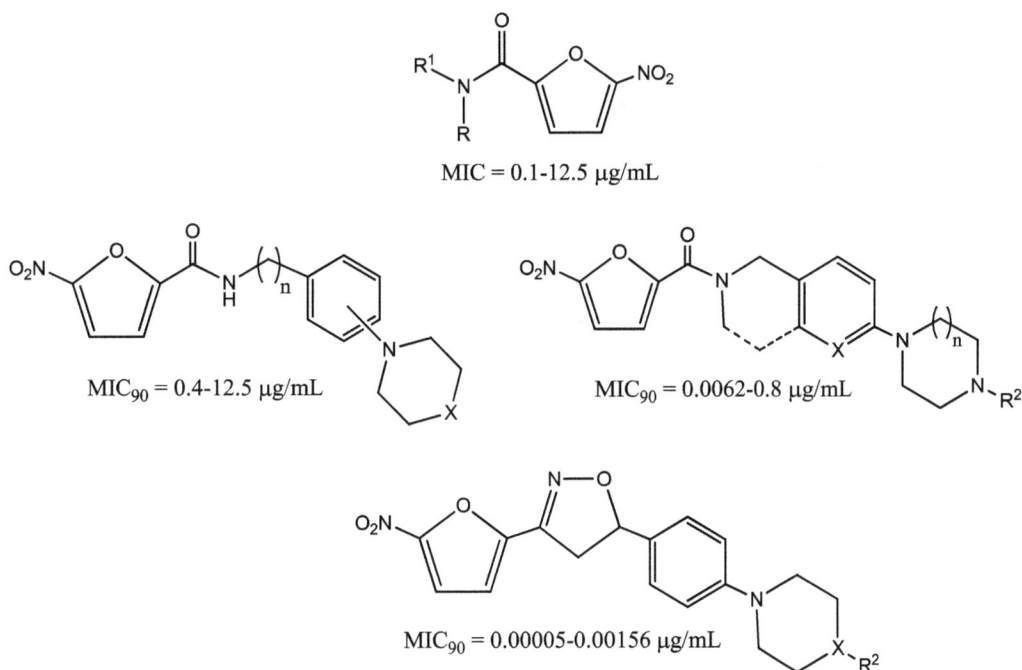

MIC = 0.1-12.5 μg/mL

MIC_{90} = 0.4-12.5 μg/mL MIC_{90} = 0.0062-0.8 μg/mL

MIC_{90} = 0.00005-0.00156 μg/mL

Figure 10: Nitrofuranyl derivatives developed by Lee and co-workers.

the hydrolytic removal of the *N*-terminal formyl group from nascent proteins being an essential bacterial metalloenzyme, which is essential in prokaryotes, however not necessary in mammalian cells (Fig. **11**). In this context this enzyme has promising perspectives as a target in drug discovery. The compounds produced by this group were base on actinonin a natural product, which is a potent

PDF inhibitor, which some of them displayed antibacterial activity against *M. tuberculosis*, including MDR strains with MIC_{90} values of <1 μM. Another important point to be considered is that pharmacokinetic studies displayed promising oral bioavailability.

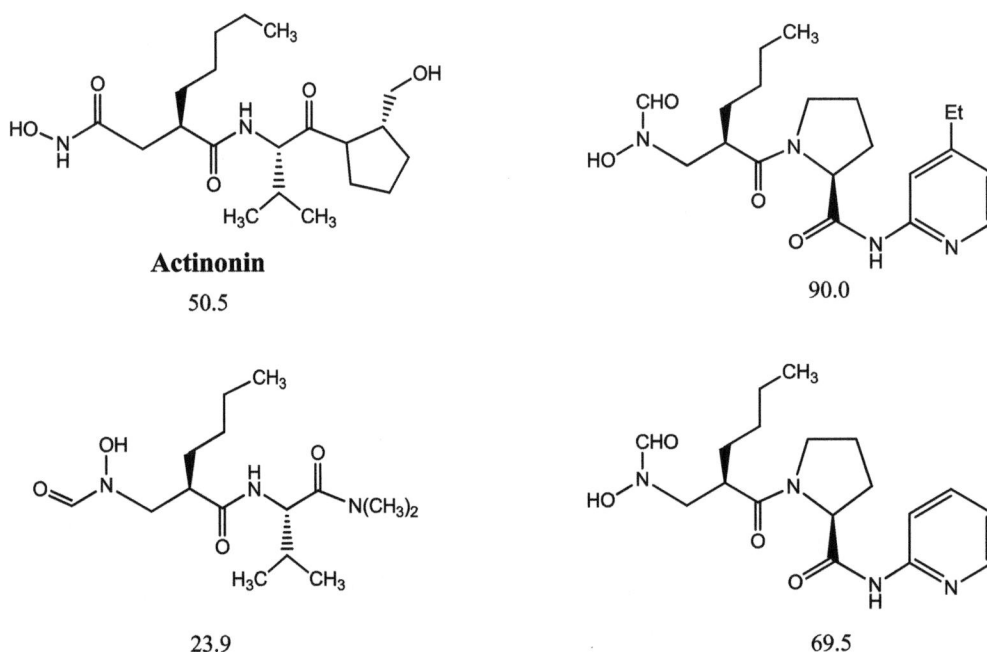

Actinonin
50.5

90.0

23.9

69.5

Effects of PDF-I on *M. tuberculosis* PDF

Figure 11: Structure of compounds able to act on peptide deformylase (PDF).

QUINOLOXALINES

The nucleus benzopyrazine also known as quinoxaline have been studied as anti-TB drug. Antonio Monge, which is involved in several works [47-54] made important contributions in this field. For example in one of his work [54] were synthesized from benzofuroxanes and β-diketones in the presence of calcium chloride and ethanolamine as catalysts, forty-three new 1,4-di-*N*-oxide-quinoxaline-carboxylic acid aryl amide derivatives and evaluated its anti-TB activity (Scheme **4**). In this context, thirteen compounds were active in the primary screening, showing an IC_{90} ≤10 μg/mL, and they were then moved on to the secondary screening level. Two of the compounds were active at this level, showing a SI ≥10. The study of the structure activity relationship indicated that the atom of chloro into quinoxaline nucleus is important for the biological activity.

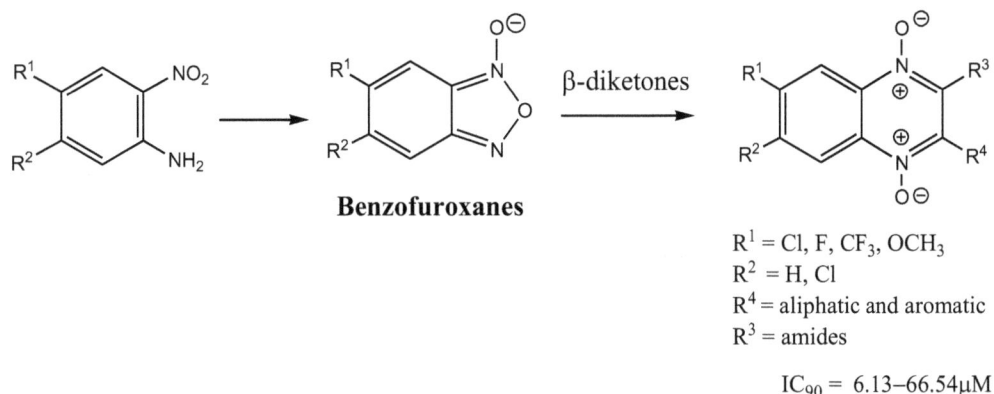

R^1 = Cl, F, CF$_3$, OCH$_3$
R^2 = H, Cl
R^4 = aliphatic and aromatic
R^3 = amides

IC$_{90}$ = 6.13–66.54μM

Scheme 4: Structure of new 1,4-di-*N*-oxide-quinoxaline-carboxylic acid aryl amide derivatives.

Das and co-workers [55] also are involved in study and the application of quinoxaline nucleus against tuberculosis. Considering that, a series of 2-(3-aryl-1-oxo-2-propenyl)-3-methylquinoxaline-1,4-dioxides and 2-acetyl-3 methyl-quinoxaline-1,4-dioxide were synthesized and evaluated, which displayed IC$_{50}$ values in the range of 1-23 μM (Fig. **12**).

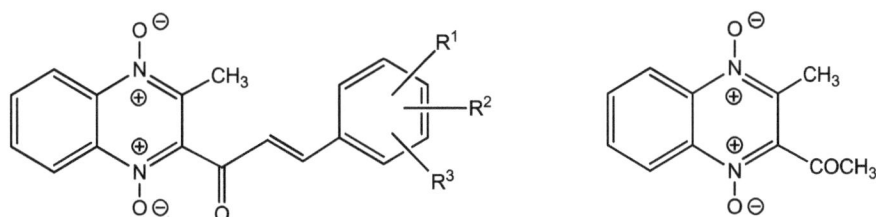

Figure 12: Structure of 2-(3-aryl-1-oxo-2-propenyl)-3-methylquinoxaline-1,4-dioxides and 2-acetyl-3 methylquinoxaline-1,4-dioxide.

CARBOHYDRATE

Carbohydrates are important constituents in the cell wall of the *Mycobacterium tuberculosis*. For example, peptidoglycan and arabinogalactan (AG) are essentials polysaccharides in the mycobacterial cell walls, which are linked by covalent attachment to arabiongalactan (AG), a polymer composed primarily of D-galactofuranosyl and D-arabinofuranosyl residues, attached to mycolic acids and is known as coreF, mycolyl-arabinogalactan–peptidoglycan (mAGP) complex (Scheme **5**) [56,57].

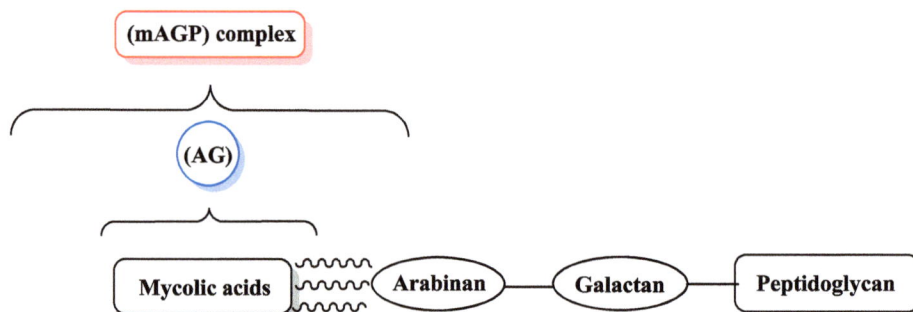

Scheme 5: Structure of (mAGP) complex [56].

The mycobacterial cell wall is also constituted of 6,6′-dimycolyltrehalose (Fig. **13**), biosynthesized by three homologous proteins, Ag85 A, B and C, which possess mycolyltransferase. The antigen 85 (Ag85) complex is a major protein component of the mycobacterial cell wall, which contribute to its biosynthesis and help maintain its integrity, catalyzing the transfer of mycolic acids into the envelope [56,58].

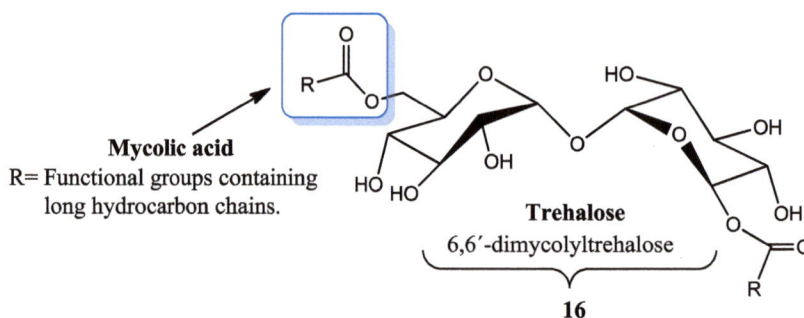

Figure 13: Structure of 6,6′-dimycolyltrehalose [56].

Due to the importance of the carbohydrates in the constitution of the *Mycobacterium tuberculosis* they represent a target in drug discovery and different research groups have been synthesized and evaluated carbohydrates with different scaffolds. Triphati and co-workers have described the synthesis and biological evaluation (Scheme **6**) of galactopyranosil amino alcohols as a new class of anti-TB agents [56,59,60]. The synthesis was based on the introduction of epichlorohydrin in the diacetonide-α-D-galactose **1** followed by regioselective oxirane ring opening with several diamines furnishing amino alcohols with two galactopyranosyl units. The compound **3** demonstrated potent *in vitro* activity against H37Rv and MDR *M. tb.* (1.56 μg/mL) when compared with ethambutol (3.25 μg/mL) (Scheme **6**).

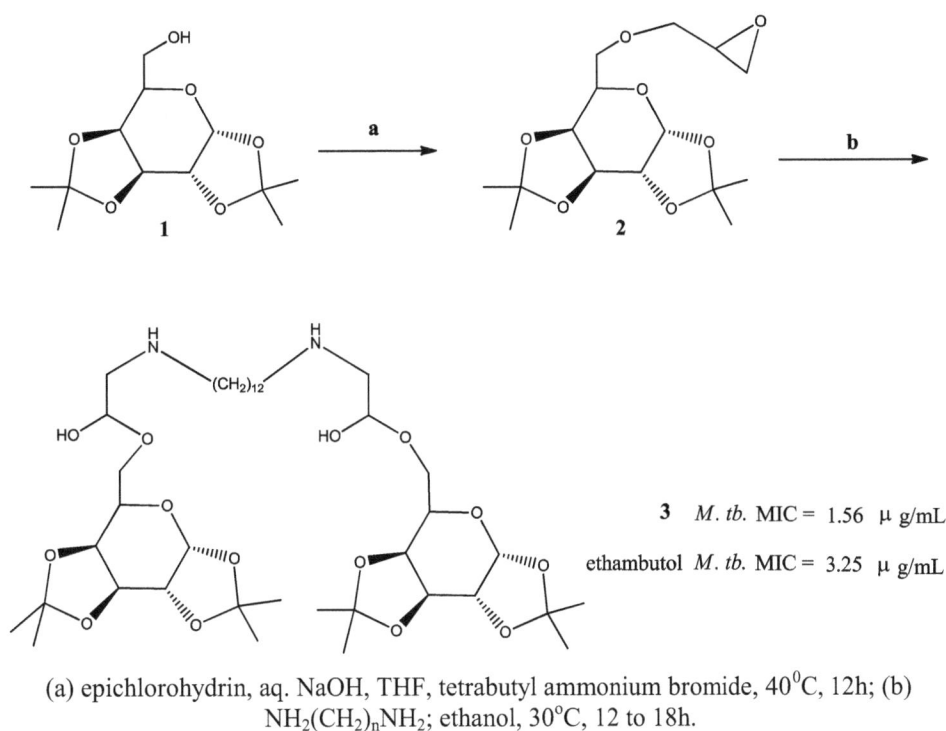

(a) epichlorohydrin, aq. NaOH, THF, tetrabutyl ammonium bromide, 40°C, 12h; (b) NH$_2$(CH$_2$)$_n$NH$_2$; ethanol, 30°C, 12 to 18h.

Scheme 6: Synthesis of galactopyranosil amino alcohols [56,59,60].

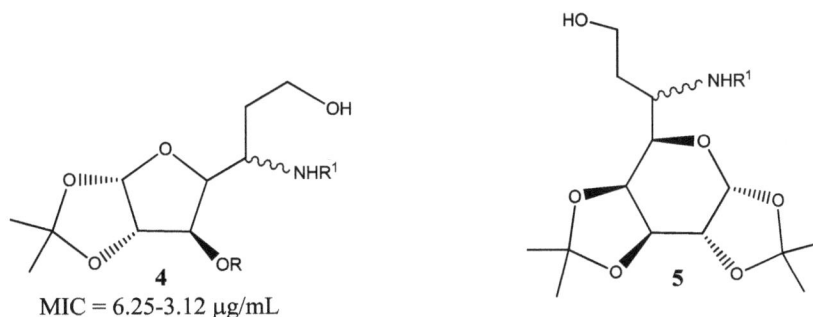

MIC = 6.25-3.12 μg/mL

Figure 14: Structure of galactopyranosil amino alcohols [56,59,60].

Triphati and co-workers have also described the synthesis of glycosylated amino alcohols by classical carbohydrate chemistry, which were evaluated (Fig. **14**) (Table **1**). The most promising compounds was **4** presenting MIC ranging from 6.25 to 3.12 µg/mL [61].

N-SUBSTITUTED GLYCOLAMIDES

Kobarfard and co-workers synthesized several *N*-substituted glycolamides by reacting glycolic acid acetonide (2,2-dimethyl-5-oxo-1,3-dioxolane) with the desired amines and evaluated against *Mycobacterium tuberculosis* [62] (Scheme **7**). The design of these compounds was based on the structural similarity with *N*-glycolyl muramic acid residues of the cell wall of *Mycobacterium tuberculosis* (Fig. **15**). The MIC of this class of compound suggested that the disubstituted amides are important for the biological activity due to the inactivity of the respective monosubstituted amides.

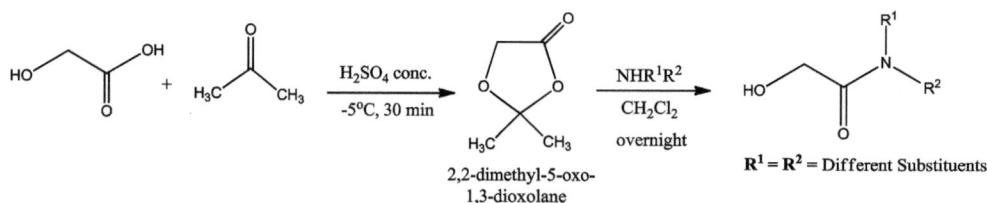

Scheme 7: Synthesis of *N*-substituted glycolamides.

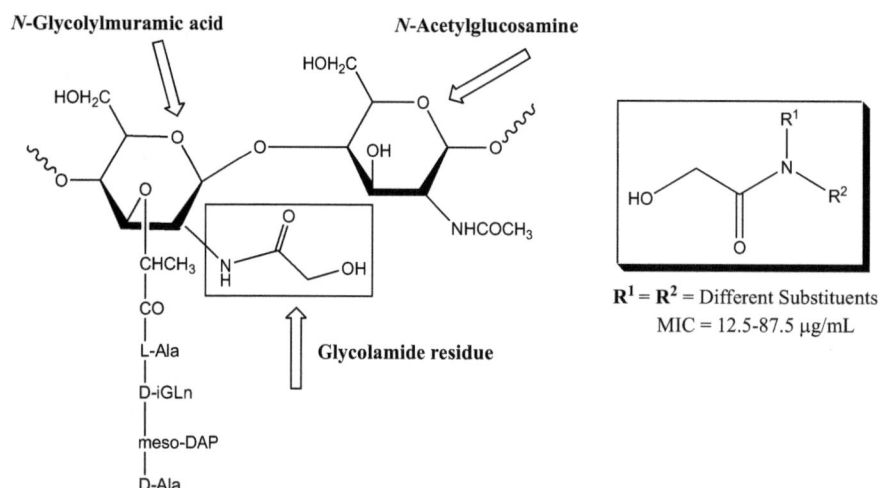

Figure 15: Structure of the basic peptidoglycan unit of mycobacterial cell wall.

ARYLOXYPHENYL CYCLOPROPYL METHANONES

A new class of aryloxyphenyl cyclopropyl methanones was discovered by Tripathi and co-workers, which was synthesized by using one-pot reaction between phenyl cyclopropyl methanones **8a-e**, prepared *in situ* by 4′-fluoro-chloro-butyrophenone **6**, and different aryl alcohols **7a-e** (Scheme **8**) [56,63]. The compounds of this class were evaluated against *M. tuberculosis* H37Rv *in vitro* and presented MICs ranging from 25 to 3.12 µg/mL. The most active compounds **10a-e** have also demonstrated activity against MDR strains and the compounds **10a** and **10c** showed low enhancement of median survival time (MST) in mice.

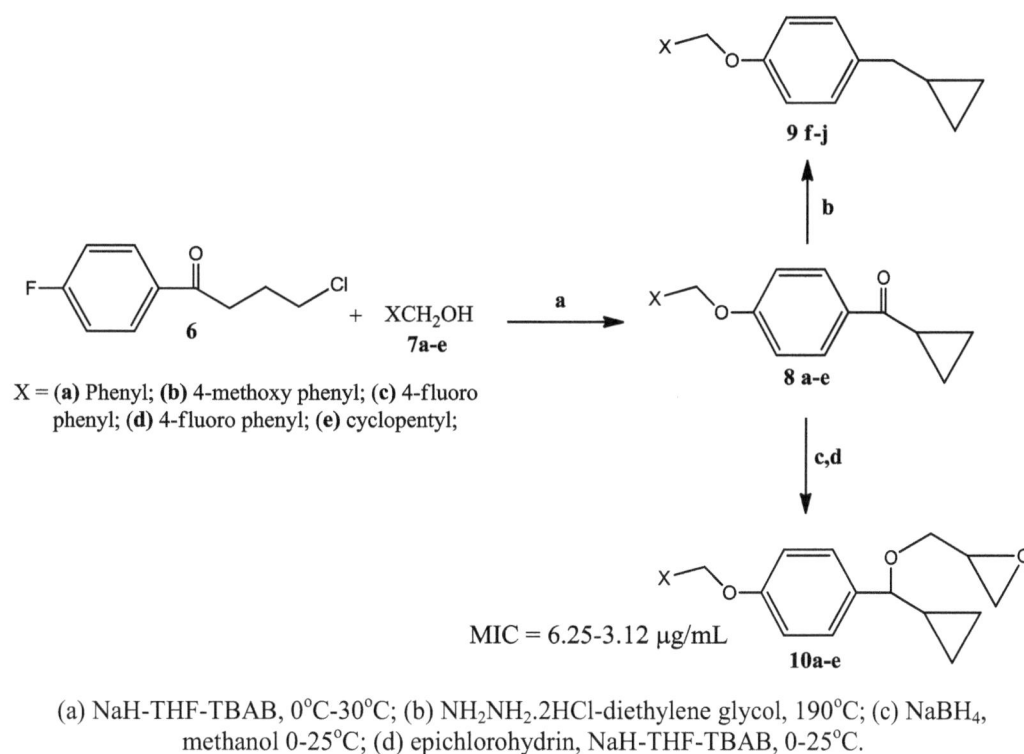

X = (**a**) Phenyl; (**b**) 4-methoxy phenyl; (**c**) 4-fluoro phenyl; (**d**) 4-fluoro phenyl; (**e**) cyclopentyl;

MIC = 6.25-3.12 µg/mL

(a) NaH-THF-TBAB, 0°C-30°C; (b) $NH_2NH_2 \cdot 2HCl$-diethylene glycol, 190°C; (c) $NaBH_4$, methanol 0-25°C; (d) epichlorohydrin, NaH-THF-TBAB, 0-25°C.

Scheme 8: Synthesis of aryloxyphenyl cyclopropyl methanones.

1,3-BENZOTHIAZIN-4-ONES

Cole and co-workers found the 1,3-benzothiazin-4-ones (BTZs) (Fig. **16**) [64], a new class of compounds able to inhibit *M. tuberculosis* by blocking the arabinan synthesis an essential component in cell wall being the enzyme decaprenylphosphoryl-β-D-ribose 2′-epimerase the most important target of this class. The selected compound nitrobenzothiazinone (BTZ043) displayed promising perspectives due to the potency and specificity for mycobacteria with a very low MIC for *M. tuberculosis* $H_{37}Rv$ (1ng/mL) being the group nitro essential for the biological activity.

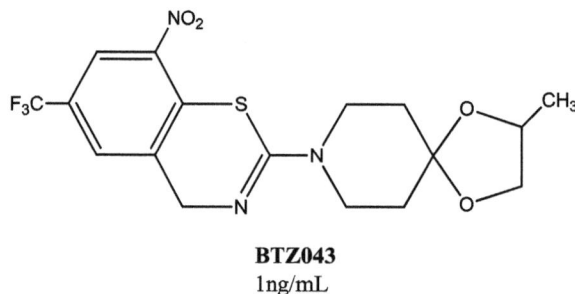

BTZ043
1ng/mL

Figure 16: Structure of the 1,3-benzothiazin-4-ones BTZ043.

3'-BROMO ANALOGUES OF PYRIMIDINE NUCLEOSIDES

Kumar and co-workers have identified a new class of compounds active against *M. tuberculosis*, 3'-bromo analogues of pyrimidine nucleosides, which were identified after the evaluation of several 3'-halogen analogues of pyrimidine nucleosides [65]. The best result found was the 3'-bromo-3'-deoxy-arabinofuranosylthymine **11** including against wild-type *M. tuberculosis* strains (MIC= 1-2μg/mL). Another important point to be considered is that the respective 5-fluorouracil displayed low potency against this bacterial compared to **11**.

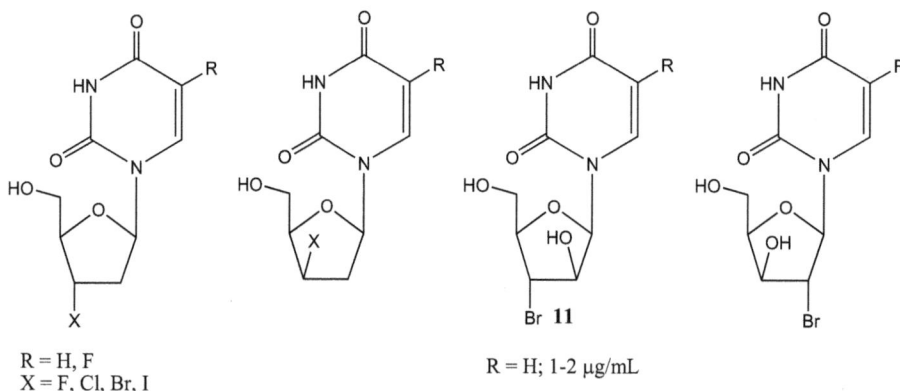

R = H, F
X = F, Cl, Br, I

R = H; 1-2 μg/mL

Figure 17: Structures of 3'-Bromo analogues of pyrimidine nucleosides.

ALPHA, OMEGA-DIAMINOALKANES

Diamines constitute a very important and versatile class of compounds with applications and roles in many fields. As a particular example in medicinal chemistry, 1,2 ethylenediamine is a pharmacophore of ethambutol, a front-line drug used to treat tuberculosis. So far, there have been no reported studies with other diamines, and this compound has motivated our group to evaluate commercial α,ω-diaminoalkanes, ($H_2N(CH_2)_nNH_2$, n = 2-12) compounds [66]. Table **1** showed that α,ω-diaminoalkanes, ($H_2N(CH_2)_nNH_2$, n = 9-12) have good activities with MIC between 3.12-2.5 µg/mL compared to that of the first line drug ethambutol 3.12 µg/mL. The good activities of the longer chain compounds and non-activity of the shorter chain compounds clearly point to the importance of the lipophilicity of the compounds: as indicated in Table **1** the Log P values of the active compounds are in the range 0.99 to 2.50. Preliminary QSAR study suggested that as well as the importance of lipophilicity, free bis amine functions are crucial for the biological activity. This can be observed by the lost of anti-TB activity when the diamines n = 9-12 are mono or disubstituted with Ac, Boc, Bz, Bn, Cbz, Me and by the fact that monoamines ($CH_3(CH_2)_nNH_2$, n = 8-11) are ineffective.

Table 1: The *in vitro* activity of compounds against *M. tuberculosis* $H_{37}Rv$ strain.

$NH_2(CH_2)_nNH_2$	MIC (µg/mL)	C Log P
(n = 12)	2.50	2.50
(n = 11)	3.12	2.00
(n = 10)	3.12	1.49
(n = 9)	3.12	0.99
(n = 8)	-	0.48
(n = 7)	-	-0.02
(n = 5)	-	-1.03
(n = 4)	-	-1.54
(n = 2)	-	-2.08

[a]Minimal Inhibition Concentration is expressed in µg/mL.
[b]Calculated by www.logp.com.

N-(ARYL)-2-THIOPHEN-2-YLACETAMIDES

Thiophene nucleus represents a very important field in drug discovery, being present in many natural and synthetic products with a wide range of pharmacological activities. Considering that, our group prepared a series of twenty one *N*-(aryl)-2-thiophen-2-ylacetamides derivatives, were synthesized (Scheme **9**) [67,68] and evaluated for their *in vitro* antibacterial activity against *Mycobacterium tuberculosis*.

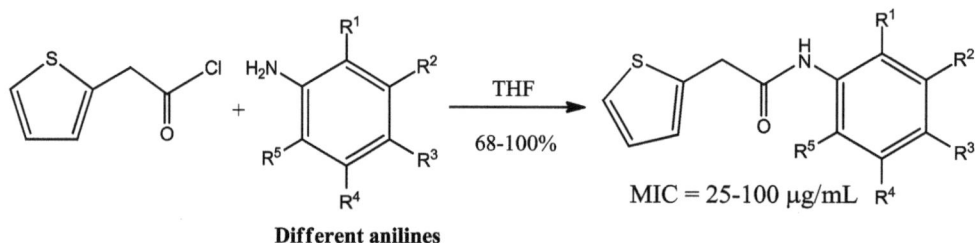

Scheme 9: Synthesis of *N*-(aryl)-2-thiophen-2-ylacetamides.

TETRAHYDROINDAZOLE

Kozikowski and co-workers identified a novel class of tetrahydroindazole, which displayed potent activity against *Mycobacterium tuberculosis*. The two lead compounds **12** and **13**, MIC = 0.6 and 1.0 µg/mL respectively, were found by High-Throughput Screening (HTS) and due to its promising activity, several modifications were made being discovered the compound **14** and **15** (MIC = 1.9 µg/mL) (Fig. **18**) [69]. The compounds **12** and **14** demonstrated good *in vitro* stability in mouse liver microsomes and also *in vivo* pharmacokinetic profiles in plasma levels.

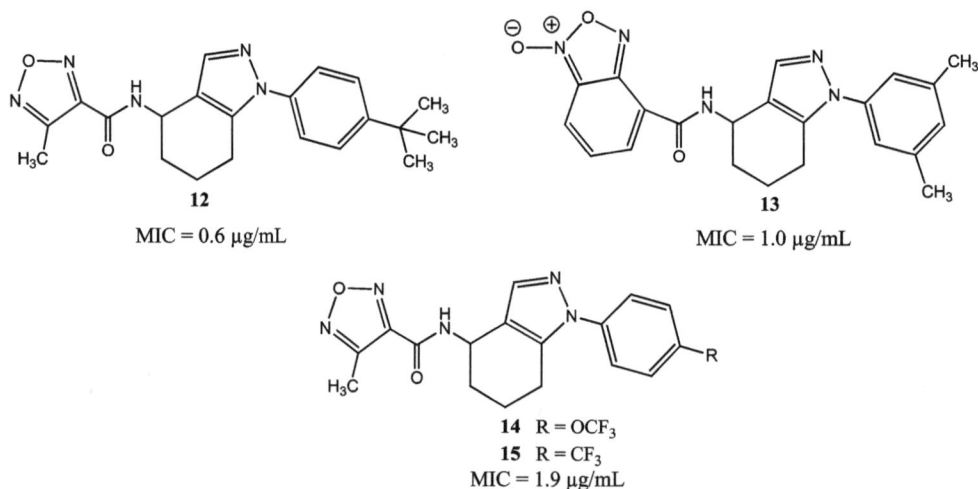

Figure 18: Structure of tetrahydroindazole derivatives.

1,4-NAPHTHOQUINONE

The nucleus 1,4-naphthoquinone is an important class, which is incorporated in different natural products displaying a wide range of biological activity. Considering that, several 1,4-naphthoquinone derivatives were synthesized and evaluated against *Mycobacterium tuberculosis* $H_{37}Rv$ strain by Mital and co-workers displaying good activity with IC_{50} values ranging from 3.9 - 0.3 µg/mL (Fig. **19**) [70].

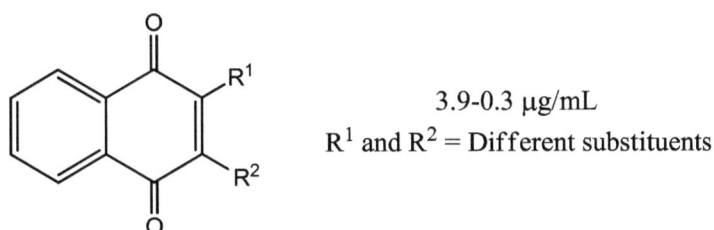

3.9-0.3 µg/mL
R^1 and R^2 = Different substituents

Figure 19: Structure of 1,4-naphthoquinone.

METAL COMPLEXES

Metal complexes have been also synthesized employing different metals and ligands and evaluated against *Mycobacterium tuberculosis*. For example, Pélinski and co-workers have synthesized (Scheme **10**) and evaluated (Table **2**) the anti-TB activity of ferrocenyl ethambutol analogues and ferrocenyl diamines [56,71]. Preliminary studies have demonstrated that the ferrocenyl diamines **16** and **17** possessed good activities against *M. tb.* $H_{37}Rv$. These ferrocenyl analogues have been synthesized by reacting ferrocene carboxaldehyde **15** with respective diamines, followed by reduction with $NaBH_4$ with 77-46% yields (two steps).

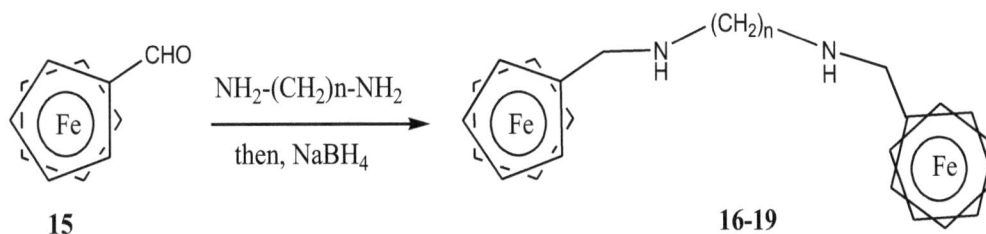

Scheme 10: Structure of ferrocenyl diamines [56].

Tabela 2: MIC values (µg/mL) of the complexes 16-19 [56].

N°	n	*M. tb.* MIC (µg/mL)	Overall Yield (%)
16	2	8	76
17	3	8	54
18	4	32	77
19	6	32	46

In the Fig. **20** there are some complexes with different metal-ligands, as well as its respective anti-TB activity.

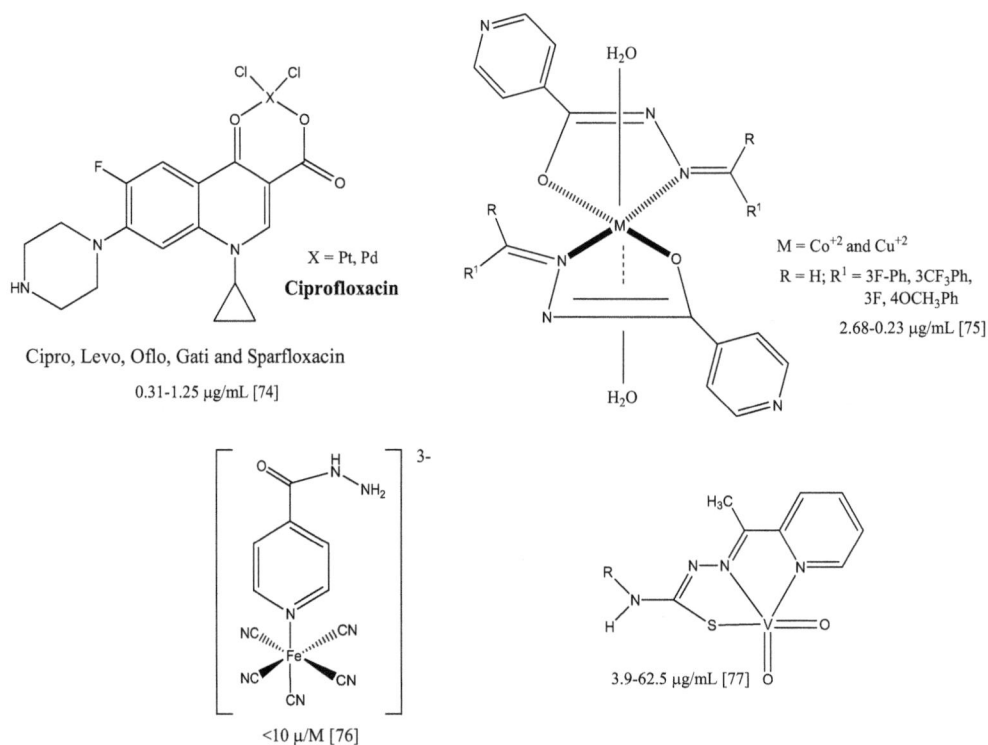

Figure 20: Structures of metal complexes active against tuberculosis.

HIGH-THROUGHPUT SCREENING AND COMBINATORIAL CHEMISTRY IN TB DRUG DISCOVERY

High-Throughput Screening (HTS) is a very important tool in drug discovery, which can quickly recognize bioactive compounds by screening large chemical libraries of compounds, bringing valuable information about drug design and interactions or function of the biological systems. This method has been also used for both, public and private research institutions in the search of new drugs and targets against TB. This technique started to be employed only in 1990s due to the lack of interest of pharmaceutical companies in TB drug discovery. In this context, the Tuberculosis Antimicrobial Acquisition and Coordinating Facility (TAACF) was established in 1994 by the National Institute of Allergy and Infectious Diseases (NIAID) to facilitate the discovery of new antitubercular drugs possessing high quality screening services (www.taacf.org) [78]. The screening of the compounds was based on assays developed by Franzblau and co-workers, which gave outstanding contributions on the development of antitubercular activity assays [79,80]. Other scientists also gave contributions on HTS for identify antimycobacterial agents, such as Duncan and co-workers [81].

Since its foundation, TAACF continue to provide a great contribution on TB drug discovery by screening compounds around the world involving scientist and institutions of different fields, as well as testing in animal models the most promising compounds found. One example of its important contribution on TB drug discovery was made by Maddry and co-workers [82] through the Molecular Libraries Screening Center Network in collaboration with TAACF, which tested a 215,110 compound library against *Mycobacterium tuberculosis* strain $H_{37}Rv$. In this evaluation several scaffolds of interest were identified such as, substituted quinolones and pyrimidines, 1,3-diaryl-4-substituted pyrazoles, 1,3,4-oxadiazoles, 2-carboxamido-1,3,4-oxadiazoles and related compounds, 1,2,4-thiadiazoles, tetrahydropyrazolo[1,5-a]pyrimidines, and also other scaffolds with good anti-TB activity, but low selectivity, such as 3-phenylpyrazolo[1,5-a]pyrimidines, 2,5-disubstituted thiazolidin-4-ones, 4(5)-phenylacetylimidazole-5(4)-carboxamides, imidazo[1,2-a]pyridine-3-amines, and amides of 3-(trifluoromethyl)-4-(piperazinylmethyl)aniline.

Another example of TAAFC contributions on TB drug discovery was the evaluation of a library containing 100,997 compounds, based on Lipinski rules, which was purchased from ChemBridge Corportation (http://www.chembridge.com) [83,84]. In this evaluation several scaffolds were identified such as, 2-aminothiazoles, substituted benzopyran-2-ones and benzopyran-4-ones, oxadiazolylthio, thiadiazolylthio and triazolylthio derivatives, phenoxyalkylimidazoles and related compounds, 8-hydroxyquinolines, 4-aminoquinolines, 2,4-Diaminoquinazolines, thieno[2,3-d]pyrimidin-4-ones, thieno[2,3-d]pyrimidin-4-amines, benzothiophene 1,1-dioxides, dihydrothiophene 1,1-dioxides and related compounds, pyrazolopyrimidinones, 1,4-naphthoquinones, piperidinamines, thioamides, ureas and thioureas, adamantyl amides and amines, and 5-nitrofuran-2-carboxamides.

Nefzi and co-workers [85] in collaboration with TAACF synthesized a library of chiral pentaamines and bis-heterocyclic compounds by using combinatorial chemistry and evaluated its anti-TB activity. Some of these compounds displayed a MIC range 2-7 µg/mL and 90–100% inhibition being more active than first line drug ethambutol (MIC = 10 µg/mL) (Scheme **11**).

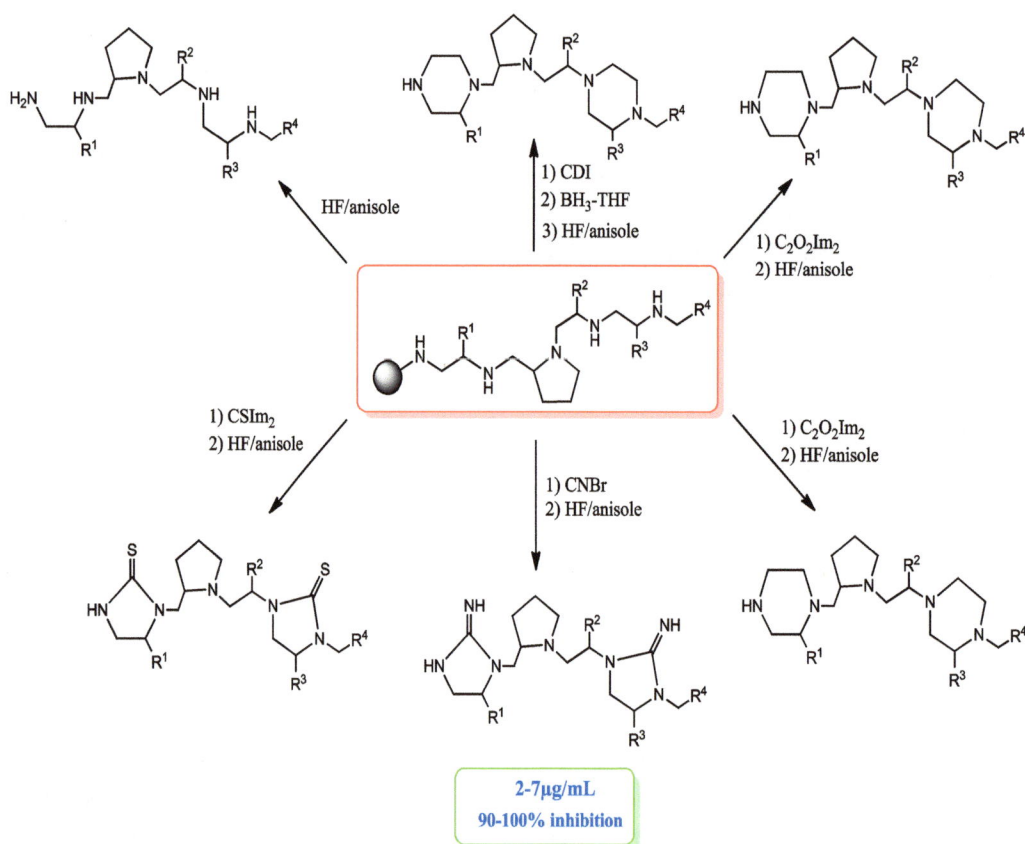

Scheme 11: Library of chiral pentaamines and bis-heterocyclic compounds.

Other evaluation of a library of compounds was made by Loughedd and co-workers [86]. In this study it was screened 1514 compounds including drugs with known anti-mycobacterial activity, and compounds and drugs used against other kind of diseases. Among of these compounds, 53 displayed activity against *M. tuberculosis* with MIC of ≤5µM, being 17 new inhibitors and 36 were known tuberculosis drugs or had been previously described as possessing anti-tuberculosis activity. Considering that, five compounds were chosen as lead compounds for the development of new anti-TB drugs. For example, nialamide, primaquine and pyrvinium were selected as the best oral drugs with anti-TB activity (Fig. **21**).

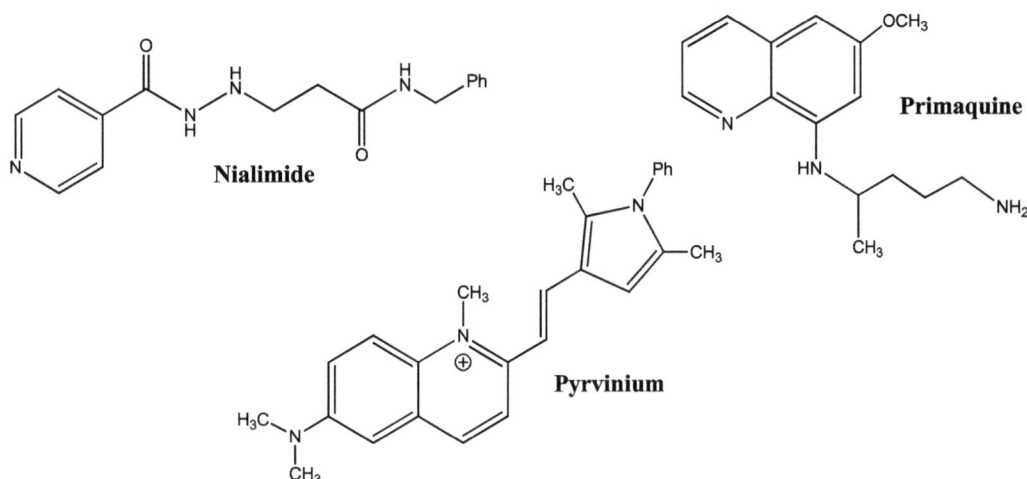

Figure 21: Structures of nialamide, primaquine and pyrvinium.

Brodin and co-workers [87] developed high throughput screening based on a phenotypic cell-based assay that uses automated confocal fluorescence microscopy. This assay was used for screening a library of 56,984 small molecules and was purchased from Timtec (26,500 molecules), Cerep (10,484) and ChemBridge™ (20,000) with the aim to evaluate its activity against *M. tuberculosis* within macrophages (Fig. **22**). The compounds were selected based on the 'rule of 5' of Lipinski, their chemical diversity and drug-like properties. Considering that, 135 compounds possessed very effective intracellular antimycobacterial activity with no cytotoxic effects in cell host. Among these the dinitrobenzamide derivatives (DNB) showed the most promising results, being active including against XDR strains. In addition, to study the structure activity relationship (SAR) of this class over 155 compounds were synthesized furnishing important information, such as the reduction of nitro or hydoxylamine inactive the compound, and the substitution of the benzyloxy nucleus by a chlorine- or fluorine atoms at position 3 were responsible for the increase of potency when compared to carboxyl substitutions. Another outstanding contribution of this work was the study of mechanism of action of this class, which was based on the inhibition of the formation of both lipoarabinomannan and arabinogalactan, attributable to the inhibition of decaprenyl-phospho-arabinose synthesis catalyzed by the decaprenyl-phosphoribose 29 epimerase. This epimerase is encoded by DprE1/DprE2 genes being close to embAC-gene cluster whose products are also involved in the biosynthesis of lipoarabinomannan and arabinogalactan and are targets of the first-line drug, ethambutol.

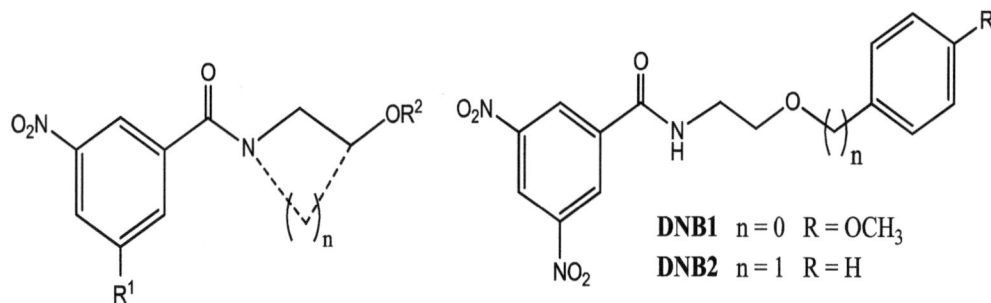

Figure 22: Structure of dinitrobenzamide derivatives (DNB).

Click chemistry reaction was developed by Karl Barry Sharpless of The Scripps Research Institute in 2001, and it was based on the 1,3-dipolar cycloaddition of azides and terminal alkynes to lead 1,2,3-triazoles being this reaction catalyzed by copper (I) [88]. This kind of reaction has versatile applications in drug discovery being able to build libraries of compounds by combinatorial chemistry techniques. Considering that, Yao and co-workers [89] used this reaction to assemble a library of over 3.500 compounds, which are bidentate inhibitors against protein tyrosine phosphatases (PTPs) (Scheme **12**). These proteins have been related with several human diseases, such as cancer, diabetes and obesity, as for example the protein tyrosine MptpB phosphatase, which is secreted by *Mycobacterium tuberculosis*. In this context, this protein has a good potential to be a target in drug discovery, due to its virulence factors for by modulating the phosphorylation and dephosphorylation of host proteins being also responsible for the survival of this bacteria in infected host macrophages. After the preparation of this new library, two very potent and selective MptpB compounds **H1-6C-W11** (*Ki* = 150 nM) and **F1S-6C-W11** (*Ki* = 170 nM) were discovered by HTS.

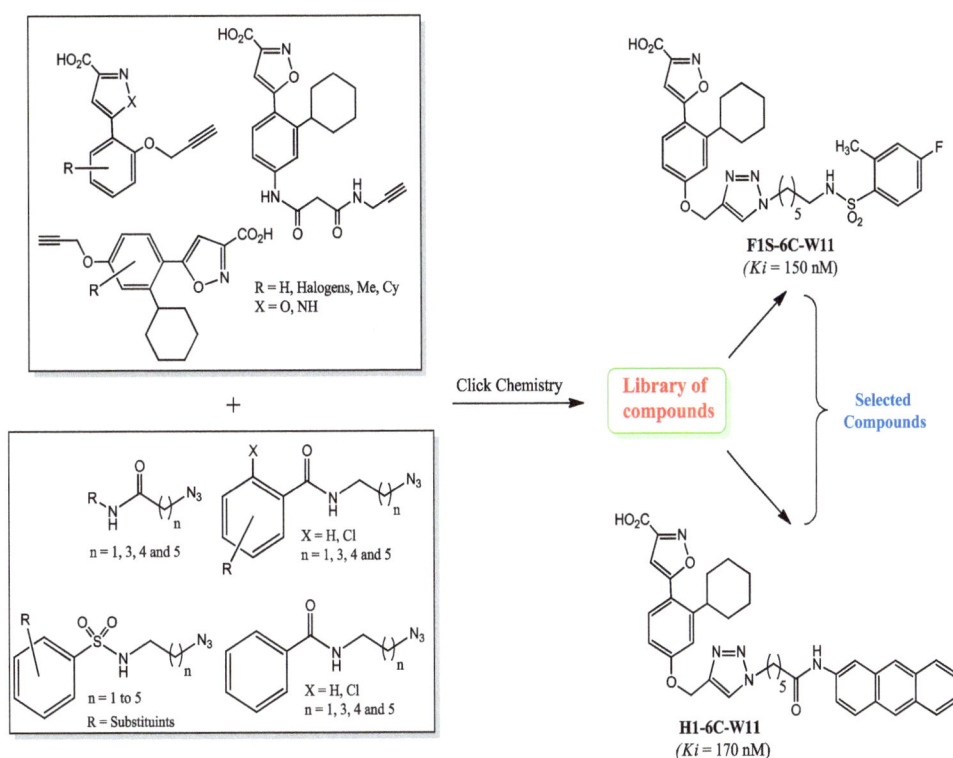

Scheme 12: Structure of bidentate inhibitors against protein tyrosine phosphatases (PTPs).

Chauhan and co-workers built a library of 80 substituted pyrimidines by using three-component solid-phase reactions leading polysubstituted pyrimidines. These pyrimidines were evaluated against *Mycobacterium tuberculosis* and six of then showed anti-TB activity at a concentration of 50 and 25μg/mL (Scheme **13**) [90].

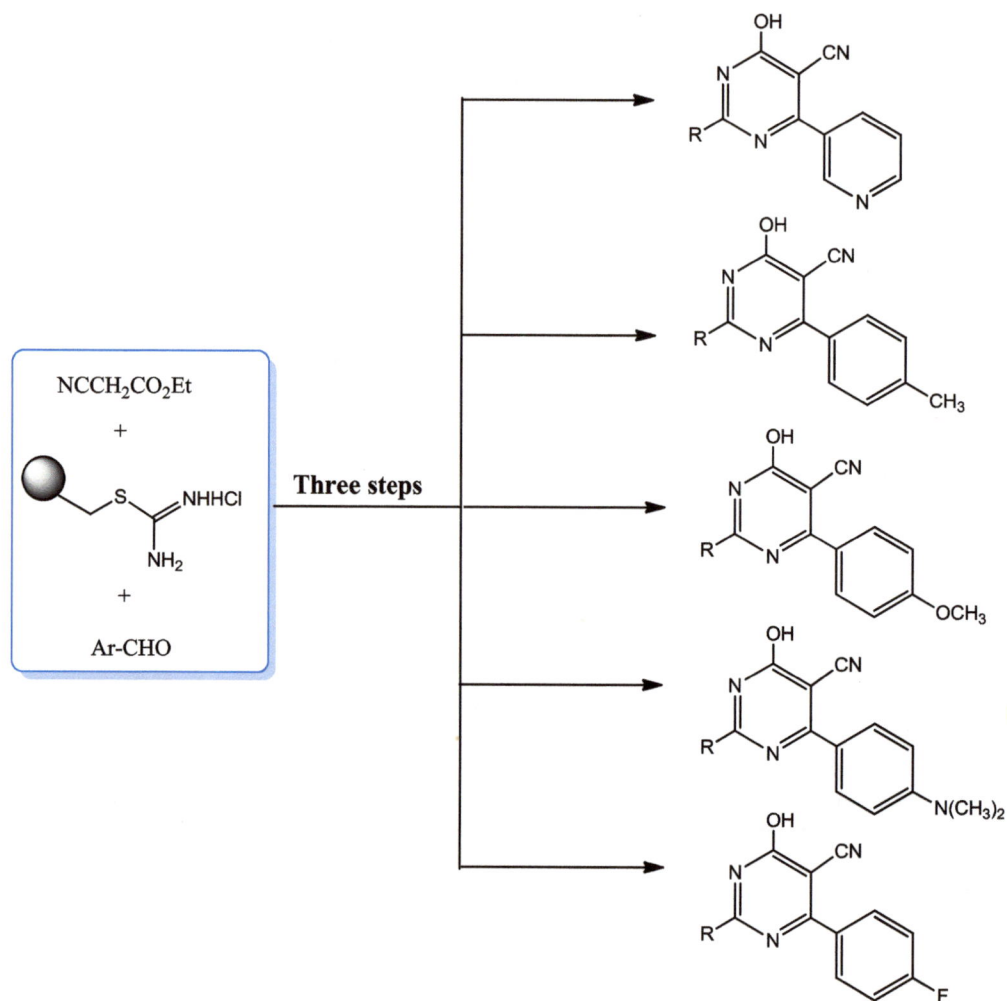

(a) $NCCH_2CO_2Et$, aromatic aldehyde, K_2CO_3/DMF 80°C, 30h; (b) MCPBA, CH_2Cl_2, rt, 18h; (c) amines, CH_2Cl_2, 40°C, 10h.

Scheme 13: Structure of polysubstituted pyrimidines.

MISCELLANEOUS

Due to the large amount of compounds evaluated against *Mycobacterium tuberculosis* by different research groups in the last five years, this section it will highlight select compounds of different class covered in the last year, with the respective structure, activity and reference. The selection was based on the potency and other promises perspectives of the compounds (Fig. **23**).

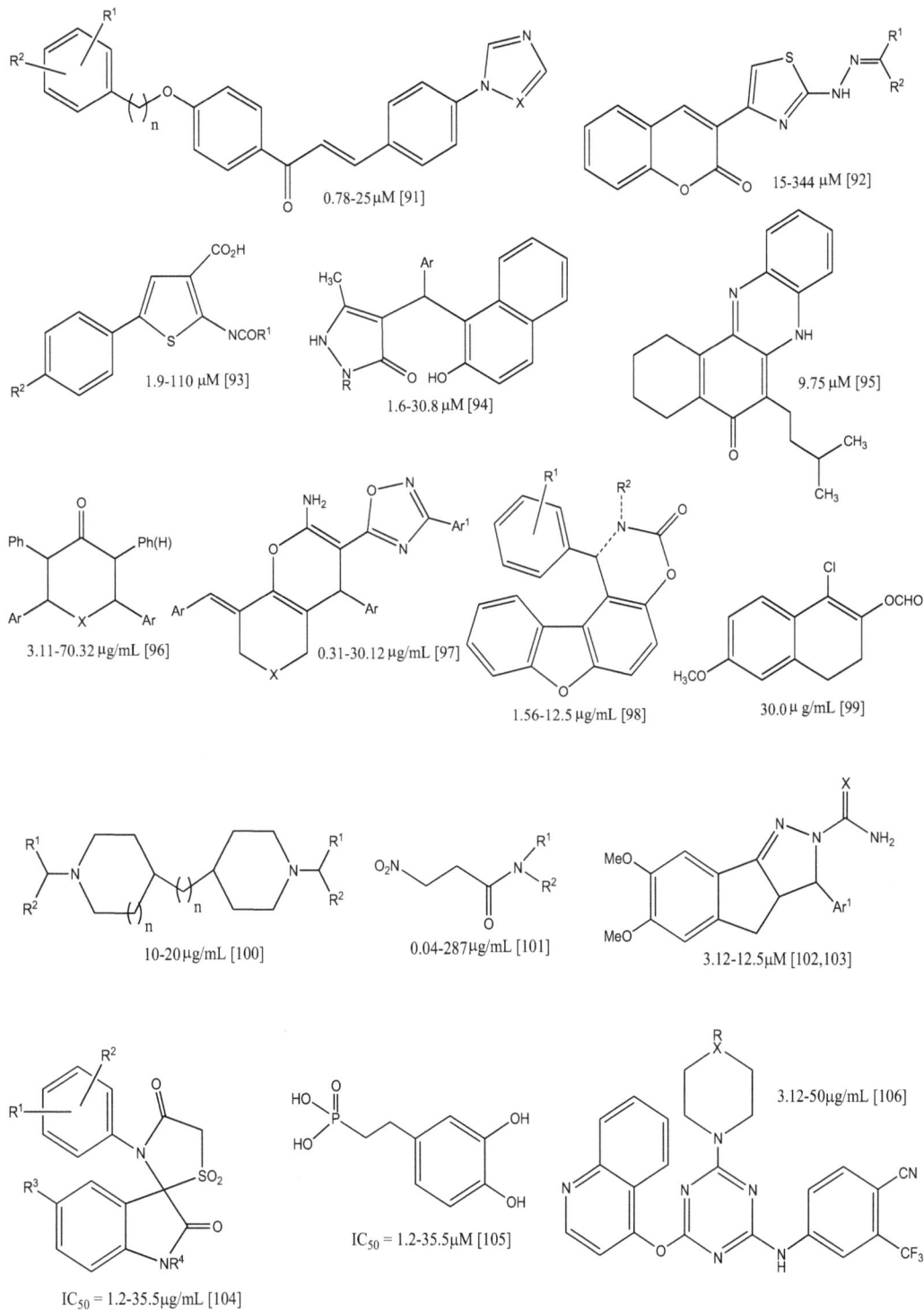

0.78-25 μM [91]

15-344 μM [92]

1.9-110 μM [93]

1.6-30.8 μM [94]

9.75 μM [95]

3.11-70.32 μg/mL [96]

0.31-30.12 μg/mL [97]

1.56-12.5 μg/mL [98]

30.0 μg/mL [99]

10-20 μg/mL [100]

0.04-287μg/mL [101]

3.12-12.5μM [102,103]

3.12-50μg/mL [106]

IC_{50} = 1.2-35.5μg/mL [104]

IC_{50} = 1.2-35.5μM [105]

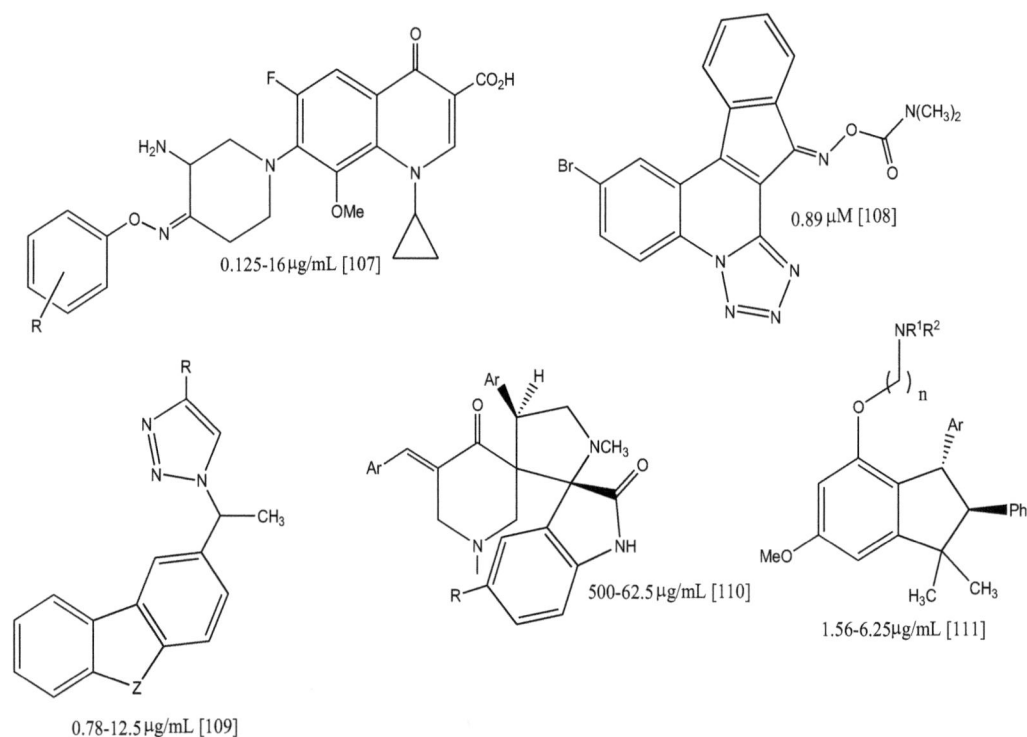

Figure 23: Selected anti-TB compounds.

ACKNOWLEDGEMENT

None Declare.

CONFLICT OF INTEREST

The author(s) confirm that this chapter content has no conflict of interest.

REFERENCES

[1]   Yves L. Janin. Antituberculosis drugs: Ten years of research. *Bioorg. & Med. Chem.* 2007;**15**:2479-2513.

[2]   De Souza MVN. *New Strategies Combating Bacterial Infection.* Iqbal A and Farrukh A. Ed.; Wiley-VCH Verlag GmbH and Co. KGaA: Weinheim **2008**; vol *3*, p. 71-87.

[3]   De Souza MVN, Gonçalves RSB, Ferreira ML. *Frontiers in Anti-Infective Drug Discovery.* Atta-ur-Rahman FRS & Iqbal CM. Ed.; Bentham **2009**; vol *9*, p. 176-201.

[4]   Gutierrez-Lugo MT, Bewley CA. Natural Products, Small Molecules, and Genetics in Tuberculosis Drug Development. *J Med Chem* 2008;**51**:2606-2612.

[5]　Goldman RC, Laughon BE. Discovery and validation of new antitubercular compounds as potential drug leads and probes. *Tuberculosis* 2009;**89**:331-333.

[6]　Murphy DJ, Brown JR. Computational biology in anti- tuberculosis drug discovery. *Infectious Disorders: Drug Targets* 2009;**9**:319-326.

[7]　Biological Activities of Hydrazone Derivatives. Sevim Rollas, Küçükgüzel SG. *Molecules* 2007;**12**:1910-1939.

[8]　Aponte, JC, Vaisberg AJ, Castillo D, Gonzalez G, Estevez Y, Arevalo J, Quiliano M, Zimic M, Verastegui M, Malaga E, Gilman RH, Bustamante JM, Tarleton RL, Wang Y, Franzblau SG, Pauli GF, Sauvain M, Hammond GB. Trypanoside, anti tuberculosis, leishmanicidal, and cytotoxic activities of tetrahydrobenzothienopyrimidines. *Bioorg Med Chem* 2010;**18**:2880-2886.

[9]　Turan-Zitouni G, Oezdemir A, Asim KZ, Benkli K, Chevallet P, Akalin G. Synthesis and antituberculosis activity of new thiazolylhydrazone derivatives. *Eur J Med Chem* 2008;**43**:981-985.

[10]　Sriram D, Yogeeswari P, Vyas DRK, Senthilkumar P, Bhat P, Srividya M. 5-Nitro-2-furoic acid hydrazones: Design, synthesis and *in vitro* antimycobacterial evaluation against log and starved phase cultures. *Bioorg Med Chem Lett* 2010;**20**:4313-4316.

[11]　Kaplancikli ZA, Turan-Zitouni G, Ozdemir A, Teulade JC. Synthesis and antituberculosis activity of new hydrazide derivatives. *Archiv der Pharmazie* 2008; **341**:721-724.

[12]　Gupta P, Hameed S, Jain R. Ring - substituted imidazoles as a new class of anti - tuberculosis agents. *Eur J Med Chem* 2004;**39**:805-814.

[13]　Banfi E, Scialino G, Zampieri D, Mamolo MG, Vio L, Ferrone M, Fermeglia M, Paneni MS, Pricl S. Antifungal and antimycobacterial activity of new imidazole and triazole derivatives. A combined experimental and computational approach. *JAC* 2006;**58**:76-84.

[14]　Mamolo MG, Zampieri D, Falagiani V, Vio L, Fermeglia M, Ferrone M, Pricl S, Banfi E, Scialino G. Antifungal and antimycobacterial activity of new *N*1-[1-aryl-2-(1H-imidazol-1-yl and 1H-1,2,4-triazol-1-yl)-ethylidene]-pyridine-2-carboxamidrazone derivatives: a combined experimental and computational approach. *ARKIVOC* 2004;**5**:231-250.

[15]　Bairwa R, Kakwani M, Tawari NR, Lalchandani J, Ray MK, Rajan MGR, Degani MS. Novel molecular hybrids of cinnamic acids and guanylhydrazones as potential antitubercular agents. *Bioorg Med Chem Lett* 2010;**20**:1623-1625.

[16]　Ferreira ML, Cardoso LNF, Goncalves RSB, Silva ET, Lourenco MCS, De Souza MVN. Synthesis and Antitubercular Evaluation of *N*'-[(E) (hydroxy, methoxy and ethoxy-substituted-phenyl) Methylidene]isonicotinohydrazide Derivatives. *LDDD* 2008;**5**:137-140.

[17]　Lourenco MC, Ferreira ML, Souza MVN, Peralta MA, Vasconcelos TA, Henrique, MGMO. Synthesis and anti-mycobacterial activity of of (*E*)-*N*-(monosubstituted-benzylidene)isonicotinohydrazide derivatives. *Euro J Med Chem* 2008;**43**:1344-1347.

[18]　Vergara FMF, Da Silva CHL, Henriques MGMO, Candéa ALP, Lourenço MCS, Ferreira ML, Kaiser CR, De Souza MVN. Synthesis and antimycobacterial evaluation of *N*-[(*E*)-(monosubstituded-benzylidene)]-2-pyrazinecarbohyrazide derivatives. *Eur J Med Chem* 2009;**44**:4954-4959.

[19]　Ferreira ML, Candéa ALP, Henrique MGMO Kaiser CR, Lima CHS, De Souza MVN. Synthesis and Cytotoxic Evaluation of Disubstituted *N*-Acylhydrazones Pyrazinecarbohydrazide Derivatives. *LDDD* 2010;**7**:275-80.

[20]　Carvalho SA, Da Silva EF, Lourenco MC, De Souza MVN, Fraga CAM. Antimycobacterial Profile of 5-phenyl-1,3,4-thiadiazole-2-arylhydrazone Derivatives. *LDDD* 2010;**7**:606-9.

[21]　De Souza MVN, Pais KC, Kaiser CR, Peralta MA, Ferreira ML, Lourenço MCS. Synthesis and *in vitro* antitubercular activity of a series of quinoline derivatives. *Bioorg Med Chem* 2009;**17**:1474-1480.

[22]   Candéa ALP, Ferreira ML, Pais KC, Cardoso LNF, Kaiser CR, Henriques MGMO, Lourenço MCS, Bezerra FAFM, De Souza MVN. Synthesis and antitubercular activity of 7-chloro-4-quinolinylhydrazones derivatives. *Bioorg Med Chem* 2009;**19**:6272-4.

[23]   De Lima FM, Candea ALP, Henriques MGMO, Lourenço MCS, Kaiser, CR, De Souza MVN. Evaluation of substituted benzaldehydes against *Mycobacterium tuberculosis*. *LDDD* 2010;**7**:754-758.

[24]   Costa MS, Boechat N, Rangel EA, Da Silva FC, De Souza AMT, Rodrigues CR, Castro HC, Junior IN, Lourenco MCS, Wardell SMSV, Ferreira VF. Synthesis, tuberculosis inhibitory activity, and SAR study of *N*-substituted-phenyl-1,2,3-triazole derivatives. *Bioorg Med Chem* 2006;**14**:8644-8653.

[25]   Dabak K, Sezer O, Akar A, Anac O. Synthesis and investigation of tuberculosis inhibition activities of some 1,2,3-triazole derivatives. *Eur J Med Chem* 2003;**38**:215-218.

[26]   Gill C, Jadhav G, Shaikh M, Kale R, Ghawalkar A, Nagargoje D, Shiradkar M. Clubbed [1,2,3] triazoles by fluorine benzimidazole: A novel approach to H37Rv inhibitors as a potential treatment for tuberculosis. *Bioorg Med Chem Lett* 2008;**18**:6244-6247.

[27]   Upadhayaya RS, Kulkarni GM, Vasireddy NR, Vandavasi JK, Dixit SS, Sharma V, Chattopadhyaya J. Design, synthesis and biological evaluation of novel triazole, urea and thiourea derivatives of quinoline against *Mycobacterium tuberculosis*. *Bioorg Med Chem Lett* 2009;**17**:4681-4692.

[28]   Patel, Navin B.; Khan, Imran H.; Rajani, Smita D. Pharmacological evaluation and characterizations of newly synthesized 1,2,4-triazoles. *Eur J Med Chem* 2010;**45**:4293-4299.

[29]   Guzeldemirci NU, Kucukbasmaci O. Synthesis and antimicrobial activity evaluation of new 1,2,4-triazoles and 1,3,4-thiadiazoles bearing imidazo[2,1-b]thiazole moiety. *Eur J Med Chem* 2010;**45**:63-68. *Eur J Med Chem* 2007;**42**:807-16.

[30]   Shiradkar M, Suresh K, Gorentla V, Dasari V, Tatikonda S, Akula KC, Shah R. Clubbed triazoles: A novel approach to antitubercular drugs. *Eur J Med Chem* 2007;**42**:807-16.

[31]   Abdel-Rahman HM, El-Koussi NA, Hassan HY. Fluorinated 1,2,4-triazolo[1,5-a]pyrimidine-6-carboxylic acid derivatives as antimycobacterial agents. *Archiv der Pharmazie* 2009;**342**:94-99.

[32]   Pandey J, Tiwari VK, Verma SS, Chaturvedi V, Bhatnagar S, Sinha A.N., Gaikwad, RP. Synthesis and antitubercular screening of imidazole derivatives. *Eur J Med Chem* 2009;**44**:3350–3355.

[33]   Zampieri D, Mamolo MG, Erik L, Giuditta S, Elena B, Vio L. Antifungal and antimycobacterial activity of 1-(3,5-diaryl-4,5-dihydro-1H-pyrazol-4-yl)-1H-imidazole derivatives. *Bioorg Med Chem* 2008;**16**:4516-4522.

[34]   Gupta P, Hameed S, Rahul J. Ring-substituted imidazoles as a new class of anti-tuberculosis agents. *Eur J Med Chem* 2004;**39**:805–814.

[35]   Sunduru N, Gupta L, Chaturvedi V, Dwivedi R, Sinha S, Chauhan PM. Discovery of new 1,3,5-triazine scaffolds with potent activity against *Mycobacterium tuberculosis* $H_{37}Rv$. *Eur J Med Chem* 2010;**45**:3335-45.

[36]   Anti-Tubercular Activity of Isatin Derivatives Fadl TA, Bin-Jubair FAS. *Int J Res Pharm Sci* 2010;**1**:113-126.

[37]   Kumar RR, Perumal S, Senthilkumar P, Yogeeswari P, Sriram D. Discovery of antimycobacterial spiro-piperidin-4-ones: an atom economic, stereoselective synthesis, and biological intervention. *J Med Chem* 2008;**51**:5731-5.

[38]   Virsodia V, Pissurlenkar RRS, Manvar D, Dholakia C. Adlakha P, Shah A, Coutinho EC. Synthesis, screening for antitubercular activity and 3D-QSAR studies of substituted *N*-phenyl-6-methyl-2-oxo-4-phenyl-1,2,3,4-tetrahydro-pyrimidine-5-carboxamides. *Eur J Med Chem* 2008;**43**:2103-2115.

[39]   Tangallapally RP, Yendapally R, Lee RE, Hevener K, Jones VC, Lenaerts AJM, McNeil MR, Wang Y, Franzblau SG, Lee RE. Synthesis and Evaluation of Nitrofuranylamides as Novel Antituberculosis Agents. *J Med Chem* 2004;**47**:5276-5283.

[40]   Kirk E. Hevener KE, Ball DM, Buolamwini JK, Lee RE. Quantitative structure-activity relationship studies on nitrofuranyl antitubercular agents. *Bioorg Med Chem.* 2008;**16**:8042–8053.

[41]   Hurdle JG, Lee RB, Budha NR, Carson EI, Qi J, Scherman MS, Cho SH, McNeil MR, Lenaerts AJ, Franzblau SG, Meibohm B, Lee RE. A microbiological assessment of novel nitrofuranylamides as anti-tuberculosis agents. *JAC* 2008;**62**:1037–1045.

[42]   Tangallapally RP, Lee REB, Lenaerts AJM, Lee RE. Synthesis of new and potent analogues of anti-tuberculosis agent 5-nitro-furan-2-carboxylic acid 4-(4-benzyl-piperazin-1-yl)-benzylamide with improved bioavailability. *Bioorg Med Chem Lett* 2006;**16**:2584–2589.

[43]   Tangallapally RP, Yendapally R, Lee RE, Lenaerts AJM, Lee, RE. Synthesis and Evaluation of Cyclic Secondary Amine Substituted Phenyl and Benzyl Nitrofuranyl Amides as Novel Antituberculosis Agents. *J Med Chem* 2005;**48**:8261-8269.

[44]   Tangallapally RP, Sun D, Budha RN, Lee REB, Lenaerts AJM, Bernd, Meibohma B, Lee, RE. Discovery of novel isoxazolines as anti-tuberculosis agents. *Bioorg Med Chem Lett* 2007;**17**:6638–6642.

[45]   Tangallapally RP, Yendapally R, Daniels AJ, Lee REB, Lee RE. Nitrofurans as Novel Anti-tuberculosis Agents: Identification, Development and Evaluation. *Curr Top Med Chem* 2007;**7**:509-526.

[46]   Teo JW, Thayalan P, Beer D, Yap AS, Nanjundappa M, Ngew X, Duraiswamy J, Liung S, Dartois V, Schreiber M, Hasan S, Cynamon M, Ryder NS, Yang X, Weidmann B, Bracken K, Dick T, Mukherjee K. Peptide deformylase inhibitors as potent antimycobacterial agents. *Antimicrob Agents Chemother* 2006;**50**:3665-73.

[47]   Vicente E, Villar R, Burguete A, Solano B, Silanes SP, Aldana I, Maddry JA, Lenaerts AJL, Franzblau SG, Cho SH, Monge A, Goldman RC. Efficacy of Quinoxaline-2-Carboxylate 1,4-Di-*N*-Oxide Derivatives in Experimental Tuberculosis. *Antimicrob Agents Chemother* 2008;**52**:3321–3326.

[48]   Jaso A, Zarranz B, Aldana I, Monge A. Synthesis of New Quinoxaline-2-carboxylate 1,4-Dioxide Derivatives as Anti-*Mycobacterium tuberculosis* Agents. *J Med Chem* 2005;**48**:2019-2025.

[49]   Vicente E, Silanes, SP, Lima LM, Ancizu S, Burguete A, Solano B, Villar R, Aldana I, Monge A. Selective activity against *Mycobacterium tuberculosis* of new quinoxaline1,4-di-*N*-oxides. *Bioorg Med Chem* 2009;**17**:385–389.

[50]   Synthesis of new 2-acetyl and 2-benzoyl quinoxaline 1,4-di-N-oxide derivatives as anti-*Mycobacterium tuberculosis* agents. Jaso A, Zarranz B, Aldana I, Monge A. *Eur J Med Chem* 2003;**38**:791-800.

[51]   Zarranz B, Jaso A, Aldana I, Monge A Synthesis and Antimycobacterial Activity of New Quinoxaline-2-carboxamide 1,4-di-*N*-Oxide Derivatives. *Bioorg Med Chem* 2003;**11**:2149-2156.

[52]   Moreno E, Ancizu S, Pérez-Silanes S, Torres E, Aldana I, Monge A. Synthesis and antimycobacterial activity of new quinoxaline-2-carboxamide 1,4-di-*N*-oxide derivatives. *Eur J Med Chem* 2010;**45**:4418-4426.

[53]   Ancizu S, Moreno E, Torres E, Burguete A, Pérez-Silanes SP, Benítez D, Villar R, Solano B, Marín A, Aldana I, Cerecetto H, González M, Monge, A. Heterocyclic-2-carboxylic Acid (3-

Cyano-1,4-di-*N*-oxidequinoxalin-2-yl)amide Derivatives as Hits for the Development of Neglected Disease Drugs. *Molecules* 2009;**14**:2256-2272.

[54]   Moreno E, Ancizu S, Pérez-Silanes S, Torres E, Aldana I, Monge A. Synthesis and antimycobacterial activity of new quinoxaline-2-carboxamide 1,4-di-*N*-oxide derivatives. *Eur J Med Chem* 2010;**45**:4418-4426.

[55]   Das U, Das S, Bandy B, Gorecki DK, Dimmock JR. *E*-2-[3-(3,4-dichlorophenyl)-1-oxo-2-propenyl]-3-methylquinoxaline-1,4-dioxide: a lead antitubercular agent which alters mitochondrial respiration in rat liver. *Eur J Med Chem* 2010;**45**:4682-6.

[56]   De Souza MVN, Ferreira ML, Pinheiro AC, Saraiva MF, Almeida MV, Valle MS. Synthesis and Biological Aspects of Mycolic Acids: An Important Target Against *Mycobacterium tuberculosis*. *The Scientific World Journal* 2008;**8**:720-751.

[57]   Crick DC, Mahapatra S, Brennan PJ. Biosynthesis of the arabinogalactan-peptidoglycan complex of *Mycobacterium tuberculosis*. *Glycobiology* 2001;**11**:107R-118R.

[58]   Content J, Cuvellerie AWL, Vicent-Levy-Frebault V, Ooms J, Bruyn J. The genes coding for the antigen 85 complexes of *Mycobacterium tuberculosis* and *Mycobacterium bovis* BCG are members of a gene family: cloning, sequence determination, and genomic organization of the gene coding for antigen 85-C of *M. Tuberculosis*. *Infect Immun* 1991;**59**:3205-12.

[59]   Tewari N, Tiwari VK, Triphati RP, Chaturvedi V, Srivastava A, Srivastava R, Shukla PK, Chatuverdi AK, Gaikwad A, Sinha S, Srivastava BS. Synthesis of galactopyranosyl amino alcohols as a new class of antitubercular and antifungal agents. *Bioorg Med Chem Lett* 2004;**14**:329-32.

[60]   Triphati RP, Tiwari VK, Tewari N, Katiyar D, Saxena N, Sinha S, Gaikwad A, Srivastava A, Chaturvedi V, Manju YK, Srivastava R, Srivastava BS. Synthesis and antitubercular activities of bis-glycosylated diamino alcohols. *Bioorg Med Chem Lett* 2005;**13**:5668-79.

[61]   Katiyar D, Tiwari VK, Tewari N, Verma SS, Sinha S, Gaikwad A, Srivastava A, Chaturvedi V, Srivastava R, Svristava BS, Tripathi RP. Synthesis and antimycobacterial activities of glycosylated amino alcohols and amines. *Eur J Med Chem* 2005;**40**:351-60.

[62]   Daryaee F, Kobarfard F, Khalaj A, Farnia P. Synthesis and evaluation of *in vitro* anti-tuberculosis activity of *N*-substituted glycolamides. *Eur J Med Chem* 2009;**44**:289-295.

[63]   Dwivedi N, Tewari N, Tiwari VK, Chaturvedi V, Manju YK, Srivastava A, Giakwad A, Sinha S, Tripathi RP. An Efficient Synthesis of Aryloxyphenyl Cyclopropyl Methanones: A New Class of Antimycobacterial Agents. *Bioorg Med Chem Lett* 2005;**15**:4526-30.

[64]   Vadim Makarov, *et al.* Benzothiazinones Kill by Blocking Arabinan Synthesis *Mycobacterium tuberculosis*. *Science* 2009;**324**:801-4.

[65]   Shakya N, Srivastav NC, Desroches N, Agrawal B, Kunimoto DY, Kumar R. 3'-Bromo Analogues of Pyrimidine Nucleosides as a New Class of Potent Inhibitors of *Mycobacterium tuberculosis*. *J Med Chem* 2010;**53**:4130-4140.

[66]   Vergara FMF, Henriques MGMO, Candea ALP, Wardell JL De Souza MVN. Antitubercular activity of α, ω-diaminoalkanes, $H_2N(CH_2)nNH_2$. *Bioorg Med Chem Lett* 2009;**19**:4937-4938.

[67]   Lourenco MC, Vicente FRC, Henrique MGMO, Candea ALP, Goncalves RSB, Nogueira TCM, Ferreira ML, De Souza MVN. Synthesis and biological evaluation of *N*-(aryl)-2-thiophen-2-ylacetamides series as a new class of antitubercular agents. *Bioorg Med Chem Lett* 2007;**17**:6895-6898.

[68]   De Souza MVN, Ferreira ML, Nogueira TCM, Goncalves RSB, Peralta MA, Lourenco MCS, Vicente FRC. Synthesis and Biological Evaluation of *N*-(Alkyl)-2-Thiophen-2- Ylacetamides Series as a New Class of Antitubercular Agents. *LDDD*, 2008;**5**:221-224.

[69] Guo S, Song Y, Huang Q, Yuan H, Wan B, Wang Y, He R, Beconi MG, Franzblau SG, Kozikowski AP. Identification, Synthesis, and Pharmacological Evaluation of Tetrahydroindazole Based Ligands as Novel Antituberculosis Agents. *J Med Chem* 2010;**53**:649–659.

[70] Mital A, Negi VS, Ramachandran U. Synthesis and biological evaluation of substituted naphthoquinone derivatives as potent antimycobacterial agents. *Arkivoc* 2008;**xv**:176-192.

[71] Razafimahefa D, Ralambomanana DA, Hammouche L, Pélinski L, Lauvagie S, Bebear C, Brocard J, Maugein J. Synthesis and antimycobacterial activity of ferrocenyl ethambutol analogues and ferrocenyl diamines. *Bioorg Med Chem Lett* 2005;**15**:2301-03.

[72] Dimby AR, Dorothée RR, Andry CR, Jeanne M, Lydie P.Synthesis and antitubercular activity of ferrocenyl diaminoalcohols and diamines. *Bioorg Med Chem* 2008;**16**:9546-9553.

[73] Moro AC, Mauro AE, Netto AVG, Ananias SR, Quilles MB, Carlos IZ, Pavan FR, Leite CQF, Horner M. Antitumor and antimycobacterial activities of cyclopalladated complexes: X-ray structure of [Pd(C^2,N-dmba)(Br)(tu)] (dmba = *N,N*-dimethylbenzylamine,tu=thiourea). *Eur J Med Chem* 2009;**44**:4611-4615.

[74] Vieira LMM, De Almeida MV, Lourenço MCS, Bezerra FAFM, Fontes APS. Synthesis and antitubercular activity of palladium and platinum complexes with fluoroquinolones. *Eur J Med Chem* 2009;**44**:4611-4615.

[75] Maccari R, Ottana R, Bottari B, Rotondo E, Vigorita MG. *In vitro* advanced antimycobacterial screening of cobalt(II) and copper(II) complexes of fluorinated isonicotinoylhydrazones. *Bioorg Med Chem Lett* 2004;**14**:5731-33.

[76] Oliveira JS, Sousa EHS, Basso LA, Palaci M, Dietze R, Santos DS, Moreira IS. An inorganic iron complex that inhibits wild-type and an isoniazid-resistant mutant 2-*trans*-enoyl-ACP (CoA) reductase from *Mycobacterium tuberculosis*. *Chem Commun* 2004; 312-313.

[77] Maia PIS, Pavan FR, Leite CQF, Lemos SSS, Gerimario F, Batista AA, Nascimento OR, Ellena J, Castellano EE, Niquet E, Deflon VM. Vanadium complexes with thiosemicarbazones: Synthesis, characterization, crystal structures and anti-*Mycobacterium tuberculosis* activity. *Polyhedron* 2009;**28**:398-406.

[78] Robert C. Goldman RC, Laughon BR. Discovery and validation of new antitubercular compounds as potential drug leads and probes. *Tuberculosis* 2009;**89**:331-333.

[79] Collins LA, Franzblau SG. Microplate Alamar Blue Assay *vs.* BACTEC 460 System for High-Throughput Screening of Compounds against *Mycobacterium tuberculosis* and *Mycobacterium avium*. *AAC* 1997;**39**:1004-9.

[80] Cho SH, Warit S, Wan B, Hwang CH, Pauli GF, Franzblau SG. Low-Oxygen-Recovery Assay for High-Throughput Screening of Compounds against Nonreplicating *Mycobacterium tuberculosis*. *AAC* 2007;**51**:1380-5.

[81] Chung GAC, Aktar Z, Jackson S, Duncan K. High-Throughput Screen for Detecting Antimycobacterial Agents. *AAC* 1995;**39**:2235-2238.

[82] Maddry JA, Ananthan S, Goldman RC, Hobrath JV, Kwong CD, Maddox C, Rasmussen L, Reynolds RC, Secrist JA, Sosa MI, White EL, Zhang W. Antituberculosis activity of the molecular libraries screening center network library. *Tuberculosis* 2009;**89**:354-363.

[83] Ananthan S, Faaleolea ER, Goldman RC, Hobrath JV, Kwong CD, Laughon BE, Maddry JA, Mehta A, Rasmussen L, Reynolds RC, Secrist III JA, Shindo N, Showe DN, Sosa MI, Suling WJ, White EL. High-throughput screening for inhibitors of *Mycobacterium tuberculosis* H37Rv. *Tuberculosis* 2009;**89**:334–353.

[84]   Goldman RC, Laughon BE, Reynolds RC, Secrist III JA, Maddry JA, Guie M-A, *et al.* Programs to facilitate tuberculosis drug discovery: the Tuberculosis Antimicrobial Acquisition and Coordinating Facility. Infect Disord – Drug Targets 2007;**7**:92-104.

[85]   Nefzi A, Appel J, Arutyunyan S, Houghten RA. Parallel synthesis of chiral pentaamines and pyrrolidine containing bis-heterocyclic libraries. Multiple scaffolds with multiple building blocks: A double diversity for the identification of new antitubercular compounds. *Bioorg Med Chem Lett* 2009;**19**:5169-5175.

[86]   Lougheed KEA, Taylor DL, Osborne SA, Bryans JS, Roger S. Buxton RS. New anti-tuberculosis agents amongst known drugs. *Tuberculosis* 2009;**89**:364-370.

[87]   Christophe T, Jackson M, Jeon HK, Fenistein D, Dominguez MC, Kim J, Genovesio A, Carralot JP, Ewann F, Kim EH, Sae SY, Kang S, Seo MJ, Park EJ, kovierova HS, Pham H, Riccardi G, Nam JY, Marsollier L, Kempf M, Guillou MLJ, Oh T, Won WK, No Z, Nehrbass U, Brosch R, Cole ST, Brodin P. High Content Screening Identifies Decaprenyl-Phosphoribose 29 Epimerase as a Target for Intracellular Antimycobacterial Inhibitors. *PLoS Pathogens* 2009;**5**:e1000645, 1-10.

[88]   Kolb HC, Sharpless KB. The growing impact of click chemistry on drug discovery. *Drug Discovery Today* 2003;**8**:1128-1137.

[89]   Tan LP, Wu H, Yang PY, Kalesh KA, Zhang X, Hu M, Srinivasan R, Yao SQ. High-Throughput Discovery of *Mycobacterium tuberculosis* Protein Tyrosine Phosphatase B (MptpB) Inhibitors Using Click Chemistry. *Org Lett* 2009;**11**:5103-5105.

[90]   Kumar A, Sinhab S, Chauhan PMS. Syntheses of Novel Antimycobacterial Combinatorial Libraries of Structurally Diverse Substituted Pyrimidines by Three-Component Solid-Phase Reactionsy. *Bioorg Med Chem Lett* 2002;**12**:667-669.

[91]   MarrapuVK, Chaturvedi V, Singh S, Singh S, Sinha S, Bhandari K. Novel aryloxy azolyl chalcones with potent activity against *Mycobacterium tuberculosis* H37Rv. *European Journal of Medicinal Chemistry* 2011;**46**:4302-4310.

[92]   Arshad A, Osman H, Bagley MC, Lam CK, Mohamad S, Zahariluddin, ASM. Synthesis and antimicrobial properties of some new thiazolyl coumarin derivatives. *Eur J Med Chem* 2011;**46**:3788-3794.

[93]   Lu X, Wan B Franzblau SG, You Q. Design, synthesis and antitubercular evaluation of new 2-acylated and 2 -alkylated amino-5-(4-(benzyloxy)phenyl)thiophene-3-carboxylic acid derivatives. Part 1. *Eur J Med Chem* 2011;**46**:3551-3563.

[94]   Gunasekaran P, Perumal S, Yogeeswari P, Sriram D. A facile four - component sequential protocol in the expedient synthesis of novel 2-aryl-5-methyl-2,3-dihydro-1H-3-pyrazolones in water and their antitubercular evaluation. *Eur J Med Chem* 2011;**46**:4530-4536.

[95]   Carneiro PF, Pinto MCFR, Coelho TS, Cavalcanti BC, Pessoa C, De Simone CA, Nunes IKC, De Oliveira NM, De Almeida RG, Pinto AV, De Moura KCG, Da Silva PA, Da Silva JEN. Quinonoid and phenazine compounds: Synthesis and evaluation against H37Rv, rifampicin and isoniazid-resistance strains of *Mycobacterium tuberculosis*. *Eur J Med Chem* 2011;**46**:4521-4529.

[96]   Raja VPA, Perumal S, Yogeeswari P, Sriram D. Synthesis and antimycobacterial activity of highly functionalized tetrahydro-4(1H)-pyridinones. *Bioorg Med Chem Lett* 2011;**21**:3881-3884.

[97]   Kumar RR, Perumal S, Menendez JC, Yogeeswari P, Sriram D. Antimycobacterial activity of novel 1, 2, 4 - oxadiazole - pyranopyridine / chromene hybrids generated by chemoselective 1,3-dipolar cycloadditions of nitrile oxides. *Bioorg Med Chem* 2011;**19**:3444-3450.

[98]   Kantevari S, Yempala T, Yogeeswari P, Sriram D, Sridhar B. Synthesis and antitubercular evaluation of amidoalkyl dibenzofuranols and 1H-benzo[2,3]benzofuro[4,5-e][1,3]oxazin-3(2H)-ones. *Bioorg Med Chem Lett* 2011;**21**:4316-4319.

[99]   Chanda D, Saikia D, Kumar JK, Thakur JP, Agarwal J, Chanotiya CS, Shanker K, Negi AS. 1 - Chloro - 2 - formyl indenes and tetralenes as antitubercular agents. *Bioorg Med Chem Lett* 2011;**21**:3966-9.

[100] Bogatcheva E, Hanrahan C, Nikonenko B, De los Santos G, Reddy VCP, Barbosa F, Einck L, Nacy C, Protopopova M. Identification of SQ609 as a lead compound from a library of dipiperidines. *Bioorg Med Chem Lett* 2011;**21**:5353-5357.

[101] Sriram D, Yogeeswari P, Methuku S, Vyas DRK, Senthilkumar P, Alvala M, Jeankumar VU. Synthesis of various 3-nitropropionamides as *Mycobacterium tuberculosis* isocitrate lyase inhibitor *Bioorg Med Chem Lett* 2011;**21**:5149–5154.

[102] Ahsan MJ, Samy JG, Dutt KR, Agrawal UK, Yadav BS, Vyas SKR, Yadav G. Design, synthesis and antimycobacterial evaluation of novel 3 - substituted -*N*-aryl-6,7-dimethoxy-3a,4-dihydro-3H-indeno[1,2-c]pyrazole-2-carboxamide analogues. *Bioorg Med Chem Lett* 2011;**21**:4451-4453.

[103] Ahsan MJ, Samy JG, Soni S, Jain N, Kumar L, Sharma LK, Yadav H, Saini L, Kalyansing RG, Devenda NS, Prasad R, Jain CB. Discovery of novel antitubercular 3a,4-dihydro-3H-indeno [1,2-c] pyrazole-2-carboxamide/carbothioamide analogues. *Bioorg Med Chem Lett* 2011;**21**:5259-5261.

[104] Vintonyak VV, Warburg K, Over B, Huebel K, Rauh D, Waldmann H. Identification and further development of thiazolidinones spiro - fused to indolin-2-ones as potent and selective inhibitors of *Mycobacterium tuberculosis* protein tyrosine phosphatase B. *Tetrahedron* 2011;**67**:6713-6729.

[105] Roy KK, Singh S, Sharma SK, Srivastava R, Chaturvedi V, Saxena, AK. Synthesis and biological evaluation of substituted 4 - arylthiazol - 2 - amino derivatives as potent growth inhibitors of replicating *Mycobacterium tuberculosis* H37Rv. *Bioorg Med Chem Lett* 2011;**21**:5589-5593.

[106] Patel RV, Kumari P, Rajani DP, Chikhalia KH. Synthesis and studies of novel 2-(4- cyano-3-trifluoromethylphenyl amino)- 4 -(quinoline- 4 -yloxy)-6-(piperazinyl/piperidinyl)-s-triazines as potential antimicrobial, antimycobacterial and anticancer agents. *Eur J Med Chem* 2011;**46**:4354-4365.

[107] Wei Z, Wang J, Liu M, Li S, Sun L, GuoH, Wang B, Lu W. Synthesis, *in vitro* atimycobacterial and antibacterial evaluation of IMB-0705593 derivatives containing a substituted benzyloxime moiety. *Molecules* 2013;**18**:3872-3893.

[108] Upadhayaya RS, Shinde PD, Sayyed AY, Kadam SA, Bawane AN, Poddar A, Plashkevych O, Földesi A, Chattopadhyaya J. Synthesis and structure of azole-fused indeno[2,1-c]quinolines and their anti-mycobacterial properties. *Org Biomol Chem* 2010;**8**:5661-73.

[109] Patpi SR, Pulipati L, Yogeeswari P, Sriram D, Jain N, Sridhar B, Murthy R, Anjana Devi T, Kalivendi SV, Kantevari S. Design, synthesis, and structure-activity correlations of novel dibenzo[b,d]furan, dibenzo[b,d]thiophene, and N-methylcarbazole clubbed 1,2,3-triazoles as potent inhibitors of *Mycobacterium tuberculosis*. *J Med Chem* 2012;**55**:3911-22.

[110] Dandia A, Jain AA, Laxkar AK.Synthesis and biological evaluation of highlyfunctionalized dispiro heterocycles. *RSC Adv.,* 2013, **3**, 8422–8430.

[111] Kumar S, Dwivedi AP, Kashyap VK, Saxena AK, Dwivedi AK, Srivastava R, Sahu DP. Synthesis and biological evaluation of *trans* 6-methoxy-1,1-dimethyl-2-phenyl-3-aryl-2,3-dihydro-1H-inden-4-yloxyalkylamine derivatives against drug susceptible, non-replicating M. tuberculosis H37Rv and clinical multidrug resistant strains. *Bioorg Med Chem Lett.* 2013;**23**:2404-7.

Send Orders for Reprints to reprints@benthamscience.net

CHAPTER 5

Compounds in Clinical Studies Based on Natural Products

Marcus V.N. de Souza[*]

Instituto de Tecnologia em Fármacos – Farmanguinhos, FioCruz – Fundação Oswaldo Cruz, R. Sizenando Nabuco, 100, Manguinhos, 21041-250, Rio de Janeiro, RJ, Brazil

Abstract: The antibiotic streptomycin was the first drug used to treat TB and illustrated well the important role of nature in the fight against diseases. For example, several natural products were discovered between 1940-60's against *Mycobacterium tuberculosis* being used nowadays in TB treatment as second-line drugs. Due to the importance of nature in the past and the present for TB treatment and drug discovery, a lot of attention has been given to new anti-TB drugs based on natural products nowadays, especially against MDR and XDR-TB. Considering that, the aim of the present chapter is to highlight promising natural product candidates in clinical trials against TB.

Keywords: Tuberculosis, *Mycobacterium tuberculosis*, natural products, semi-synthesis, drug development, treatment, multi-drug-resistant tuberculosis (MDR TB), extensive-drug-resistant tuberculosis (XDR TB), target, mechanism of action, biological evaluation, clinical studies.

INTRODUCTION

The first drug used in TB treatment appeared in 1946 with the introduction of the antibiotic streptomycin, an aminoglycoside isolated from the actinobacterium *Streptomyces griseus*, identified in 1943 by Selman Abraham Waksman and his student Albert Schatz at Rutgers University. This discovery was 61 years after the identification of the etiologic agent of tuberculosis, the *Mycobacterium tuberculosis* by R. Koch in 1882, and illustrated well the important role of nature in the fight against diseases. After the streptomycin discovery, nature still played a

*Adress correspondence to Marcus V.N. de Souza: Instituto de Tecnologia em Fármacos – Farmanguinhos, FioCruz – Fundação Oswaldo Cruz, R. Sizenando Nabuco, 100, Manguinhos, 21041-250, Rio de Janeiro, RJ, Brazil; E-mail: marcos_souza@far.fiocruz.br

crucial role in drug discovery against TB. For example, other aminoglicosides such as kanamycin from *Streptomyces capreolus,* the semisynthetic amikacin produced from kanamycin A and capreomycin from *Streptomyces kanamyceticus,* as well as D-cycloserine from *Streptomyces* sps were discovered between 1940-60′s being used nowadays in TB treatment as second-line drugs. In the twenty first century serious attention is being paid to the discovery of new molecules from nature with unexploited modes of action in special against MDR (multidrug-resistant) and XDR (extensively drug resistant) tuberculosis [1-7]. Considering that, the aim of the present chapter is to highlight promising natural product candidates in clinical trials against TB.

RIFAMYCINS

Due to the importance of rifampicin in TB treatment and the problem rifampicin-resistance several research groups and pharmaceutical companies have been searched for more potent drugs with lesser side effects. In this context, other semisynthetic rifampin analogues have been introduced for clinical use, such as rifapentine, rifalazil, rifabutin and rifametane. The semisythetic production of rifampin and its analogues were obtained from fermentation broth of *Streptomyces mediterranei* and chemical reactions (Scheme **1**) [8-10].

Mechanism of Action

Rifampin became clinical available in 1966 and it is responsible for the reduction of the duration of therapy, from 12 to 6 months, when combined with others drugs, as well as from 9 to 2 or 3 months in latent infection. Its mechanism of action is based on the inhibition of bacterial DNA-dependent RNA polymerase, which produces essential proteins and it is responsible to copy their own genetic information, the DNA. Despite the importance of rifampin in the TB treatment, the emergence of different rifampicin-resistant bacteria, increase the problems to global tuberculosis control [9,10]. This resistance occurs during therapy against active tuberculosis and normally arises from mutations in the beta subunit of the ribosomal polymerase gene (*rpoB*). The inactivation of rifampicin by different rifampicin-resistant bacteria is due to the glycosilation or phosphorylation of rifampicin and 3-formylrifamycin SV in the C_{21} and C_{23} position (Scheme **2**) [9,10].

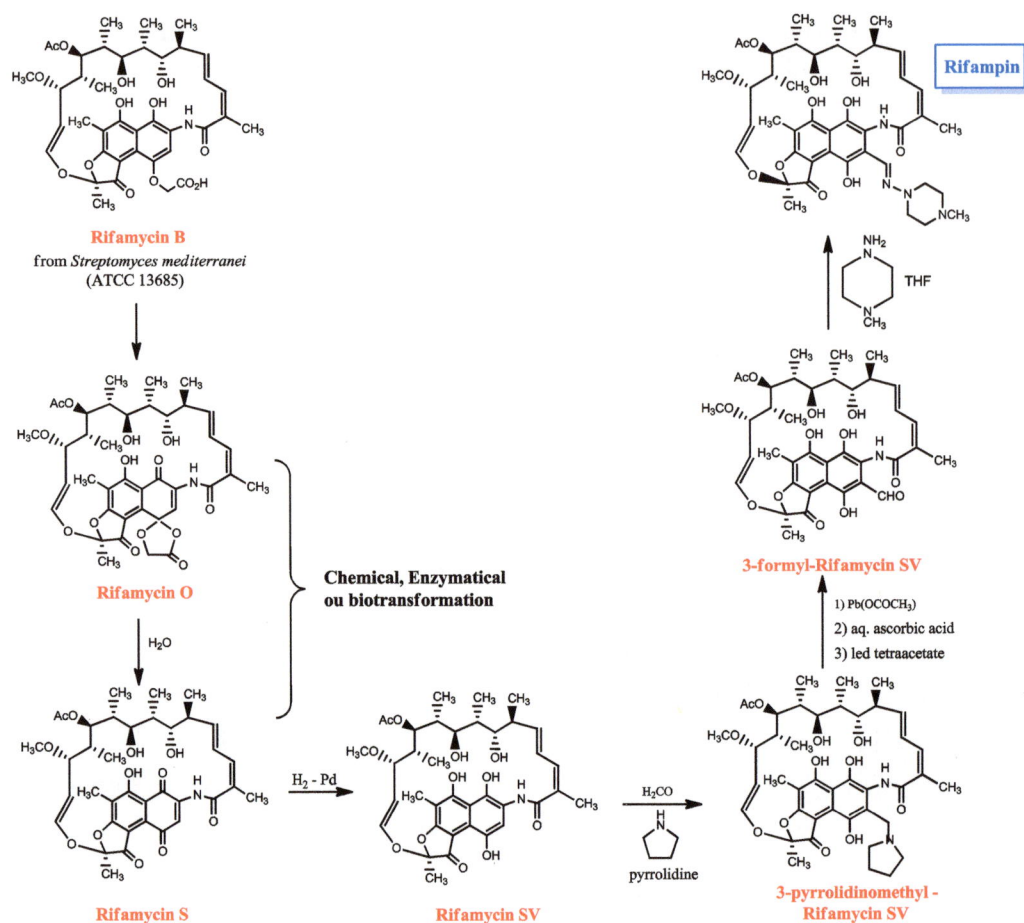

Scheme 1: Semisynthetic synthesis of rifampin.

Rifapentine

After a thirty years gap, in which no new TB drug was introduced in the market, Rifapentine (Fig. **1**) [10] was developed by Hoechst Marion Roussel under the trade name Priftin. This cyclopentyl-substituted rifampicin was approved by FDA in 1998 and it possesses the same broad spectrum activity than rifampin. However an important difference between both rifamycins is the elimination half-life of rifapentine, which is almost 4 fold greater in humans than rifampin. This can be explained by the higher lipophilicity, which facilitates tissue penetration of this drug, as well as the lack of biotransformation to antimicrobially inactive metabolites.

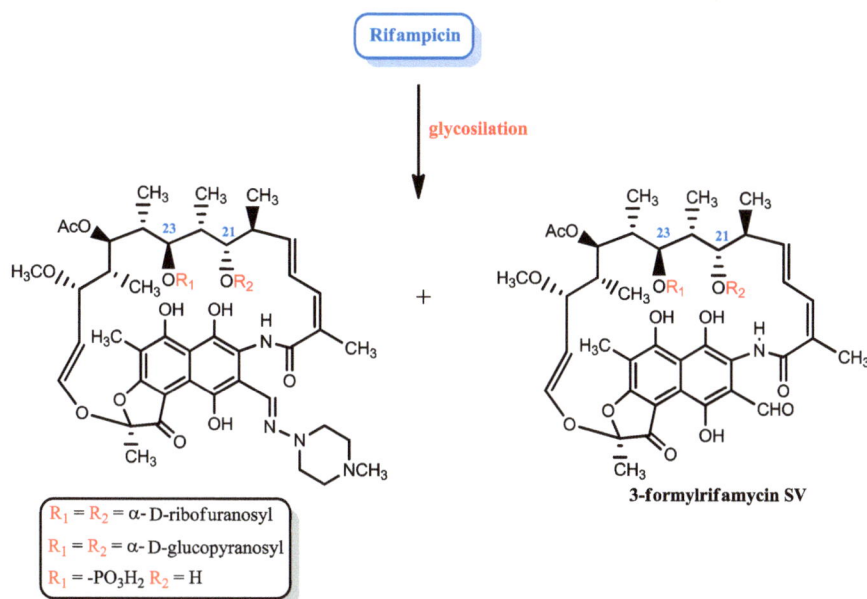

Scheme 2: Inactivation of rifampicin by different rifampicin-resistant bacteria.

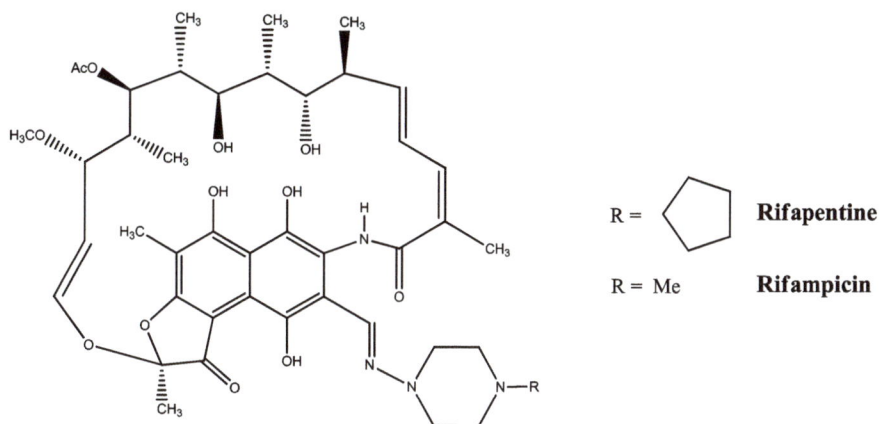

Figure 1: Structure of rifapentine.

Rifalazil

The benzoxazinorifamycin, common known as Rifalazil or (KRM 1648) (Fig. **2**) is also a semi-synthetic analogue of rifampin [10,11] produced by Kaneka Corporation that possesses potent bactericidal activity against *M. tuberculosis in vitro* and *in vivo*. Studies *in vitro* have shown that rifalazil is 64-fold more active than rifampin against different *M. tuberculosis* strains. Rifalazil also presents good oral activity against *M. tuberculosis* both in animal and humans with a long half-life of about 60h. This rifamycin was in Phase II clinical trials, however, due to severe side effects in the fourth day of Phase II trial, the development of rifalazil was aborted.

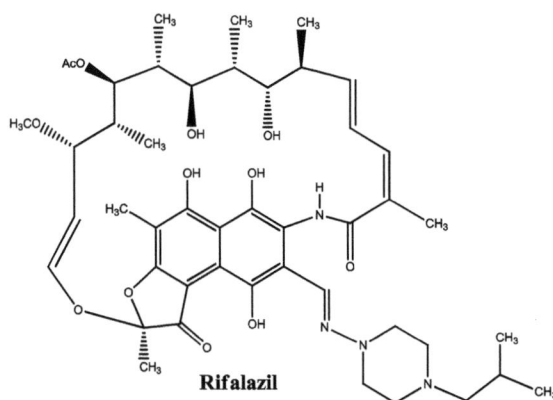

Figure 2: Structure of rifalazil.

Rifabutin

Rifabutin (Fig. **3**) [10,12] is the first rifamycin approved by FDA for the prevention of MAC (*Mycobacterium avium* complex) disease in people with advanced HIV infection. People with MAC present fatigue, weight loss, abdominal pain, night sweats, fever, and liver dysfunction and it can contribute to death. This rifamycin is used in combination with others drugs, such as ciprofloxacin, ethambutol, amikacin, azithromycin and clarithromycin. Rifabutin is manufactured by Adria Laboratories, Columbius, Ohio, with the brand name Mycobutin.

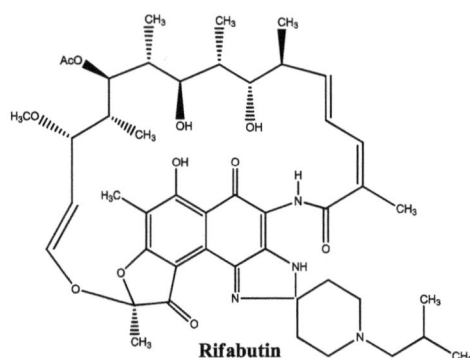

Figure 3: Structure of rifabutin.

Rifametane

The semi-synthetic analogue of rifampin, rifametane (SPA-S-565) (Fig. **4**) have been developed by Societa Prodotti Antibiotici (SPA), Milan, Italy. In the phase I pharmacokinetic study of rifametane was conducted in 8 healthy male volunteers with a 300 mg single oral compared with 300 mg of conventional ripampicin [10,13]. The pharmacokinetic profiles of rifametane were significantly more favorable than those of rifampicin. Currently SPA is collaborating with Glaxo India to advance rifametane into phase II trials.

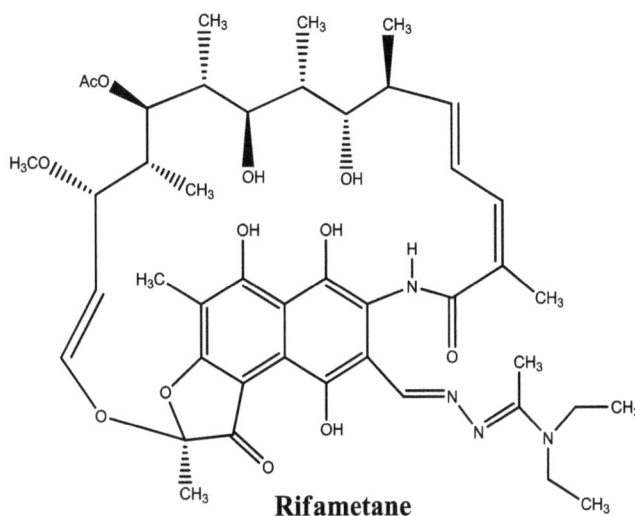

Figure 4: Structure of rifametane.

PLEUROMUTILIN

Natural product pleuromutilin and its derivatives have a potent activity against drug-resistant Gram-positive bacteria and mycoplasmas [14,15], favorable pharmacokinetic and pharmacodynamic properties and do not show target-specific cross-resistance to other antibiotics [14,16-18]. For example, pleuromutilin is under development by the TB Global Alliance (Fig. **5**) [19], who are also investigating several others promising analogues in the search of new drugs against MDR-TB. One advantage of pleuromutilin as a TB-drug is its unique mechanism of action, which seems not to have any specific cross-resistance with other antibacterial classes, and then has promising perspective against MDR-TB.

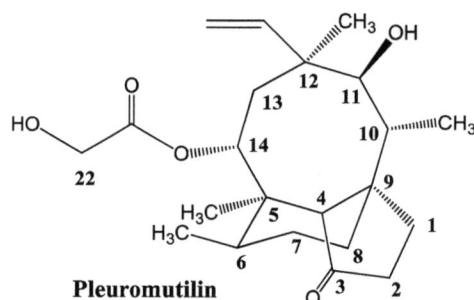

Figure 5: Pleuromutilin structure.

Pleuromutilin (Figure **5**) was first described in 1951 by Kavanagh and colleagues [14,20], who isolated the substance in a crystalline form from cultures of two species of basidiomycetes, *Pleurotus mutilus* and *P. passeckerianus*. In this work, pleuromutilin had its biological activity evaluated against several kinds of microorganisms and sarcoma, and attracted considerable attention as a consequence of its significant *in vitro* antibiotic activity against Gram-positive bacteria and its low animal toxicity.

In the early 1950's, Anchel started the chemical and structural studies of pleuromutilin. He determined the molecular formula as $C_{22}H_{34}O_5$ and demonstrated the presence of two hydroxyl groups, a hindered carbonyl group and an isolated double bond into pleuromutilin structure [14,21]. Only 10 years later did pleuromutilin have its complete structure elucidated, first, by Arigoni [14,22], and one year later, by Birch [14,23]. Both came independently to the same structure and demonstrated that pleuromutilin is a diterpene, constituted of a rather rigid 5-6-8 tricyclic carbon skeleton with eight stereogenic centers.

The pioneer works of Arigoni and Birch allowed the development of the initial structure-activity relationships (SARs) studies in pleuromutilin, started in the middle of the 1970's by Riedl [14,24] and Egger and Reinshagen [14,25,26].

In the early reports, pleuromutilin obtained by fermentation was used as start material and a number of semisynthetic pleuromutilin analogues were prepared and tested against *S. aureus*, *Mycoplasma hominis*, *M. gallisepticum* and *M. hyorhinis*. The molecular modifications of pleuromutilin were focused essentially on the functional groups such as the 11-OH group, the carbonyl group at the five-membered ring, the terminal methylene group and mainly at the C-14 glycolic acid chain (Fig. **6**). In these studies, it was verified that the esterification or oxidation of the C-11 hydroxyl group yielded inactive compounds and the reaction of the carbonyl group at the five-membered ring with hydroxylamine yielding an oxime which also furnished an inactive compound (Fig. **6**). When the terminal methylene was hydrogenated, the activity of pleuromutilin remained inalterable (Fig. **6**). Two modifications at the C-14 position furnished inactive compounds, the oxidation of the hydroxyl group at the C-14 glycolic acid chain yielding a carboxylic acid and the cleavage of the ester group yielding a compound named mutilin (Fig. **6**). The most relevant results were obtained when the ester group was maintained and variations on the side chain were realized. All compounds were active, however the activity varied widely with the substitution. When neutral side chains were utilized, a little effect in comparison with the original compound was observed. Side chains containing a carboxylic group reduced the activity. Better activities were reached by substitution for side chains containing a thioether and an aromatic or an amino group (Fig. **6**).

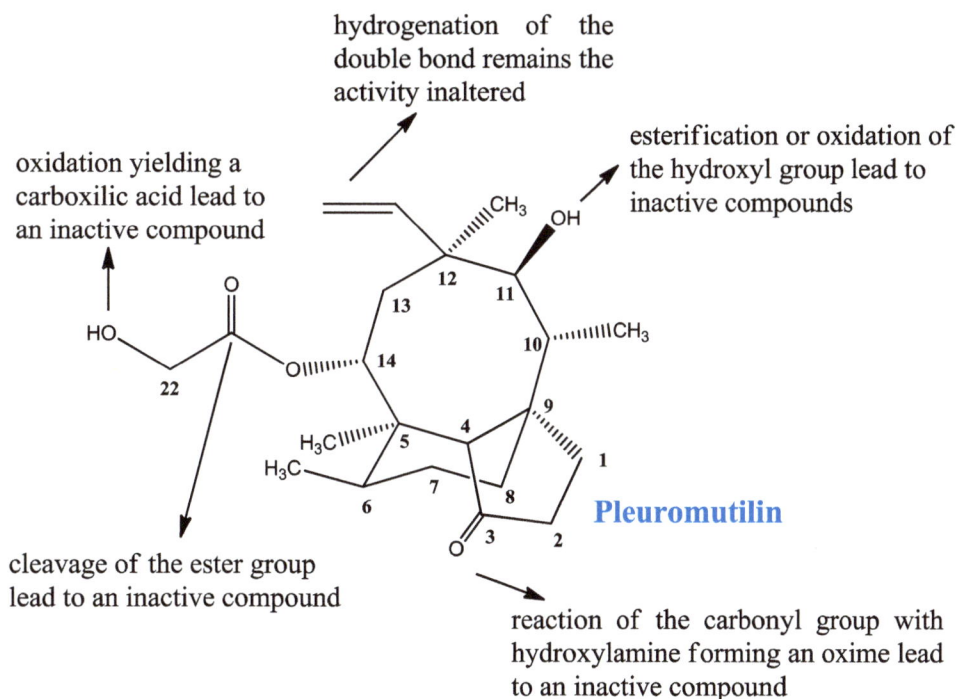

Figure 6: SARs studies in pleuromutilin.

These preliminary works lead to the development of tiamulin and valnemulin (Fig. **7**), actually used as therapeutic veterinary agents [27]. The discovery of more active derivates stimulated the beginning of mechanisms of action studies.

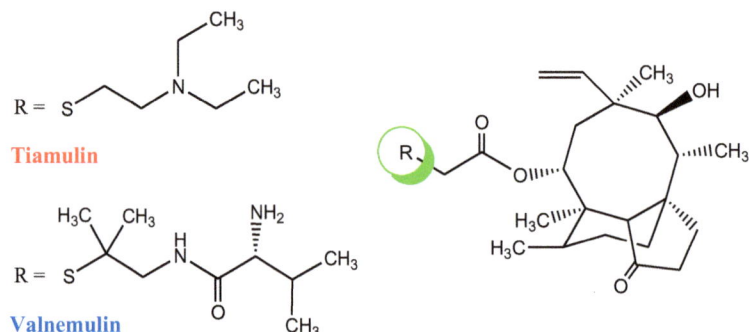

Figure 7: Tiamulin and valunemulin.

Mechanism of Action

Studies utilizing tiamulin, valnemulin and others chemically related substances demonstrated that pleuromutilins act as bacterial protein biosynthesis inhibitors [14,28-32]. These substances bind to 70S ribosome which is composed of two subunits, a small (30S) and a large (50S) [14,33,34]. The specific target in the ribosome is the domain V of 23S rRNA at the peptidyl transferase centre, where the pleuromutilins prevent the correct positioning of the tRNAs for peptide transfer, inhibiting the peptidyl trasferase [14,35]. Crystallography studies utilizing a structure of the 50S ribosomal subunit from *Deinococcus radiodurans* in complex with tiamulin showed that this drug binds to 23S rRNA through an extensive network of hydrophobic interactions involving exclusively nucleotides of domain V and through hydrogen bonds to G2061 and U2585 [14,36]. The tricyclic nucleus of tiamulin is located inside a cavity at the A-tRNA binding site, confined by the residues G2061, A2451, C2452, A2503, U2504, G2505 and U2506 and its positioning is stabilized by a hydrogen bond between the hydroxyl group at C-11 position of tiamulin and the G2505 residue. Another important interaction occurs with the G2061 of the 23S rRNA, since this residue promotes hydrophobic contacts with groups of the tiamulin cyclo-octane ring and a hydrogen bond with the sulfur atom of the side chain [14,36]. It is important to mention that the binding site of pleuromutilins is different from erythromycin

(Fig. **8**), which is a ribosome targeted antibiotic. However, other antibiotics such as chloramphenicol (Fig. **8**), puromycin and carbomycin A (Fig. **8**) compete with pleuromutilins for binding to the ribosome.

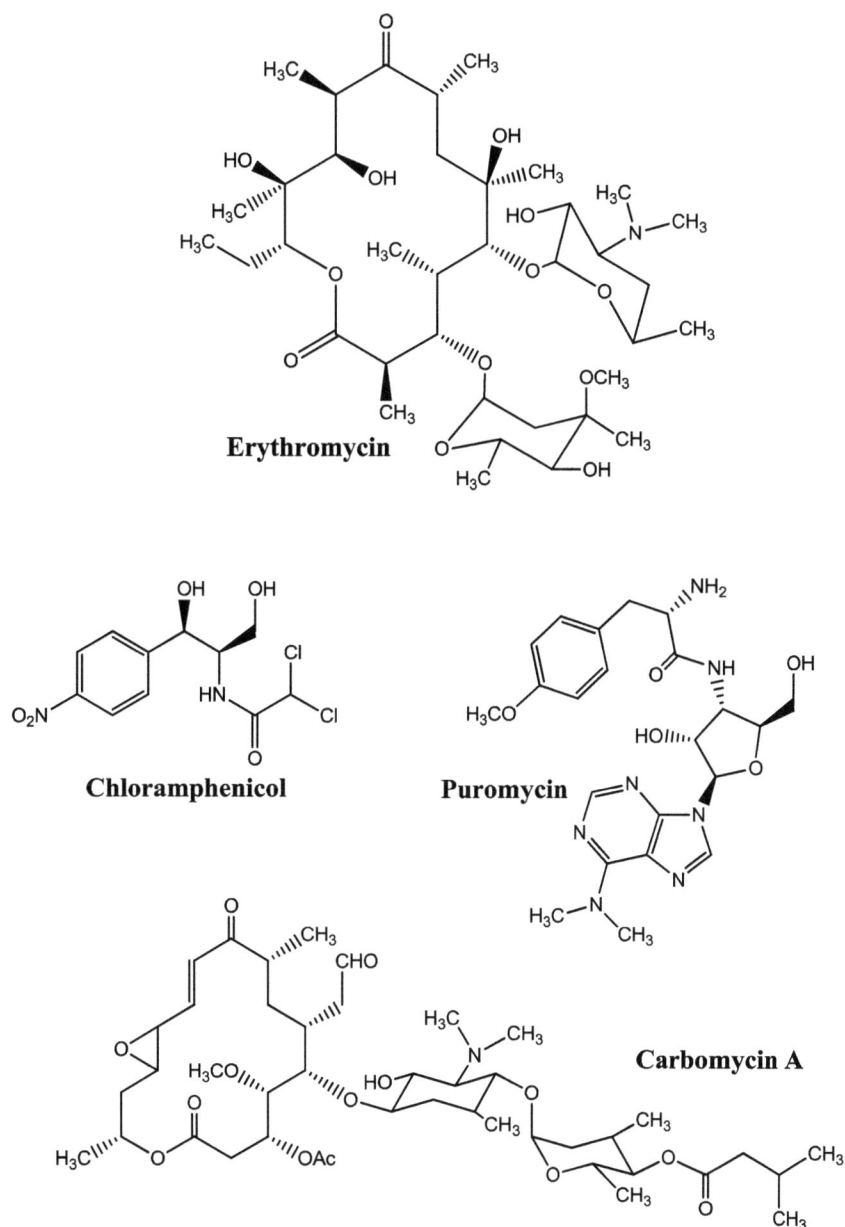

Figure 8: Structures of erythromycin, chloramphenicol puromycin and carbomycin A.

The knowledge about the mechanism of action and the drug interactions at the binding site compose very important tools in rational design of new pleuromutilin derivatives. Associated with SARs studies, both have allowed the development of new substances. One important example is retapamulin (Fig. **9**) introduced to the market in 2007 [14].

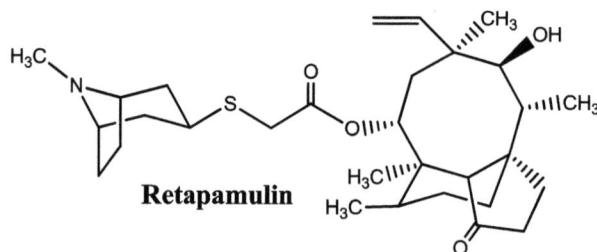

Figure 9: Structure of retapamulin.

ERYTHROMYCIN

Another natural product under development by the TB Global Alliance is the well known macrolide antibiotic erythromycin (Fig. **8**) [4,37], which is usually used in patients having an allergy to penicillin antibiotics. This 14-membered lactone, isolated from a strain of the actinomycete *Saccharopolyspora* at the beginning of the 1940's, possesses ten asymmetric centers and two carbohydrates (L-cladinose and D-desoamine). Franzblau and co-workers [4,38] evaluated *in vitro* and *in vivo* several macrolides of different sizes. They investigated also the structure-activity relationships and made important contributions to the development of new anti-TB macrolides.

CAPURAMYCIN

Another promising natural product able to efficiently inhibit translocase I inhibitors is capuramycin, isolated in 1986 by Yamaguchi and co-workers (Fig. **10**) [4,39] from the culture of *Streptomyces griseus* 446-S3. Capuramycin possesses a uracil nucleoside and a caprolactam subunit. Several analogues of capuramycin have been synthesized and evaluated against MDR-TB. One of these is (RS-118641), identified by Koga and co-workers [4,40], and synthesized at the Lead Discovery Research Laboratories of Sankyo Co. Ltd. (Tokyo, Japan). In 2004, Sequella, Inc. licensed the

Capuramycin class of antibacterials from Daiichi-Sankyo and RS-118641, now SQ641 is currently under Phase I study (Fig. **10**) [4,40,41].

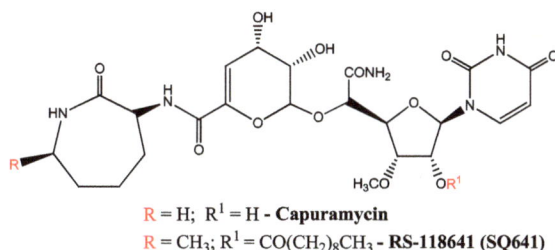

R = H; R^1 = H - **Capuramycin**
R = CH$_3$; R^1 = CO(CH$_2$)$_8$CH$_3$ - **RS-118641 (SQ641)**

Figure 10: Structure of capuramycin and RS-118641 (SQ641).

CAPRAZAMYCINS

Caprazamycins A-G (CPZs) (Fig. **11**), like Capuramycins belong to the class of nucleoside natural products first isolated from a fermentation of *Streptomyces sp.* MK730-62F2 by Igarashi and co-workers in 2003 [42-44]. This liponucleoside antibiotics displayed promising activity *in vitro* against Gram-positive bacteria, especially against *Mycobacteria* by acting in the translocase I enzyme. Several analogues have been synthesized and evaluated against TB building a SAR of this class of compounds, which identified CPZEN-45, a simplify analogue with potent anti-TB activity including against XDR strains being in preclinical studies [45,46].

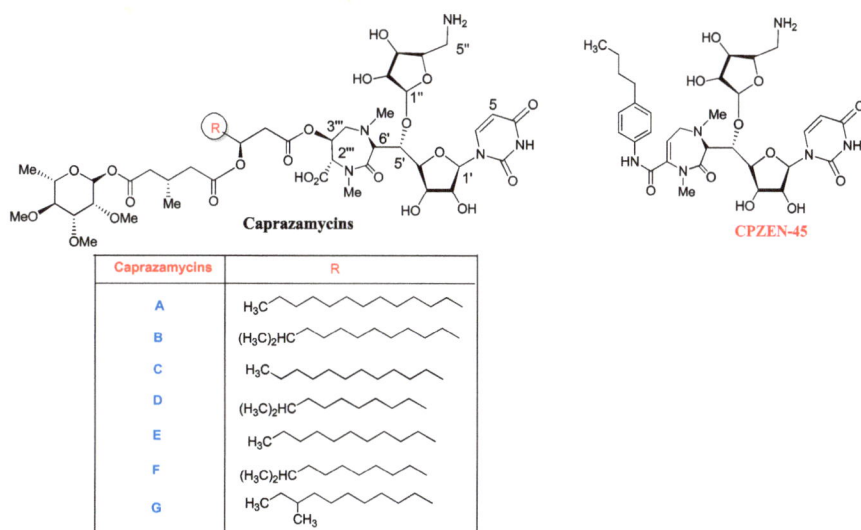

Figure 11: Structure of caprazamycins A-G and CPZEN-45 [42].

FAS20013

Compound FAS20013 (Fig. **12**) is a promising synthetic β-sulfonylcarboxamide developed by FASgen, Inc. and shows a good activity against MDR and latent TB [4,47]. The design of this compound was based on the natural products thiolactomycin and cerulenin (Fig. **12**), acting in β-ketoacyl synthase. Due to its promising results, FAS20013 is under preclinical development and demonstrating once more the importance of the study of natural products in TB field.

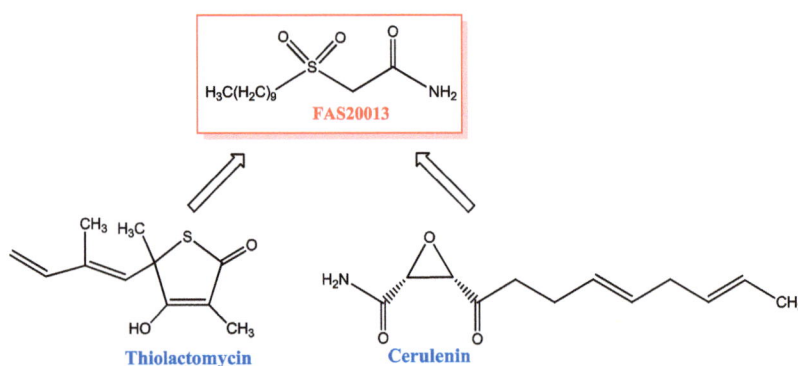

Figure 12: Structure of FAS20013, cerulenin and thiolactomycin.

CERULENIN

Cerulenin (Fig. **12**) is a natural product isolated from the fungus *Cephalosporium caerulens*. It was isolated for the first time from the culture broth of the fungal strain KF-140 by Omura and co-workers in 1967 and was identified as an antimicrobial agent. The activity of cerulenin against *Mycobacterium tuberculosis* [4,48-51] is based on the inhibition of the biosynthesis of fatty acids, which are important for its survival. These acids help in the fight against hydrophobic drugs and dehydration, and also allow this bacterium to be more effective in the host´s immune system by growing inside macrophages. The target of this natural product for inhibition of the bacterial growth is the enzyme fatty acid synthase (FAS). This enzyme is known as type I FAS, present in animals, fungi and some bacteria (eukaryotic cells) and type II FAS, present in plants, some bacteria and mitochondria (prokaryotic cells) [4,48]. In both enzymes, cerulenin is able to irreversible block β-ketoacyl synthase, which is a condensing enzyme necessary for the production of fatty acids [4,49].

THIOLACTOMYCIN

The antibiotic thiolactomycin (TLM) (Fig. **2**) exhibits a broad-spectrum of activity against several bacterial species, including laboratory strains of *Mycobacterium tuberculosis*. However, despite its modest MIC (62,5 μg/ml) against *Mycobacterium tuberculosis* this natural product, found in a Japanese soil sample and described for the first time in 1982 by Oishi and co-workers [52,53], has several advantages as lead compound, such as good pharmacokinetic and physical properties. In this context it can be mention good oral absorption, water solubility, lipophilicity and low toxicity *in vivo* [54,55]. Another advantage of TLM is its activity against several resistant strains of *Mycobacterium tuberculosis* being its mechanism of action based on the inhibition of KasA and KasB, two KAS enzymes that are components of the specialized FASII system involved in synthesis of the very long-chain meromycolic acids, constituent of building blocks for bacterial cell walls [4,50,56-60].

Synthetic Studies of TLM

Due to the promising perspectives of TLM several groups increased the efforts towards the synthesis of even more effective agents, leading to the current list of compounds that present a good level of activity, in the search for more potent TLM derivatives.

An efficient strategy for the synthesis of TLM core was developed by Wang and Salvino (Scheme **3**) [50,61], and it was based on Claisen self ester condensation of methyl propionate **1** using KH to generate ß-keto ester **2**. The selective bromination **3**, followed by nucleophilic substitution of bromine with thioacetic acid lead thioester **4**, and finally, cyclization furnished the 3,5-dimethylthiotetronic acid **5**, the key intermediate for the synthesis of thiolactomycin and its analogues.

Based on the key intermediate **5** Kamal and co-workers have synthesized (Scheme **4**) and evaluated (Table **1**) the anti-TB activity of a series of thiolactomycin analogues [50,62]. The compounds **6** and **7** were synthesized from **5** by the etherification of 4-hydroxy group with alkyl dihalides. The bromo ether derivative **7** when reacted with methyl thioglycolate, produced compound **8**. The anti-TB evaluation of the analogues **7** and **8** indicated that they have moderate activities against *M. tuberculosis* $H_{37}Rv$ and clinical isolates (sensitive strains), however significant activity against MDR strains (Table **2**).

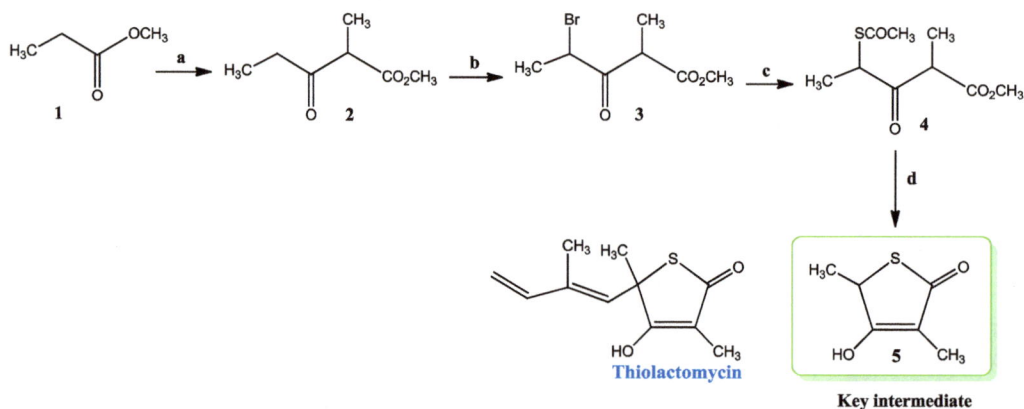

(a) anhydrous KH, THF; (b) $PyHBr_3$, acetic acid; (c) AcSH, EtN_3, CH_2Cl_2; (d) KOH, H_2O-EtOH.

Scheme 3: Analogues of thiolactomycin.

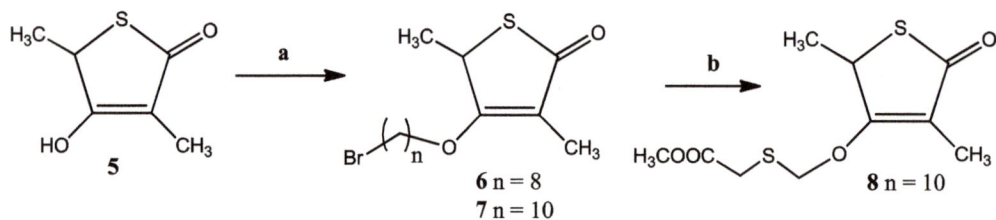

(a) $Br(CH_2)_nBr$, anhyd K_2CO_3, acetone, reflux; (b) CH_3OCOCH_2SH, anhyd K_2CO_3, acetone, reflux.

Scheme 4: Analogues of thiolactomycin [50].

Table 1: MIC values (µg/mL) of the compounds 7 and 8 and isoniazid [50].

Compound	M. tb. MDR	M. tb. Clinical Sensitive	M. tb. $H_{37}Rv$
7	4.0-16.0	4.0-16.0	4.0
8	1.0-4.0	1.0-4.0	1.0
Isoniazid	8->16	0.12-0.25	0.25

Senior and co-workers [50,63] described a series of TLM analogues (Scheme **5**) also based on the key intermediate **5** using Sonogashira coupling reaction between

9 and aryl iodine to produce compounds **10a-c** in 47-86% yields. The biological evaluation of these compounds indicated that they exhibit higher *in vitro* inhibitory activity against the recombinant *Mycobacterium tuberculosis* ß-ketoacyl-ACP synthase mtFabH condensing enzyme when compared to TLM.

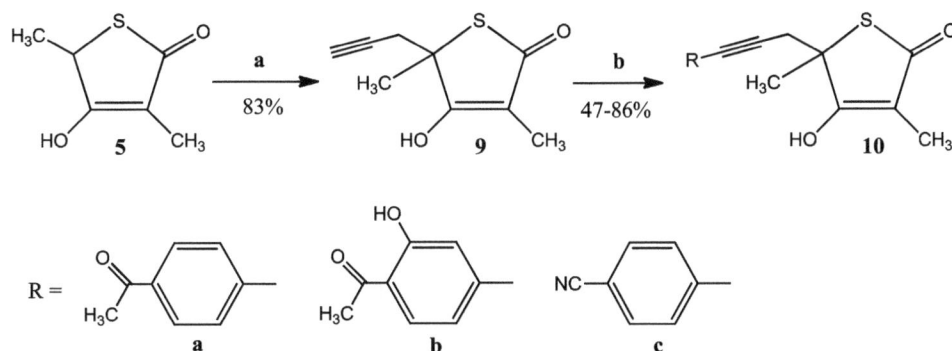

(a) LHMDS, THF, HCCCH₂Br, -78°C; (b) DMF, Et₃N, CuI, (PPh₃)₂PdCl, R-I.

Scheme 5: Analogues of thiolactomycin [50].

ACKNOWLEDGEMENT

None Declare.

CONFLICT OF INTEREST

The author(s) confirm that this chapter content has no conflict of interest.

REFERENCES

[1]   Copp BR, Pearce AN. Natural product growth inhibitors of *Mycobacterium tuberculosis Nat. Prod Rep* 2007;**24**:278–97.

[2]   Copp BR. Antimycobacterial natural products *Nat Prod Rep* 2003;**20**:535–557.

[3]   De Souza MVN. Plants and Fungal Products with activity against Tuberculosis. *The Scientific World Journal* 2005;**5**:609-628.

[4]   De Souza MVN. Promising candidates in clinical trials against multidrug-resistant tuberculosis (MDR-TB) based on natural products *Fitoterapia* 2009;**80**:453–460.

[5]   Liu X, Chen C, He W, Huang P, Liu M, Wang Q, Guo H, Bolla K, Lu Y, Song F, Dai H, Liu M, Zhang L Exploring anti-TB leads from natural products library originated from marine microbes and medicinal plants. *Antonie Van Leeuwenhoek* 2012;**102**:447-61.

[6]   Salomon CE, Schmidt LE. Natural products as leads for tuberculosis drug development. *Curr Top Med Chem* 2012;**12**:735-65.

[7] García A, Bocanegra-García V, Palma-Nicolás JP, Rivera G. Recent advances in antitubercular natural products. *Eur J Med Chem* 2012;**49**:1-23.

[8] Cahisson RE. Treatment of chronic infections with rifamycins: Is resistance likely to follow? *Antimicrobi Agents Chemother* 2003;**47**:3037-9.

[9] Floss HG, Yu TW. Rifamycin – Mode of action, resistence and biosynthesis. *Chem Rev* 2005;**105**:621-32.

[10] Souza MVN. Promising drugs against tuberculosis. *Rec Pat Anti-Infect Drug Discov* 2006;**1**: 33-45.

[11] Yamne T, Hashizume T, Yamashida K, Hosoe K, Kuze F, Watanabe K. US4983602 (**1991**).

[12] Marsili L, Rossetti V, Pasqualucci C. US4219478 (**1980**).

[13] Potkar C, Gogtav N, Kshirsagar NA, Ajav S, Cooverji ND, Bruzzese, T. Phase I pharmacokinetic study of a new 3-azinomethyl-rifamycin (rifametane) as compared to rifampicin. *Chemotherapy* 1999;**45**:147-53.

[14] Gonçalves RBS, Souza MVN. Recent developments in pleuromutilin derivatives, a promising class against bacterial respiratory disease. *Current Respiratory Medicine Reviews* 2010;**6**:91-101.

[15] Drews J, Georgopoulos G, Laber G, Schutze E, Unger J. Antimicrobial activity of 81.723 hfu, a new pleuromutilin derivative. *Antimicrob Agents Chemother* 1975;**7**:507-16.

[16] Berner H, Schultz G, Fisher G. Chemistry of pleuromutilins, 3. Synthesis of 14-O-acetyl-19,20-dihydro-A-nor-mutilins. *Monatsh Chem* 1981;**112**:1441-50.

[17] Poulsen SM, Karlsson M, Johansson LB, Vester B. The pleuromutilin drugs tiamulin and valnemulin bind to the RNA at the peptidyl transferase centre on the ribosome. *Mol Microbiol* 2001;**41**:1091–99.

[18] Hunt E. Pleuromutilin antibiotics. *Drugs Fut* 2000;**25**:1163–8.

[19] http://www.iom.edu/Object.File/Master/59/970/Ginsberg.pdf. Accessed August 27, 2010.

[20] Kavanagh F, Hervey A, Robbins WJ. Antibiotic substances from basidiomycetes. VIII. *Pleurotus multilus* (Fr.) Sacc. and *Pleuotus passeckerianus* Pilat. *Proc Natl Acad Sci* 1951; **37**:570-4.

[21] Anchel M. Chemical studies with pleuromutilin. *J Biol Chem* 1952;**199**:133–40.

[22] Arigoni D. Structure of a new type of terpene. *Gazz Chim Ital* 1962;**92**:884–901.

[23] Birch AJ, Cameron DW, Holzapfel CW, Richards RW. Diterpenoid nature of pleuromutilin. *Chem Ind* 1963;374–5.

[24] Riedl K. Studies on pleuromutilin and some of its derivatives. *J Antibiotics* 1976;**29**:132–9.

[25] Egger H, Reinshagen H. New pleuromutilin derivatives with enhanced antimicrobial activity I. Synthesis. *J Antibiotics* 1976;**29**:915–22.

[26] Egger H, Reinshagen H. New pleuromutilin derivatives with enhanced antimicrobial activity II. Structure-activity correlations. *J Antibiotics* 1976;**29**:923–27.

[27] Hannan PCT, Windsor HM, Ripley PH. *In vitro* susceptibilities of recent field isolates of *Mycoplasma hyopneumoniae* and *Mycoplasma hyosynoviae* to valnemulin (Econor®), tiamulin and enrofloxacin and the *in vitro* development of resistance to certain antimicrobial agents in *Mycoplasma hyopneumoniae*. *Res Vet Sci* 1997;**63**:157–160.

[28]   Hodgin LA, Högenauer G. The mode of action of pleuromutilin derivatives. *Eur J Biochem* 1974;**47**:527–33.

[29]   Högenauer G. The mode of action of pleuromutilin derivatives. *Eur J Biochem* 1975;**52**:93–8.

[30]   Dornhelm P, Högenauer G. The effects of tiamulin, a semisynthetic pleuromutilin derivative, on bacterial polypeptide chain initiation. *Eur J Biochem* 1978;**91**:465–73.

[31]   Högenauer G, Ruf C. Ribosomal binding region for the antibiotic tiamulin: stoichiometry, subnit location, and affinity for various analogs. *Antimicrob Agents Chemother* 1981;**19**: 260–265.

[32]   Högenauer G, Egger H, Ruf C, Stumper B. Affinity labeling of Escherichia coli ribosomes with a covalently binding derivative of the antibiotic pleuromutilin. *Biochemistry* 1981;**20**: 546–52.

[33]   Schuwirth BS, Borovinskaya MA, Hau CW, *et al*. Structures of the bacterial ribosome at 3.5 Å resolution. *Science* 2005;**310**:827–34.

[34]   Selmer M, Dunham CM, Murphy FV, *et al*. Structure of the 70S ribosome complexed with mRNA and tRNA. *Science* 2006;**313**:1935–42.

[35]   Poulsen SM, Karlsson M, Johansson LB, Vester B. The pleuromutilin drugs tiamulin and valnemulin bind to the RNA at the peptidyl transferase centre on the ribosome. *Mol Microbiol* 2001;**41**:1091–99.

[36]   Schlünzen F, Pyetan E, Fucini P, Yonath A, Harms JM. Inhibition of peptide bond formation by pleuromutilins: the structure of the 50S ribosomal subunit from *Dinococcus radiodurans* in complex with tiamulin. *Mol Microbiol* 2004;**54**:1287–94.

[37]   A. Hudson, T. Imamura, W. Gutteride, T. Kanyok and P. Nunn http://www.who.int/tdr/publications/publications/antitb_drug.htm. Accessed August 27, 2010.

[38]   Falzari K, Zhu Z, Pan D, Liu H, Hongmanee P, Franzblau SG. *In vitro* and *in vivo* activities of macrolide derivatives against Mycobacterium tuberculosis. *Antimicrob Agents Chemother* 2005;**49**:1447–54.

[39]   Yamaguchi H, Sato S, Yoshida S, Takada K, Itoh M, Seto H, *et al*. Capuramycin, a new nucleoside antibiotic. Taxonomy, fermentation, isolation and characterization. *J Antibiot* 1986;**39**:1047–53.

[40]   Koga T, Fukuoka T, Doi N, Harasaki T, Inoue H, Hotoda H, *et al*. Activity o capuramycin analogues against Mycobacterium tuberculosis, Mycobacteriu avium and Mycobacterium intracellulare *in vitro* and *in vivo*. *J Antibiot Chemother* 2004;**54**:755–60.

[41]   Nikonenko BV, Reddy VM, Protopopova M, Bogatcheva E, Einck L, Nacy CA. Activity of SQ641, a capuramycin analog, in a murine model of tuberculosis. *Antimicrobial Agents and Chemotherapy* 2009;**53**:3138-3139.

[42]   De Souza MVN, Facchinetti V, Cardinot D, Gomes C. Natural Products with Translocase I inhibitory activity, as new lead compounds against tuberculosis. *Bol Latinoam Caribe Plant Med Aromat* 2010;**9**:1-12.

[43]   Igarashi M, Nakagawa N, Doi N, Hattori S, Naganawa H, Hamada M. Caprazamycin B, a novel anti-tuberculosis antibiotic, from Streptomyces sp. *The Journal of antibiotics* 2003;**56**:580-3.

[44] Igarashi M, Takahashi Y, Shitara T, Nakamura H, Naganawa H, Miyake T, Akamatsu Y. Caprazamycins, novel lipo-nucleoside antibiotics, from Streptomyces sp. II. Structure elucidation of caprazamycins. *The Journal of antibiotics* 2005;**58**:327-37.

[45] http://www.newtbdrugs.org/project.php?id=92 Accessed August 27, 2011.

[46] Miyake T, Takahashi Y, Igarashi M. Synthesis and activity of CPZEN-45, a new antituberculous drug candidate. Abstracts of Papers, *235th ACS National Meeting*, New Orleans, LA, United States, April 6-10, 2008, CARB-104.

[47] Sano Y, Nomura S, Kamio Y, Omura S, Hata T. Studies on cerulenin. III. Isolation and physico-chemical properties of cerulenin. *J Antibiot Ser A* 1967;**20**:344–8.

[48] D'Agnolo G, Rosenfeld IS, Awaya J, Omura S, Vagelos PR. Inhibition of fatty acid synthesis by the antibiotic cerulenin. Specific inactivation of beta-ketoacyl-acyl carrier protein synthetase. *Biochim Biophys Acta* 1973;**326**:155–6.

[49] Omura S. The antibiotic cerulenin, a novel tool for biochemistry as an inhibitor of fatty acid synthesis. *Bacteriol Rev* 1976;**40**:681–97.

[50] Souza MVN, Ferreira M, Pinheiro AC, Saraiva MF, Almeida MV, Valle MS. Synthesis and biological aspects of mycolic acids: an important target against Mycobacterium tuberculosis. *TSWJ* 2008;**8**:720–51.

[51] Mani NS, Townsend CAA. A concise synthesis of (+)-cerulenin from a chiral oxiranyllithium. *J Org Chem* 1997;**62**:636–40.

[52] Oishi H, Noto T, Sasaki H, Suzuki K, Hayashi T, Okazaki H, Ando K, Sawada M. Thiolactomycin, a new antibiotic I. taxonomy of the producing organism, fermentation and biological properties *J Antibiot* 1982;**35**:391-5.

[53] Noto T, Miyakawa S, Oishi H, Endo H, Okazaki H. Thiolactomycin, anew antibiotic III. *In vitro* antibacterial activity. *J Antibiot* 1982;**35**:401-10.

[54] Miyakawa S, Suzuki K, Noto T, Harada Y, Okazaki, H. Thiolactomycin, a new antibiotic IV. Biological properties and chemotherapeutic activity in mice. *J Antibiot* 1982;**35**:411-19.

[55] Lipinski CA, Lombardo F, Dominy BW, Feeney PJ. Experimental and computational approaches to estimate solubility and permeability in drug discovery and development settings. *Adv Drug Delivery Rev* 2001;**46**:3-26.

[56] Kremer L, Douglas JD, Baulard AR, Morehouse C, Guy MR, et al. Thiolactomycin and Related Analogues as Novel Anti-mycobacterial Agents Targeting KasA and KasB Condensing Enzymes inMycobacterium tuberculosis. *J Biol Chem* 2000;**275**:16857-64.

[57] Slayden RA, Lee RE, Armour JW, Cooper AM, Orme, IM, et al. Antimycobacterial action of thiolactomycin: an inhibitor of fatty acid and mycolic acid synthesis *Antimicrob Agents Chemother* 1996;**40**:2813-19.

[58] Nishida I, Kawaguchi A, Yamada M. Effect of Thiolactomycin on the Individual Enzymes of the Fatty Acid Synthase System in Escherichia coli *J Biochem* 1986;**99**:1447-54.

[59] De Souza MVN. *New Strategies Combating Bacterial Infection*. Iqbal A and Farrukh A. Ed.; Wiley-VCH Verlag GmbH and Co. KGaA: Weinheim **2008**; vol *3*, p. 71-87.

[60] Kapilashrami K, Bommineni GR, Machutta CA, Kim P, Lai CT, Simmerling C, Picart F, Tonge PJ. Thiolactomycin-based β-ketoacyl-AcpM synthase A (KasA) inhibitors:

fragment-based inhibitor discovery using transient one-dimensional nuclear overhauser effect NMR spectroscopy. *J Biol Chem* 2013;**288**:6045-52.

[61]   Wang CLJ, Salvino JM. Total synthesis of (±) thiolactomycin. *Tetrahedron Lett* 1984;**25**:5243-6.

[62]   Kamal A, Shaik AA, Sinha R, Yadav, JS, Arora SK. Antitubercular agents. Part 2: New thiolactomycin analogues active against *Mycobacterium tuberculosis*. *Bioorg Med Chem Lett* 2005;**15**:1927-9.

[63]   Senior SJ, Illarionov PA, Gurcha SS, Campbell IB, Schaeffer ML, Minnikin DE, Besra GS. Total synthesis of (±) thiolactomycin. *Bioorg Med Chem Lett* 2004;**14**:373-6.

CHAPTER 6

Anti-TB Evaluation of Natural Products From Plants

Marcus V.N. de Souza[*]

Instituto de Tecnologia em Fármacos - Farmanguinhos, FioCruz - Fundação Oswaldo Cruz, R. Sizenando Nabuco, 100, Manguinhos, 21041-250, Rio de Janeiro, RJ, Brazil

Abstract: Natural products represent an outstanding source of compounds able to play an important role in the treatment of several human diseases. For example, plants are an incredible source of bioactive compounds isolated from different species with an impressive structural diversity, representing a field of inspiration for the development of new drugs. The importance of natural products in drug discovery can be noted in the large number of drugs derived from plants available against different classes of disease. Due to the importance of the plants in drug discovery, several compounds have been isolated and evaluated from different species against *Mycobacterium tuberculosis*, which some of the most promising it will be described in this chapter.

Keywords: Tuberculosis, *Mycobacterium tuberculosis*, natural products, plants, semi-synthesis, synthesis, analogues, treatment, multi-drug-resistant tuberculosis (MDR TB), extensive-drug-resistant tuberculosis (XDR TB), target, mechanism of action, biological evaluation, drug development.

INTRODUCTION

The plants are an incredible source of bioactive compounds isolated from different species with an impressive structural diversity, representing a field of inspiration for the development of new drugs. The importance of natural products in drug discovery can be noted in the large number of drugs derived from plants available against different classes of diseases. As examples, it can be mention the narcotic analgesic morphine extracted from the opium poppy *Papaver Somniferum*; the antimalarial quinine and artemisinin found in *Cinchona officinalis* and *Artemisia annua L.*, respectively; the anticancer vincristine and

---

*Adress correspondence to **Marcus V.N. de Souza**: Instituto de Tecnologia em Fármacos - Farmanguinhos, FioCruz - Fundação Oswaldo Cruz, R. Sizenando Nabuco, 100, Manguinhos, 21041-250, Rio de Janeiro, RJ, Brazil; E-mail: marcos_souza@far.fiocruz.br

paclitaxel extracted from *Catharanthus roseus* and *Taxus brevifolia* Nutt, respectively; and the antiasthma ephedrine, isolated from the Ma huang herb (Fig. **1**) [1]. Due to the importance of the plants in drug discovery, several compounds have been isolated and evaluated from different species against *Mycobacterium tuberculosis*, which some of the most promising are described below.

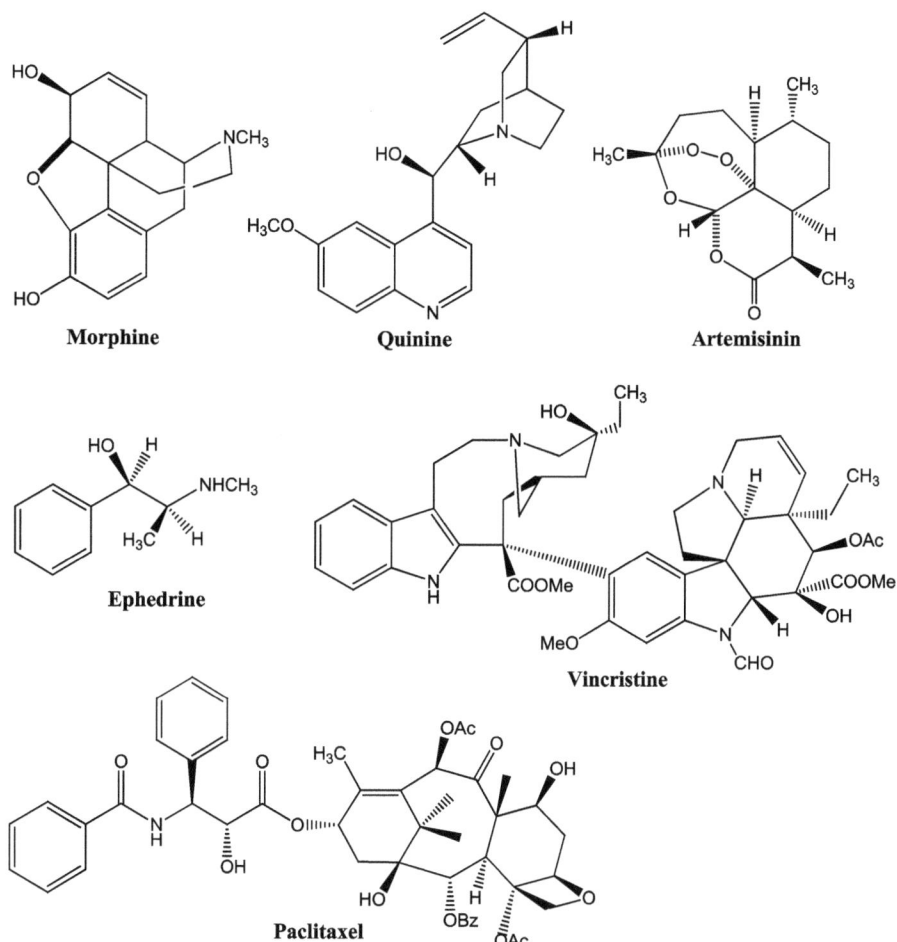

Figure 1: Structure of important natural products from plants [1].

ALKALOIDS

Bidebiline E

Bidebiline E (Fig. **2**) is a new dimer aporphine alkaloid isolated by Kanokmedhakul and co-workers [2] from the roots of *Polyalthia cerasoides*

(Roxb.) Benth. ex Bedd (Annonaceae). This specie is a tree 5-15 m in height, which is very common in Thailand being used in traditional medicine as a tonic and a febrifuge by a water decoction of the roots. The anti-TB evaluation of this compound is MIC = 6.25 μgmL^{1-}.

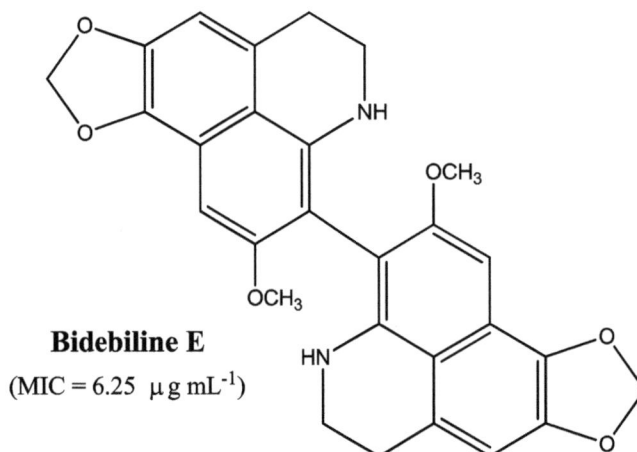

Bidebiline E

(MIC = 6.25 $\mu g\ mL^{-1}$)

Figure 2: Structure of Bidebiline E.

Liriodenine and 6-Methoxy-Dihydrochelirubine

Corona and co-workers evaluated thirty five plant-derived secondary metabolites against sensitive and MDR *Mycobacterium tuberculosis* [3]. Among all the compounds tested, liriodenine was the most active MIC = 3.12 μgmL^{-1}. In the three MDR strains used the best result was the natural product 6-methoxy-dihydrochelirubine MIC = 12.5 μgmL^{-1} (Fig. **3**).

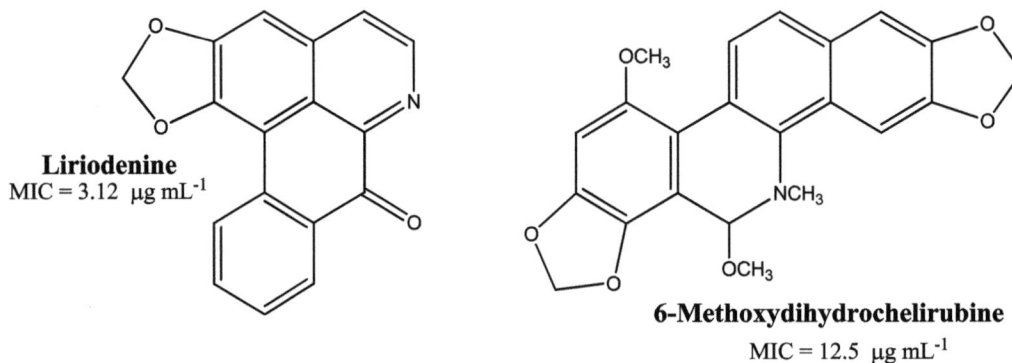

Liriodenine
MIC = 3.12 $\mu g\ mL^{-1}$

6-Methoxydihydrochelirubine
MIC = 12.5 $\mu g\ mL^{-1}$

Figure 3: Liriodenine and 6-methoxy-dihydrochelirubine.

Tryptanthrin

Tryptanthrin (Fig. **4**) is an indoloquinazolinone alkaloid with potent anti-TB activity MIC = 1.0 μgmL^{-1}. This natural indigo dye is a constituent of the Chinese and Taiwanese medicinal plants *Strobilanthes cusia*, *Polygonum tinctorium* and *Isatis tinctoria* used as topical fungicide. Due to the important perspective of this natural product demonstrated by Franzblau's experiments, his co-workers prepared and evaluated at Phatogenic corporation a series of synthetic tryptanthrins [4,5]. These derivatives were prepared by using isatoic anhydrides (synthesized from anilines and anthranilic acids) and isatins leading the PA-505, one of the best derivatives with MIC = 0.015 μgmL^{-1}. However, in despite of the potent anti-TB activity tryptanthrin and PA-505 demonstrated poor results in animal models.

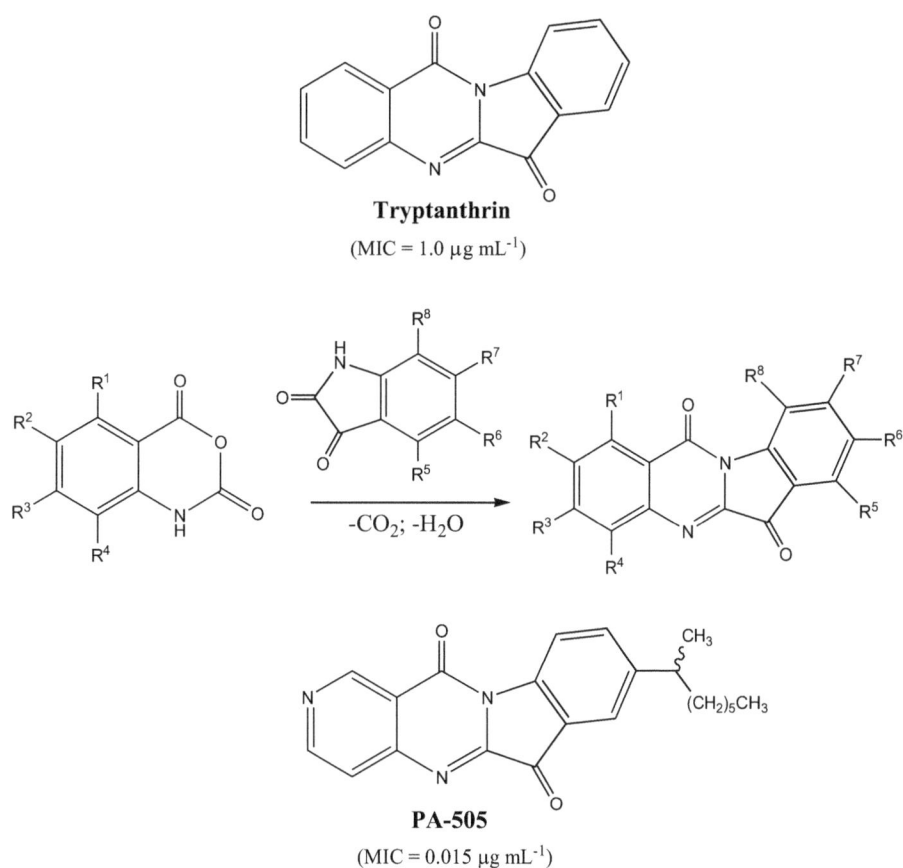

Tryptanthrin

(MIC = 1.0 $\mu g\ mL^{-1}$)

PA-505

(MIC = 0.015 $\mu g\ mL^{-1}$)

Figure 4: Structure of tryptanthrin and PA-505.

COUMARINS

(+)-Calanolide A

Calanolide A (Fig. **5**) belongs to the class of coumarin and it was first isolated from *Calophyllum lanigerum* trees in Malaysia and evaluated against cancer by National Cancer Institute. Although no antitumor activity have been found this natural product proved to be very effective against the AIDS virus being a non-nucleoside reverse transcript inhibitor. In addition to its potent anti-HIV activity compounds of this class displayed promising perspectives against *Mycobacterium tuberculosis* as demonstrated Xu and co-workers [6]. It is important to mention that the ring A, its substituents and stereogenic centers are critical to anti-TB activity.

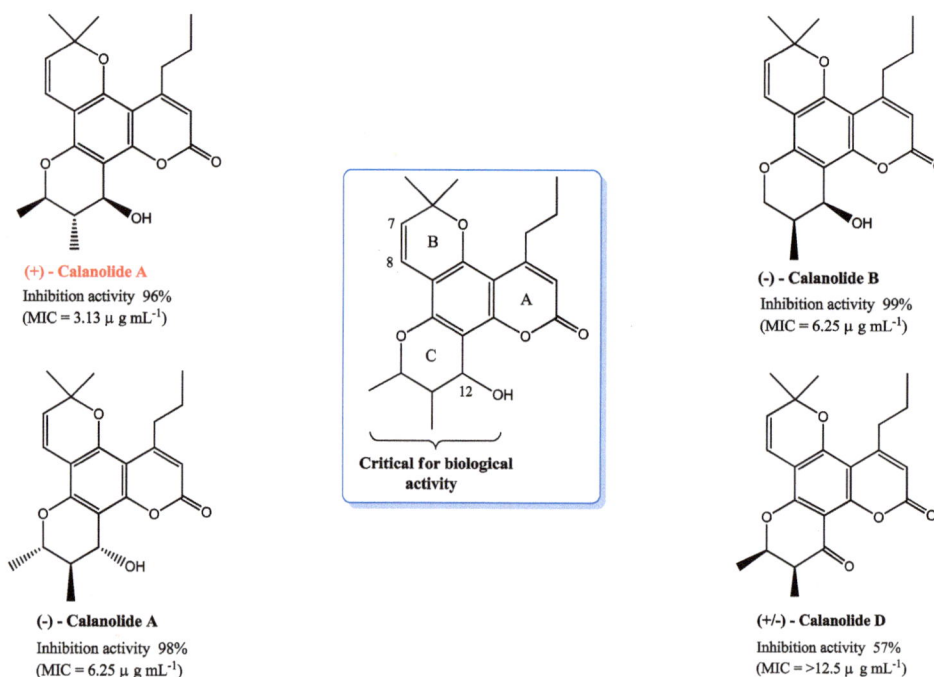

(+) - Calanolide A
Inhibition activity 96%
(MIC = 3.13 µ g mL^{-1})

Critical for biological
activity

(-) - Calanolide B
Inhibition activity 99%
(MIC = 6.25 µ g mL^{-1})

(-) - Calanolide A
Inhibition activity 98%
(MIC = 6.25 µ g mL^{-1})

(+/-) - Calanolide D
Inhibition activity 57%
(MIC = >12.5 µ g mL^{-1})

Figure 5: Structures of different coumarins.

CHALCONES

Licochalcone A

Traditional Chinese medicine is an important source of study on drug discovery. For example, Moller and co-workers used Licorine roots, which are largely used in China in the treatment of different diseases, such as bronchial asthma, inflammation, and gastric and duodenal ulcers to isolate licochalcone A (Fig. **6**). This natural product was tested on 62 clinical isolates *Mycobacteria* sp[6] [7].

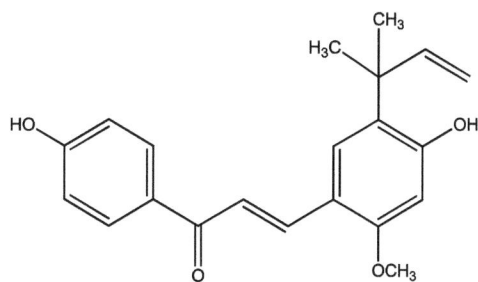

Licochalcone A

Figure 6: Structure of licochalcone A [1].

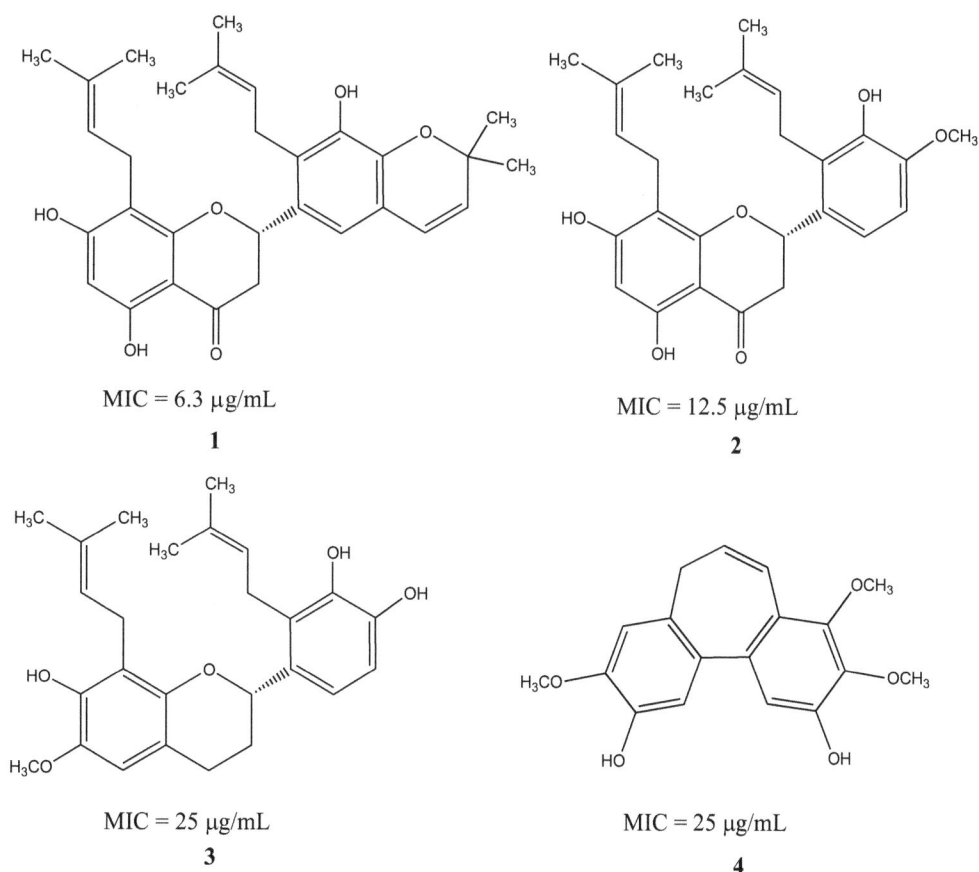

MIC = 6.3 µg/mL

1

MIC = 12.5 µg/mL

2

MIC = 25 µg/mL

3

MIC = 25 µg/mL

4

Figure 7: Compounds isolated from the plant *Dendrolobium lanceolatum* [1].

FLAVONONE

In Thai medicine the plant *Dendrolobium lanceolatum* is used traditionally as a diuretic and for urinary disease. This plant is a shrub 1-3 m in height and known in Thailand as "Kraduk-Khiat" or "Kraduk-Ueng", where it is present in the northeastern part. These four new compounds **1-4** have been tested by Kanokmedhakul and co-workers [1,8] against *Mycobacterium tuberculosis* H37Rv with MIC values of 6.3, 12.5, 25 and 25 μg/mL respectively (Fig. **7**).

LACTONE

Micromolide

Micromolide (Fig. **8**) is a γ-lactone derivative of oleic acid, (-)-Z-9-octadecene-4-olide from the dichloromethane extract of the stem bark o *Micromelum hirsutum*, which was isolated, elucidated and evaluated against *Mycobacterium tuberculosis* by Pauli and co-workers [9,10] with others alkaloids. This compound displayed potent anti-TB activity MIC=1.5 μg/mL and a selectivity index (SI) of 63, which is comparable for example, with the first line anti-TB drug ethambutol.

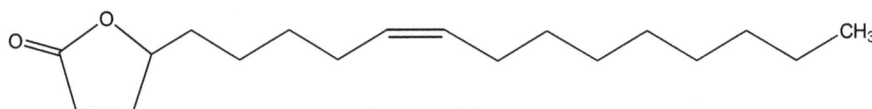

Micromolide
MIC = 1.5 μg/mL

Figure 8: Structure of micromolide.

POLYYNES

Pauli and co-workers [11] isolated five polyynes from the roots of *Angelica sinensis* and evaluated its anti-TB proprieties. This herb commonly called Dang Gui or Dong Quai is usually found to northwest China and used in traditional medicine in Asia especially for women's disorders, including anemia, dysmenorrhea, amenorrhea, premenstrual and menopausal syndromes. The most potent anti-TB constituents were falcarindiol (**5**), 9Z,17-octadecadiene-12,14-diyne-1,11,16-triol,1-acetate (**6**), exhibiting MIC values of 1.4-26.7 μg/mL (Fig. **9**).

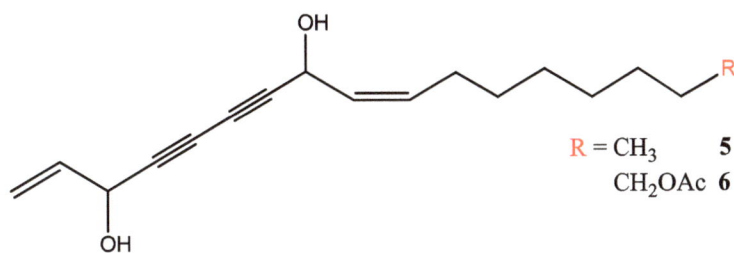

Figure 9: Structures of falcarindiol, *9Z*,17-octadecadiene-12,14-diyne-1,11,16-triol,1-acetate.

PYRONES

Compounds from *Piper sanctum*

Mata and co-workers [12] have isolated 14 new compounds from the leaves of *Piper sanctum*, which is a common specie in the southcentral region of Mexico, where it is commonly known as "acuyo", "hierba santa", and "hoja santa". In the traditional medicine this tree is used for treat colds, bronchitis, tuberculosis, stomach cramps, skin irritations, arthritis and toothaches. The 14 compounds isolated were evaluated against *Mycobacterium tuberculosis* with MIC values ranging from 4 to 64 µg/mL with the best results for the substances **7**, **8** and **9** with 4 and 6.25 respectively (Fig. **10**).

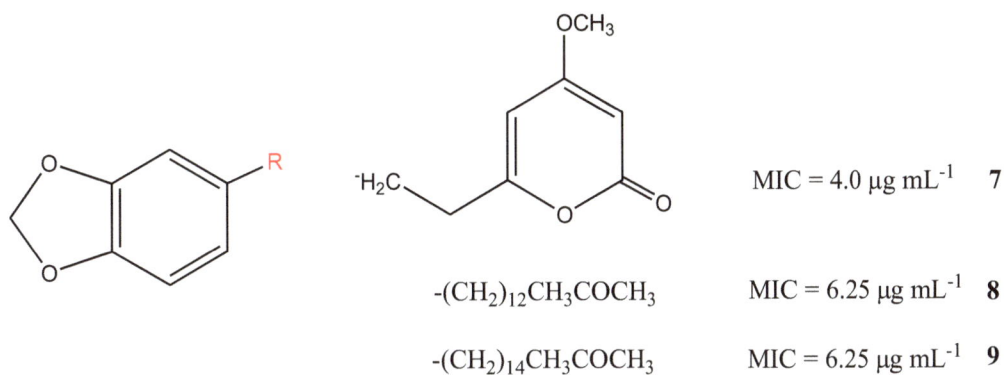

	MIC = 4.0 µg mL^{-1} **7**
-(CH$_2$)$_{12}$CH$_3$COCH$_3$	MIC = 6.25 µg mL^{-1} **8**
-(CH$_2$)$_{14}$CH$_3$COCH$_3$	MIC = 6.25 µg mL^{-1} **9**

Figure 10: Structures of compounds isolated from the leaves of *Piper sanctum*.

Quinquangulin and Rubrofusarin

The naphthopyrone natural products quinquangulin and rubrofusarin (Fig. **11**) [13] were extracted from stem and fruits of *Senna oblique, a* Peruvian plant by

Farnsworth and co-workers, which evaluated their anti-TB activity having both a MIC of 12 µg/mL.

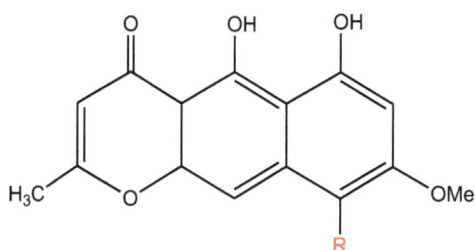

R = CH₃ Quinquangulin
R = H   Rubrofusarin
Inhibition activity at 50 µg mL^{-1} = 99%
(MIC = 12.5 µg mL^{-1})

Figure 11: Structures of quinquangulin and rubrofusarin [1].

STEROLS

Aguinaldo and co-workers [14] have investigated the anti-TB proprieties of the constituents from the hexane fraction of *Morinda citrifolia* Linn. (Rubiaceae). This specie is a abundant plant of the Indo-Pacific, for example in Philippine archipelago, being used in traditional medicine for different purposes, such as diabetic, dysentery, heartburn, liver problems, analgesic effects, hypotensive and health tonic. The best anti-TB activity found in the hexane fraction was the lipid **10** MIC = 2.5 µg/mL, obtained by autoxidation of the compound **11** (Fig. **12**).

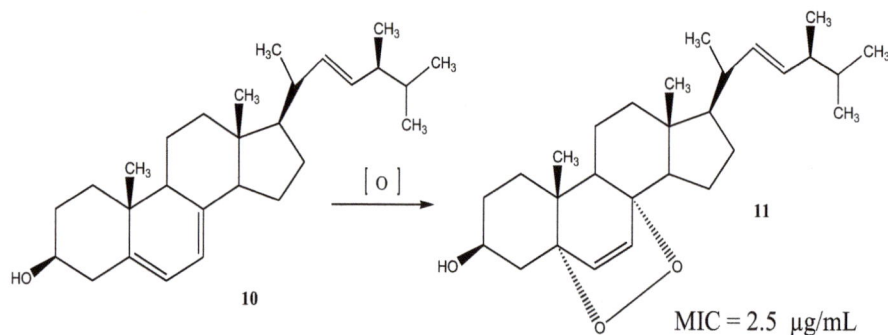

Figure 12: Structure of the sterols **10** and **11**.

TERPENES

Diterpenes

Argentinean and Chilean plants

Timmermann *et al.* have also reported anti-TB activity of several sterol and terpenoids from Argentinean and Chilean plants [1,15,16]. For example, the Argentinean plants *Ruprenchtia triflora* Griseb. (Polygonaceae) and *Calceolaria pinnifolia* Cav. (Scrophulariaceae) were examined against *M. tuberculosis* [1,17]. The *R. triflora* is found in the semiarid Chaco region of South America and is used by indigenous peoples as a sedative. The CH_2Cl_2/MeOH extract furnished several sterols and a triterpene as the active components against *M. tuberculosis*, such as the unknown sterol **12** with a MIC value of 2.0 µg/mL (Fig. **14**). The plant *C. pinnifolia* was also found in a semi-arid and mountainous region of northwestern Argentina, where it was used as an astringent. Among the ten diterpenes isolated from the diterpenes, **13** and **14** were the most active, each with a MIC of 4.0 µg/mL (Fig. **15**).

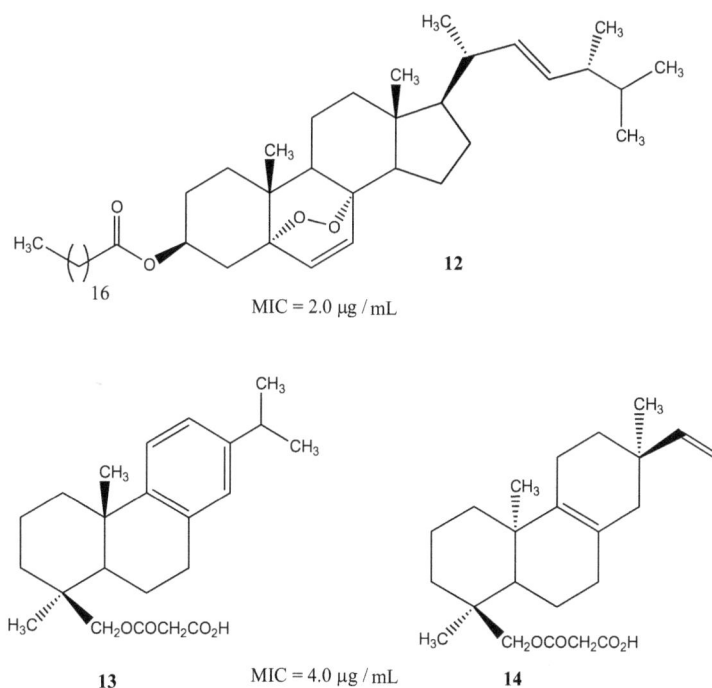

Figure 13: Structures of the diterpenes 12-14 [1].

Compounds from the roots of Turkish *Salvia multicaulis*

Ulubelen and co-workers [18] have been identified several compounds from the roots of Turkish *Salvia multicaulis*. This specie has been widely used as traditional medicine in different parts of the world for different purposes, such as menstrual disorders, and miscarriage, heart diseases, hepatitis, and treatment of hemorrhage. They are also used as anti-TB, antibacterial, antiseptic, diuretic, spasmolytic, carminative, hemostatic and antiphlogistic activities treatment of hemorrhage. The compounds isolated were evaluated against *Mycobacterium tuberculosis* being the most potent the diterpenoid **16** (MIC = 0.46 μgmL^{-1}) (Fig. **13**).

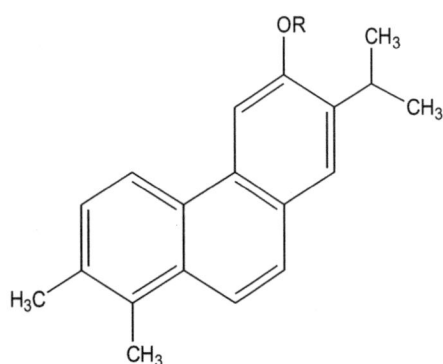

15 R = CH$_3$ MIC = 5.60 μg mL^{-1}
16 R = H   MIC = 0.46 μg mL^{-1}

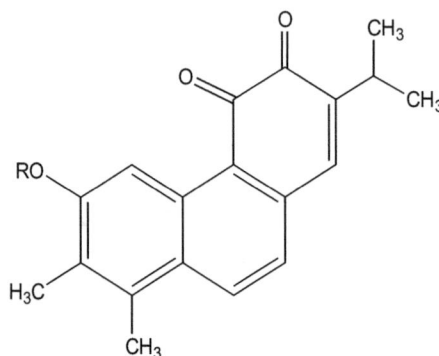

17 MIC = 2.0 μg mL^{-1}

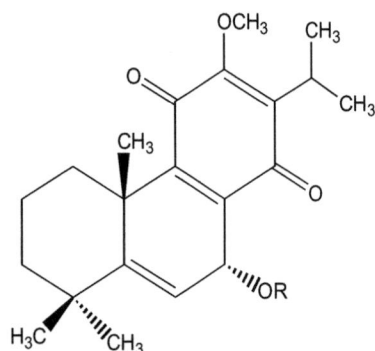

18 R = H   MIC = 1.2 μg mL^{-1}
19 R = Ac

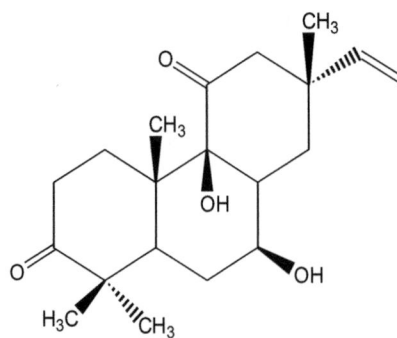

20 MIC = 7.3 μg mL^{-1}

Figure 14: Structures of compounds from the roots of Turkish *Salvia multicaulis*.

21 R^1 = (CH₃)₂CHCH₂CO; R^2 = CH₃   MIC = 12.5 µg/mL

22 R^2 = CH₃CH₂CH(CH₃)CO; R^2 = CH₃ MIC = 12.5 µg/mL

23 R^2 = CH₃CH₂CH(CH₃)CO; R^2 = H   MIC = 12.5 µg/mL

24 MIC = 25.0 µg/mL

25 MIC = 12.5 µg/mL

26 MIC = 12.5 µg/mL

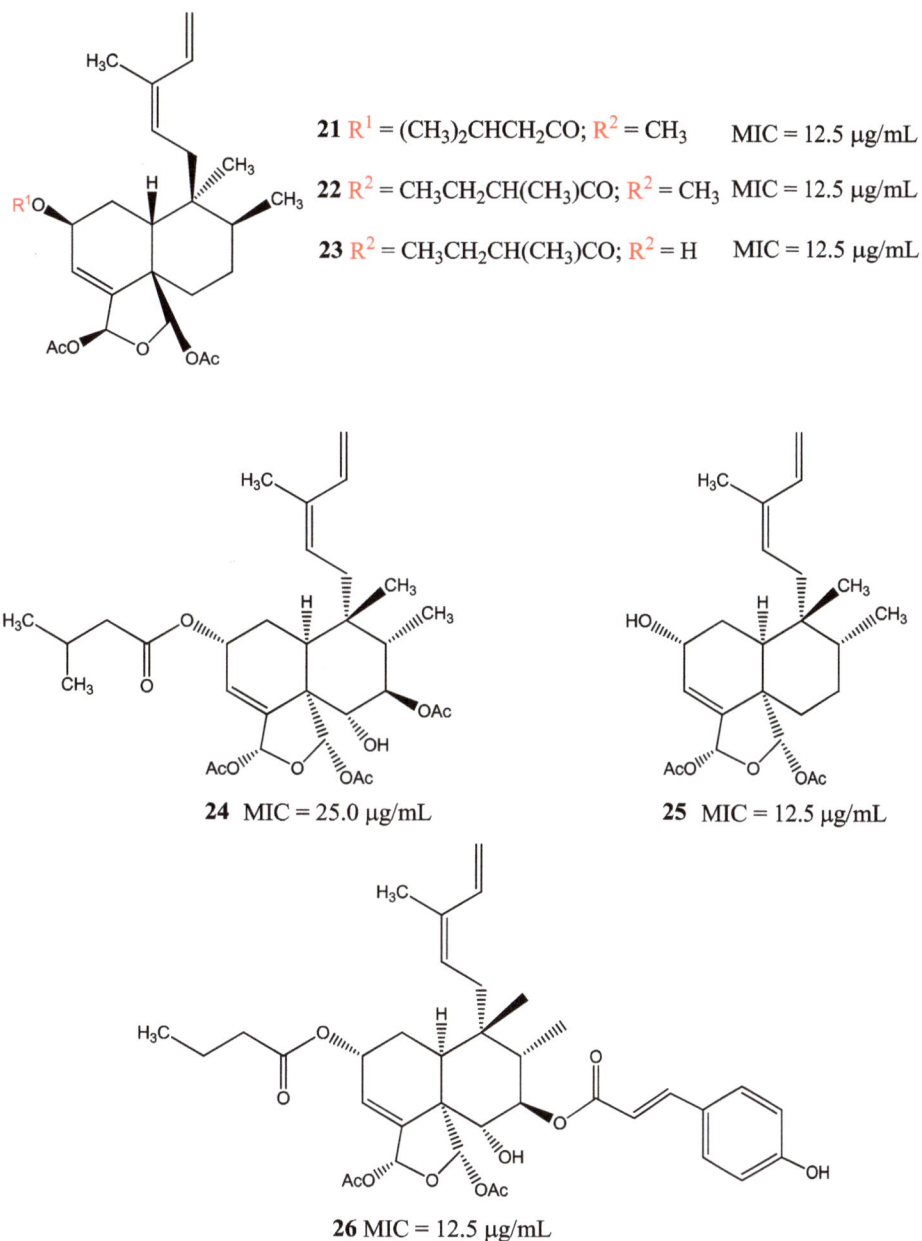

Figure 15: Structures of the compounds isolated from Thailand plant.

Compounds from Thailand plant

Kanokmedhakul and coworkers [19] have also isolated new diterpenes **21-26** from *Casearia grewiifolia* Vent. (Flacourtiaceae) commonly known in Thailand as

"Kruai pa" or "Pha sam" (Fig. 15). This plant is a shrubby tree 3-10 m in height, present in the northern and northeastern parts of Thailand, and decoctions of the bark and flowers are used traditionally as a tonic and a febrifuge, respectively. The four new terpenoids and the known terpenoids (22 and 23) were evaluated against *M. tuberculosis* and shown to possess promising antimycobacterial activities with MIC of 12.5 µg/mL for 21-23, 25, and 26, and 25 µg/mL for 24.

Lachenerol A and B

Timmermann and coworkers [1,20] have isolated and evaluated four new constituents of *Sapium haematospermum* against *M. tuberculosis*. This species is a plant native to drier regions of South America, commonly known in Argentina as "lecheryn", which is traditionally used in dental care. The most active compound was the new pimarane, lachenerol A (Fig. 16), which showed a MIC value of 4 µg/mL. The presence of the hydroxyl group in C-19 in the pimarane, lachenerol B decreased the biological activity with a MIC of 128 µg/mL (Fig. 16).

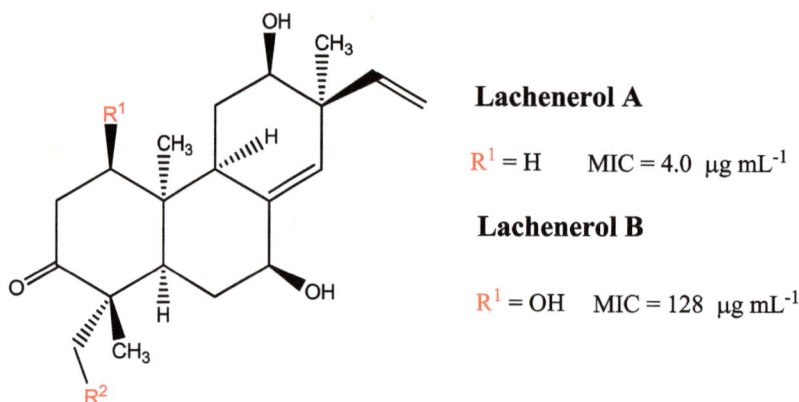

Lachenerol A

R^1 = H   MIC = 4.0 µg mL^{-1}

Lachenerol B

R^1 = OH   MIC = 128 µg mL^{-1}

Figure 16: Structures of lachenerol A and B [1].

Phorbol Esters

Based on their chemical studies of Thai medical plants, Chantrapromma and co-workers [1,21] have elucidated three new compounds (27, 28 and 34) and evaluated with the other six known phorbol esters against *Mycobacterium tuberculosis* H37Rv (Fig. 17). This plant, *Sapium indicum* L., is a mangrove plant belonging to the family Euphorbiceae, which is a widely present in the coastal areas of countries of Southeast Asia bordering the Indian Ocean and different phytochemical studies have resulted in the isolation of several phorbol esters. The minimum inhibitory concentration (MIC) showed antimycobacterial activity between 3.12-200 µg/mL, however no activity was found in the compound **30** and **32** (MIC >200 µg/mL). The best result was found in the compound **29**, and it is interesting to observe that 4β-isomers showed higher activity than 4α-isomers.

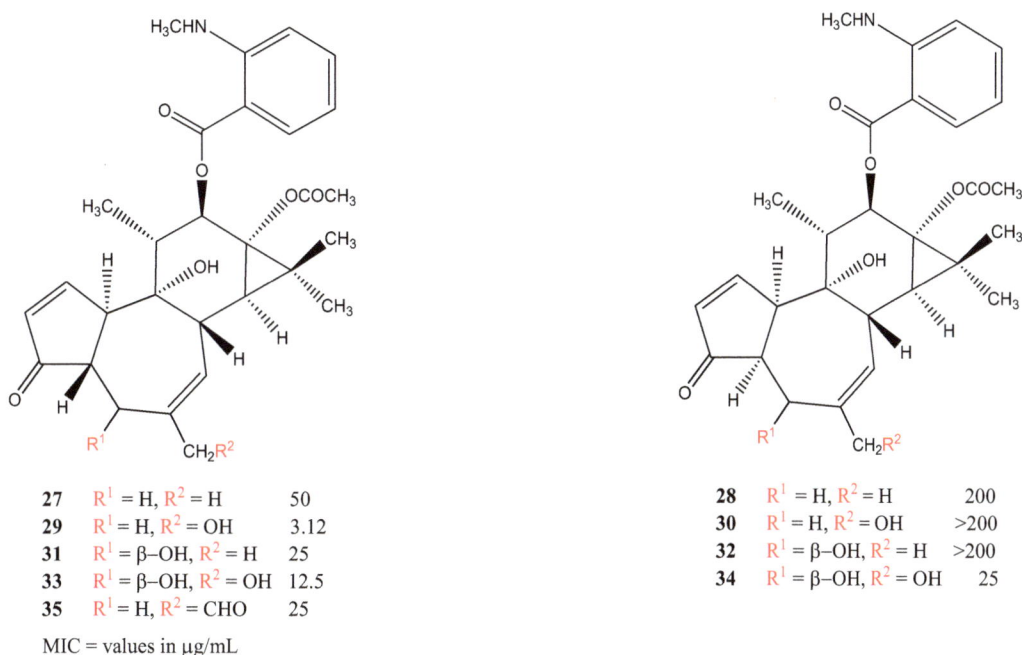

27	R^1 = H, R^2 = H	50
29	R^1 = H, R^2 = OH	3.12
31	R^1 = β–OH, R^2 = H	25
33	R^1 = β–OH, R^2 = OH	12.5
35	R^1 = H, R^2 = CHO	25

MIC = values in µg/mL

28	R^1 = H, R^2 = H	200
30	R^1 = H, R^2 = OH	>200
32	R^1 = β–OH, R^2 = H	>200
34	R^1 = β–OH, R^2 = OH	25

Figure 17: Structure of compounds isolated from *Sapium indicum L.*, a Thai plant.

8,9-Secokaurane

The plant species of the genus *Croton* (Euphorbiaceae) is common in Thailand being used in traditional medicine against gastric ulcers, dysmenorrhea, gastric cancers, and dysentery. Kittakoop and co-workers have found two new 8,9-secokaurane diterpenes **37** and **38** and the known **36** from *Croton kongensis*, which displayed MICs of 25.0, 6.25, and 6.25 µg/mL, respectively (Fig. **18**) [22].

(+)-Totarol

Karchesy and coworkers have isolated the new constituent (+)-totarol (Fig. **19**) from *Chamaecyparis nootkatenses* outerbark, which was active against *M. tuberculosis* H$_{37}$Rv with a MIC of 16 µg/mL [1,23]. This plant was collected from the Western slopes of the Olympic peninsula and it is used in traditional medicine by indigenous peoples in sweat baths for arthritis and rheumatism, infusions to sores, and swellings.

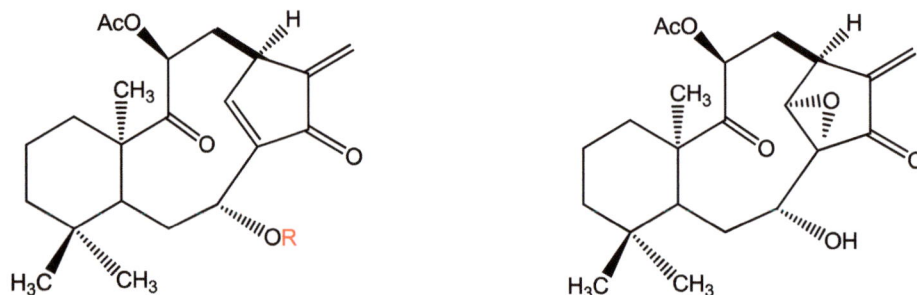

36 R = Ac MIC = 25.0 μg/mL

38 R = H MIC = 6.25 μg/mL

37 MIC = 6.25 μg/mL

Figure 18: Structures of the 8,9-secokaurane diterpenes 36-38.

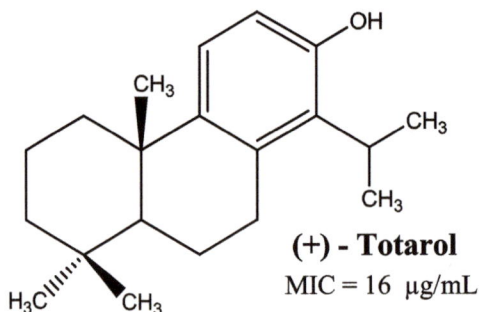

(+) - Totarol
MIC = 16 μg/mL

Figure 19: Structure of (+)-totarol [1].

Sesquiterpenes

Dehydrocostus Lactone

A contribution made by Fischer and co-workers was the structure-activity relationship (SAR) of dehydrocostus lactone, a major constituent of *Saussurea lappa* Clark (Asteraceae) MIC = 2μg/mL. Aiming to improve the anti-TB activity of this natural product several oxidative modifications have been done, however these modifications displayed significantly lower activities against *M. tuberculosis* (MIC = 32 - >128μg/mL) (Fig. **20**) [24].

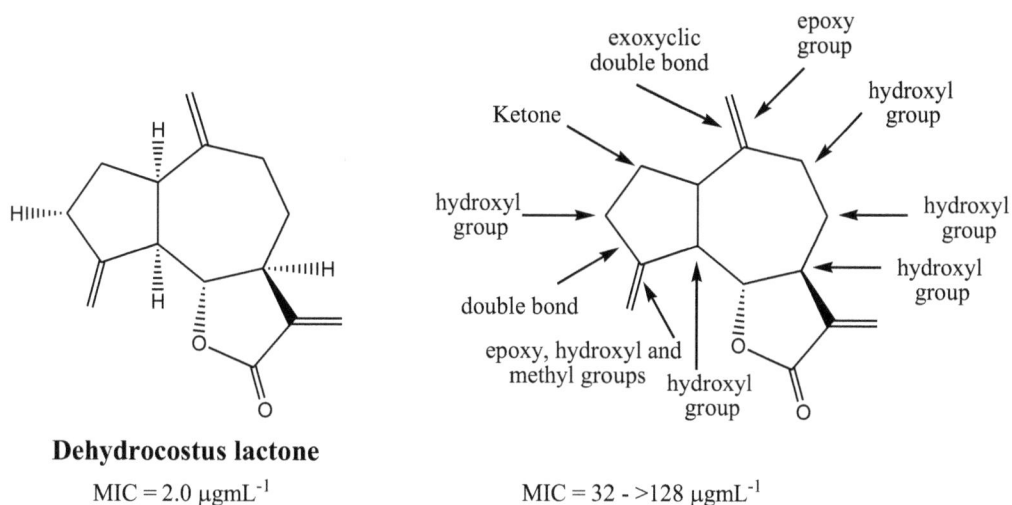

Dehydrocostus lactone

MIC = 2.0 µgmL^{-1} MIC = 32 - >128 µgmL^{-1}

Figure 20: Structure and SAR of dehydrocostus lactone.

Phytol

Phytol (Fig. **21**) is an acyclic terpenoid found in several species of plants being an extremely common natural product, including found in petroleum sediments. This compound have several applications, for example is used for the synthesis of vitamins E and K, it is used as ingredient of fragrances, beauty care product, detergent, soap, and household product. Rajab and co-workers [25] evaluated (*E*)-phytol as the principal anti-TB constituent (MIC = 2.0 µgmL^{-1}) of a methanol extract of the Kenyan shrub *Leucas volkensii*. Negi and co-workers evaluated several semisynthetic analogues of phytol (MIC 15.6-50 µg/mL) with better results when compare to this natural product (MIC 100 µg/mL) [26].

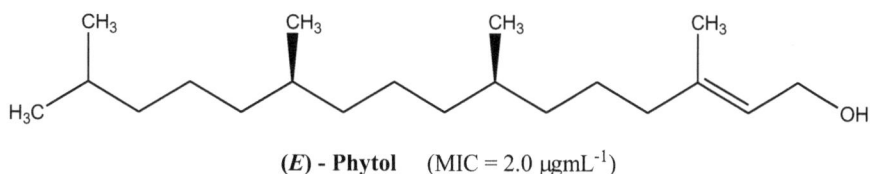

(*E*) - **Phytol**   (MIC = 2.0 µgmL^{-1})

Figure 21: Structure of phytol.

Triterpenes

Fischer and co-workers [27] isolated from methanolic extracts of seeds of *Melia volkensii* Gürke (Meliaceae), two new natural products 12β-hydroxykulactone **39** and 6β-hydroxykulactone **40** and the known substances kulactone **41** and kulonate **42**. This tree is found in dry areas of East Africa and used in traditional medicine to alleviate pain having also antifeedent and larvicide activities. The natural products **39**, **40**, **41** and **42** were evaluated against *M. tuberculosis* $H_{37}Rv$ possessing MIC of 16, 4, inactive and 16μg/mL, respectively (Fig. **22**).

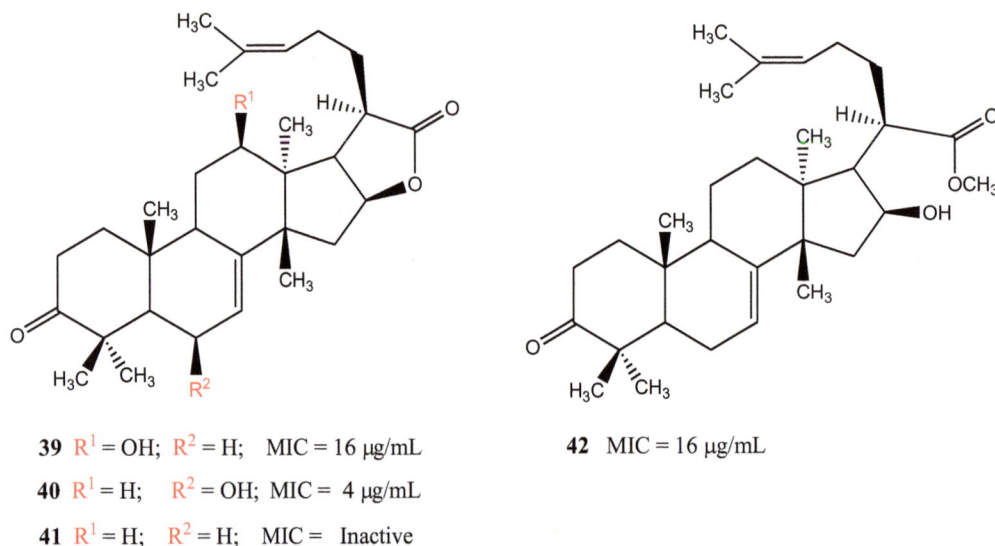

39 R^1 = OH; R^2 = H; MIC = 16 μg/mL

40 R^1 = H; R^2 = OH; MIC = 4 μg/mL

41 R^1 = H; R^2 = H; MIC = Inactive

42 MIC = 16 μg/mL

Figure 22: Structure of compounds isolated from methanolic extracts of seeds of *Melia volkensii* Gürke (Meliaceae).

MISCELLANEOUS

N-trans-Feruloylmethoxytyramine

Chen and co-workers [28] have isolated and evaluated against *Mycobacterium tuberculosis* several new and known compounds from the roots of *Litsea hypophaea* Hay (Lauraceae) a tree that grows in Taiwan forest. Among the compounds tested the known *N-trans*-feruloylmethoxytyramine shows a potent *in vitro* activity MIC = 1.6 μgmL^{-1} (Fig. **23**).

Shinanolone and (-)-4-Hydroxy-1-Tetralone

Lall and co-workers have identified in an ethanolic extract of *Euclea natalensis* root several compounds and the known compound shinanolone (Fig. **24**) [29]. This species occurs in different habitats, such as coastal and inland forests and bushveld. For example, it is widely present in tropical and subtropical Africa as well as on the east coast of South Africa and it is important in African medicine. For example, the root bark is used by the Zulus to treat bronchitis, pleurisy and chronic asthma [30]. This compound showed activity against different Gram-positive bacterial strains and a drug-sensitive strain of *Mycobacterium tuberculosis* (strain no. H37Rv ATCC 25923) at a concentration of 0.1 mg/mL. Another analogue of shinanolone is (-)-4-hydroxy-1-tetralone (Fig. **24**), which was found in the root extracts of the Formosan plant *Engelhardia roxburghiana* and displayed a MIC of 4.0 µg/mL [31].

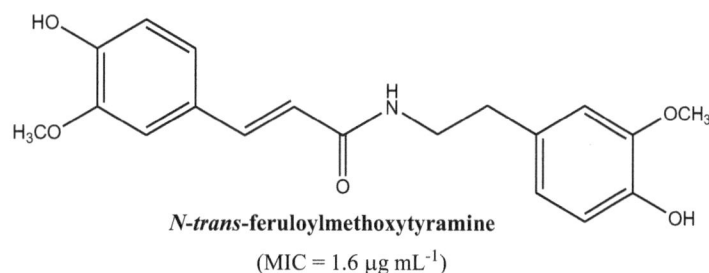

N-*trans*-feruloylmethoxytyramine
(MIC = 1.6 µg mL^{-1})

Figure 23: Structure of *N-trans*-feruloylmethoxytyramine.

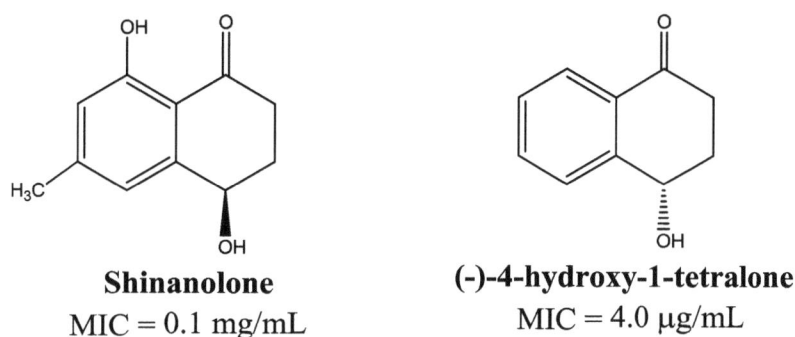

Shinanolone
MIC = 0.1 mg/mL

(-)-4-hydroxy-1-tetralone
MIC = 4.0 µg/mL

Figure 24: Structure of shinanolone and (-)-4-hydroxy-1-tetralone.

SELECTED ANTI-TB NATURAL PRODUCTS FOUND FROM PLANTS BETWEEN 2010 AND 2013

This section it will highlight select natural products of different class covered in this year, with the respective structure, activity and reference. The selection was based on the potency and other promises perspectives of the compounds (Fig. **25**).

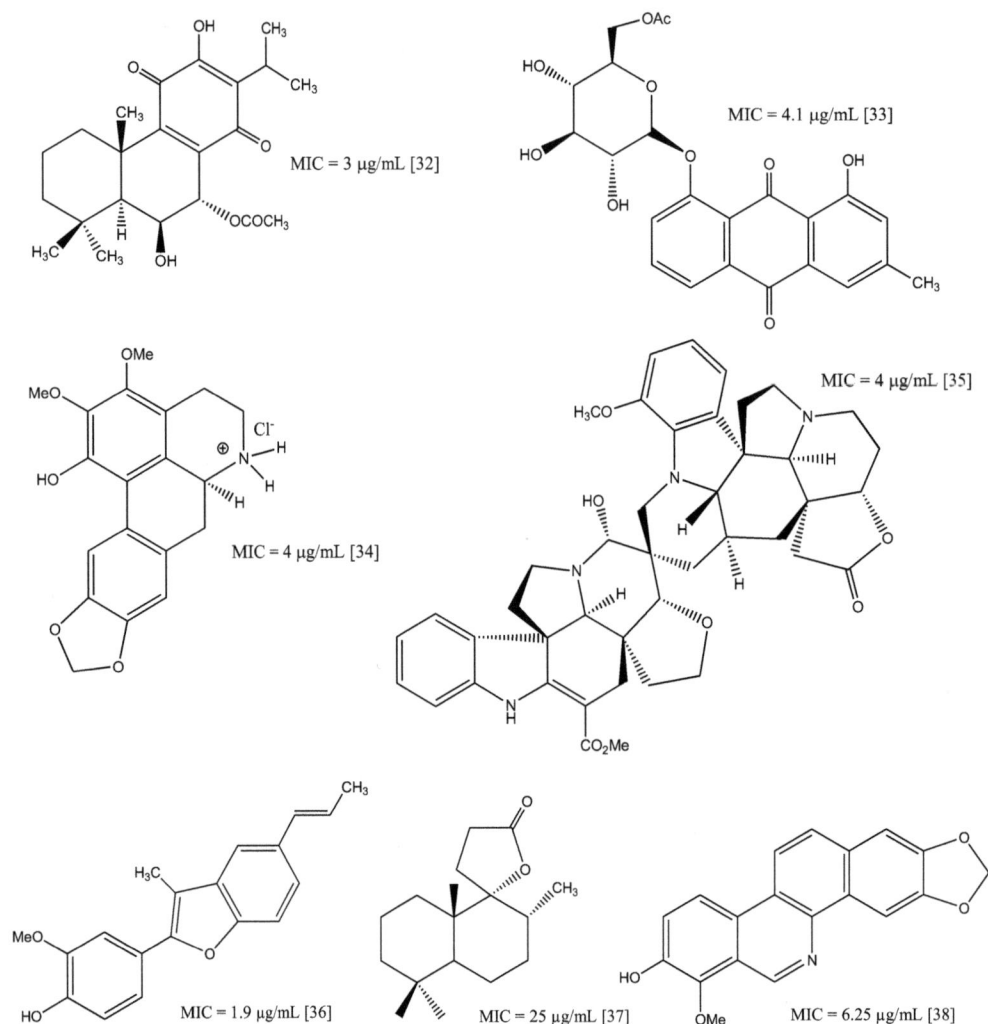

MIC = 3 µg/mL [32]

MIC = 4.1 µg/mL [33]

MIC = 4 µg/mL [35]

MIC = 4 µg/mL [34]

MIC = 1.9 µg/mL [36]

MIC = 25 µg/mL [37]

MIC = 6.25 µg/mL [38]

Figure 25: Natural products from plants between 2010-2013.

ACKNOWLEDGEMENT

None Declare.

CONFLICT OF INTEREST

The author(s) confirm that this chapter content has no conflict of interest.

REFERENCES

[1]   De Souza MVN. Plants and Fungal Products with activity against Tuberculosis. *The Scientific World Journal* 2005;**5**:609-628.

[2]   Kanokmedhakul S, Kanokmedhakul K, Lekphrom R. Bioactive Constituents of the Roots of Polyalthia cerasoides. *J Nat Prod* 2007;**70**:1536-1538.

[3]   Corona M del R, Hernández JMJF, Santiago OG, González EG, Salinas GMM, Fernández SS, Delgado G, Herrerae JL. Evaluation of Some Plant-derived Secondary Metabolites Against Sensitive and Multidrugresistant *Mycobacterium tuberculosis J Med Chem Soc* 2009;**53**:71-75.

[4]   Lester A. Mitscher LA, Baker, WR. A search for novel chemotherapy against tuberculosis amongst natural products *Pure & Appl Chem* 1998;**70**:365-371.

[5]   Hwang JM, Oh T, Kaneko T, Upton AM, Franzblau SG, Ma Z, Cho SN, Kim P. Design, synthesis, and structure-activity relationship studies of tryptanthrins as antitubercular agents. *J Nat Prod* 2013;**76**:354-67.

[6]   Xu ZQ, Barrow WW, Suling WJ, Westbrook L, Barrow E, Lin YM, Flavin MT. Anti-HIV natural product (+)-calanolide A is active against both drug-susceptible and drug-resistant strains of *Mycobacterium tuberculosis*. *Bioorg Med Chem* 2004;**12**:1199-1207.

[7]   Moller AF, Chen M, Fuursted K, Chirstensen SB, Kharazmi A. *In Vitro* Antimycobacterial and Antilegionella Activity of Licochalcone A from Chinese Licorice Roots. *Planta Med.* 2002;**68**:416.

[8]   Kanokmedhakul S, Kanokmedhakul K, Nambuddee K, Kongsaeree P. New Bioactive Prenylflavonoids and Dibenzocycloheptene Derivative from Roots of *Dendrolobium lanceolatum*. *J Nat Prod* 2004;**67**:968-72.

[9]   Ma C, Case RJ, Wang Y, Zhang HJ, Tan GT, Hung NV, Cuong NM, Franzblau SG, Soejarto DD, Fong HHS, Pauli GF. Anti-tuberculosis constituintes from the stem bark of *Micromelum hirsutum*. *Planta Medica* 2005;**71**:261-267.

[10]   Yuan H, He R, Wanb B, Wangb Y, Pauli GF, Franzblau SG, Kozikowski AP. Modification of the side chain of micromolide, an anti-tuberculosis natural product. *Bioorg & Med Chem Lett* 2008;**18**:5311-5315.

[11]   Deng S, Wang Y, Inui T, Chen SN Norman R. Farnsworth NR, Cho S, Franzblau SG Pauli GF. Anti-TB Polyynes from the Roots of *Angelica sinensis*. *Phytother Res* 2008;**22**:878-882.

[12]   Mata R, Morales I, Perez O, Cruz IR, Acevedo L, Mendoza, LE, Bye R, Franzblau SG, Timmermann B. Antimycobacterial Compounds from *Piper sanctum*. *J Nat Prod* 2004;**67**:1961-1968.

[13]   Grahan JG, Zhang H, Pendland SL, Santarsiero BD, Mesecar AD, Cabieses F, Farnsworth NR. Antimycobacterial Naphthopyrones from *Senna oblique*. *J Nat Prod* 2004;**67**:225.

[14]   Jonel P. Saludes JP, Mary J. Garson MJ, Scott G. Franzblau SG, Alicia M. Aguinaldo AM. Antitubercular Constituents from the Hexane Fraction of *Morinda citrifolia* Linn. (Rubiaceae) *Phytother Res* 2002;**16**:683-685.

[15]   Wachter G, Franzblau SG, Montenegro G, Hoffmann JJ, Maiese WM, Timmermann BN. Inhibition of *Mycobacterium tuberculosis* Growth by Saringosterol from *Lessonia nigrescens*. *J Nat Prod* 2001;**64**:1463-4.

[16]   Wachter G, Valcic S, Flagg ML, Franzblau SG, Montenegro G, Suarez E, Timmermann, BN. Antitubercular activity of pentacyclic triterpenoids from plants of Argentina and Chile. *Phytomedicine* 1999;**6**:341-5.

[17]   Woldemichael GM, Franzblau SG, Zhang F, Wang Y, Timmermann, BN. Inhibitory effect of sterols from Ruprechtia triflora and diterpenes from Calceolaria pinnifolia on the growth of Mycobacterium tuberculosis. *Planta Med* 2003;**69**:628-631.

[18]   Ulubelen A, Topcu G, Johansson CB. Norditerpenoids and Diterpenoids from *Salvia multicaulis* with Antituberculous Activity *J Nat Prod* 1997;**60**:1275-1280.

[19]   Kanokmedhakul S. Kanokmedhakul K. Kanarsa T. Buayairaksa M. New Bioactive Clerodane Diterpenoids from the Bark of *Casearia grewiifolia*. *J Nat Prod* 2005;**68**:183-8.

[20]   Woldemichael GM, Gutierrez-Lugo MT, Franzblau SG, Wang Y, Suarez E, Timmermann BN. *Mycobacterium tuberculosis* Growth Inhibition by Constituents of *Sapium haematospermu*. *J Nat Prod* 2004;**67**:598-603.

[21]   Chumkaew P, Karalai C, Ponglimanont C, Chantrapromma K. Antimycobacterial Activity of Phorbol Esters from the Fruits of *Sapium indicum*. *J Nat Prod* 2003;**66**:540-3.

[22]   Thongtan J, Kittakoop P, Ruangrungsi N, Saenboonrueng J, Thebtaranonth, Y. New Antimycobacterial and Antimalarial 8,9-Secokaurane Diterpenes from *Croton kongensis J Nat Prod* 2003;**66**:868-870.

[23]   Constantine GH, Karchesy JJ, Franzblau SG, LaFleur LE. (+)−Totarol from *Chamaecyparis nootkatensis* and activity against *Mycobacterium tuberculosis*. *Fitoterapia* 2001;**72**:572-4.

[24]   Cantrell CL, Nunez IS, Acosta, JC, Foroozesh M, Fronczek, FR, Fischer NH, Franzblau SG. Antimycobacterial Activities of Dehydrocostus Lactone and Its Oxidation Products. *J Nat Prod* 1998;**61**:1181-1186.

[25]   Rajab MS, Cantrell CL, Franzblau SG, Fischer NH. Antimycobacterial activity of (*E*)-phytol and derivatives: a preliminary structure-activity study. *Planta Med* 1998;**64**:2-4.

[26]   Saikia D, Parihar S, Chanda D, Ojha S, Kumar JK, Chanotiya CS, Shanker K, Negi AS. Antitubercular potential of some semisynthetic analogues of phytol. *Bioorg Med Chem Lett* 2010;**20**:508-12.

[27]   Charles L, Cantrell, Rajab CMS, Franzblau SG, Fischer NH. Antimycobacterial Triterpenes from Melia volkensii. *J Nat Prod* 1999;**62**:546-548.

[28]   Pan PC, Cheng MJ, Peng CF, Huang HY, Chen JJ, Chen IS. Secondary metabolites from the roots of Litsea hypophaea and their antitubercular activity. *J Nat Prod* 2010;**73**:890-6.

[29]   Weigenand O, Hussein AA, Lall N, Meyer JJM. Antibacterial Activity of Naphthoquinones and Triterpenoids from *Euclea natalensis* Root Bark. *J Nat Prod* 2004;**67**:1936.

[30]   Wky BV, Wky PV *Field Guide to Trees of Southern Africa*; Struik, Cape Town (**1997**). p. 184.

[31]   Lin, WY, Peng, CF, Tsai, IL, Chen, JJ, Cheng MJ, Chen, IS. Antitubercular Constituents from the Roots of Engelhardia roxburghiana. *Planta Med* 2005;**71**:171-5.

[32]   Rijo P, Simões MF, Francisco AP, Rojas R, Gilman RH, Vaisberg AJ, Rodríguez B, Moiteiro C. Antimycobacterial metabolites from Plectranthus: royleanone derivatives against *Mycobacterium tuberculosis* strains. *Chem Biodivers* 2010;**7**:922-32.

[33] Liang HX, Dai HQ, Fu HA, Dong XP, Adebayo HA, Zhang LX, Cheng YX, Bioactive compounds from Rumex plants. *Phytochem Lett* 2010;**3**:181-184.

[34] Guzman JD, Gupta A, Evangelopoulos D, Basavannacharya C, Pabon LC, Plazas EA, Muñoz DR, Delgado WA, Cuca LE, Ribon W, Gibbons S, Bhakta S. Anti-tubercular screening of natural products from Colombian plants: 3-methoxynordomesticine, an inhibitor of MurE ligase of *Mycobacterium tuberculosis*. *J Antimicrob Chemother* 2010;**65**:2101-7.

[35] Macabeo AP, Vidar WS, Chen X, Decker M, Heilmann J, Wan B, Franzblau SG, Galvez EV, Aguinaldo MA, Cordell GA. *Mycobacterium tuberculosis* and cholinesterase inhibitors from Voacanga globosa. *Eur J Med Chem* 2011;**46**:3118-23.

[36] Scodro RB, Pires CT, Carrara VS, Lemos CO, Cardozo-Filho L, Souza VA, Corrêa AG, Siqueira VL, Lonardoni MV, Cardoso RF, Cortez DA. Anti-tuberculosis neolignans from Piper regnellii. *Phytomedicine* 2013;**20**:600-4.

[37] Tiwari N, Thakur J, Saikia D, Gupta MM. Antitubercular diterpenoids from Vitex trifolia. *Phytomedicine* 2013;**20**:605-10.

[38] Luo X, Pires D, Aínsa JA, Gracia B, Duarte N, Mulhovo S, Anes E, Ferreira MJ. Zanthoxylum capense constituents with antimycobacterial activity against Mycobacterium tuberculosis *in vitro* and *ex vivo* within human macrophages. *J Ethnopharmacol* 2013;**146**:417-22.

Send Orders for Reprints to reprints@benthamscience.net

CHAPTER 7

Anti-TB Evaluation of Natural Products From Fungus

Marcus V.N. de Souza*

Instituto de Tecnologia em Fármacos - Farmanguinhos, FioCruz - Fundação Oswaldo Cruz, R. Sizenando Nabuco, 100, Manguinhos, 21041-250, Rio de Janeiro, RJ, Brazil

Abstract: For six decades, natural products have taken a central role in the discovery of new antimicrobial agents. The structural diversity of these compounds and its ability for interacting specifically with biological target molecules has laid an ideal foundation in the development of new drugs. The importance of fungus in TB treatment can be observed in several aminoglycosides isolated from different *Streptomyces* species, which are used as second line drug. Due to the fundamental importance of fungi in the past and present of TB treatment, several research groups isolated and evaluated a number of compounds from different fungal species against *Mycobacterium tuberculosis*, which will be described in this chapter.

Keywords: Tuberculosis; *Mycobacterium tuberculosis*; natural products; fungus; semi-synthesis; synthesis; analogues; treatment; multi-drug-resistant tuberculosis (MDR TB); extensive-drug-resistant tuberculosis (XDR TB); target; mechanism of action; biological evaluation; drug development.

INTRODUCTION

Despite the large number of synthetic drugs used to treat tuberculosis, natural products were of fundamental importance to the development of tuberculosis treatment. For example streptomycin, an aminoglycoside isolated from the actinobacterium *Streptomyces griseus*, identified in 1943 by Selman Abraham Waksman was the first drug used to treat TB, which is still being used as second-line drugs. After this remarkable discovery from the 1940s and 60 different natural products were isolated from fungal species and evaluated against this

*Adress correspondence to Marcus V.N. de Souza: Instituto de Tecnologia em Fármacos - Farmanguinhos, FioCruz - Fundação Oswaldo Cruz, R. Sizenando Nabuco, 100, Manguinhos, 21041-250, Rio de Janeiro, RJ, Brazil; E-mail: marcos_souza@far.fiocruz.br

disease such as, kanamycin from *Streptomyces capreolus*, the semisynthetic amikacin produced from kanamycin A and capreomycins, from fermentation of *Streptomyces capreolus*, which also is still being used against TB as second-line drugs [1]. Due to the fundamental importance of the fungi on the past and present of TB treatment several research groups have isolated and evaluated a number of compounds from different fungal species, which it will be highlight in this chapter.

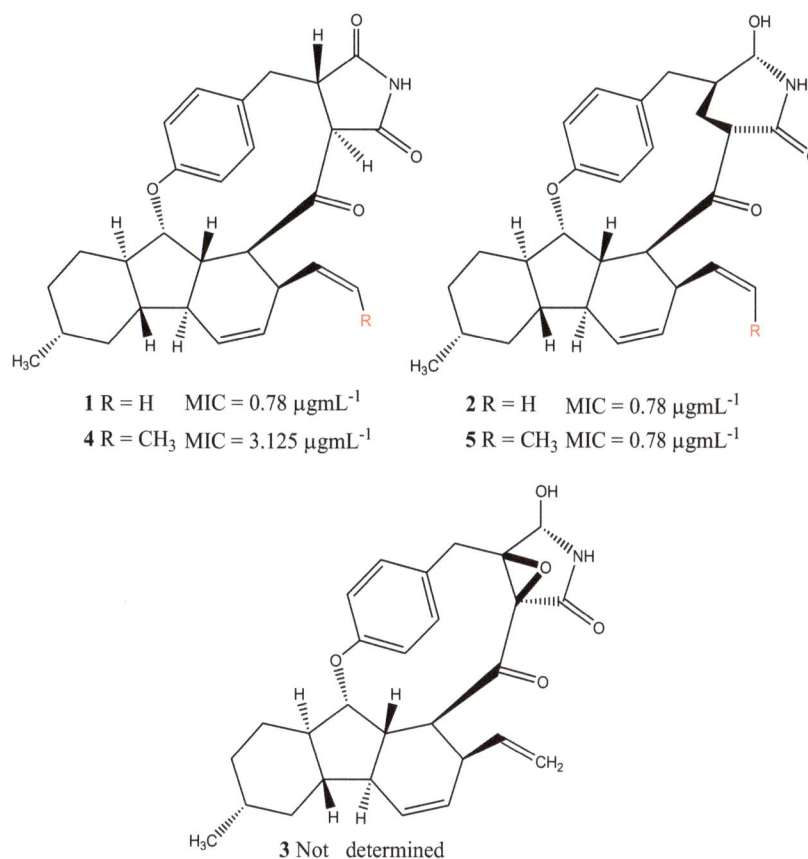

1 R = H   MIC = 0.78 μgmL^{-1}
4 R = CH$_3$ MIC = 3.125 μgmL^{-1}

2 R = H   MIC = 0.78 μgmL^{-1}
5 R = CH$_3$ MIC = 0.78 μgmL^{-1}

3 Not determined

Figure 1: Structures of hirsutellones (1-5).

ALKALOIDS

Hirsutellones (1-5)

The alkaloid class named hirsutellone is a very strained 12 or 13-membered ring possessing a succinimide or lactam, a *para*-substituted phenyl ether, and a tricyclic polyketide moieties. Isaka and co-workers [2] have isolated, elucidated and evaluated against *M. tuberculosis* five new hirsutellone A-E (**1-5**) from the insect pathogenic fungus *Hirsutella nivea* BCC 2594, which showed potent anti-TB activity (MIC = 0.78-3.25 μgmL^{-1}) (Fig. **1**).

CARBOHYDRATE

Mycothiol

The natural product mycothiol (Fig. **2**) was isolated for the first time by Sakuda and co-workers [3] from *Streptomyces sp* AJ9463 being synthesized by Rosazza and co-workers in 2004 [4]. This compound, which has in its structure acethylcysteine, glucosamine and inositol is found in the majority of actinomycetes and has several functions such as, remove toxins, alkylating agents, antibiotics and oxidative stress playing a similar function of glutathione in eukaryotes [5-10]. Considering that mycothiol could be a critical role in the protection and growth of *Mycobacterium tuberculosis* being an important target in anti-TB drug discovery.

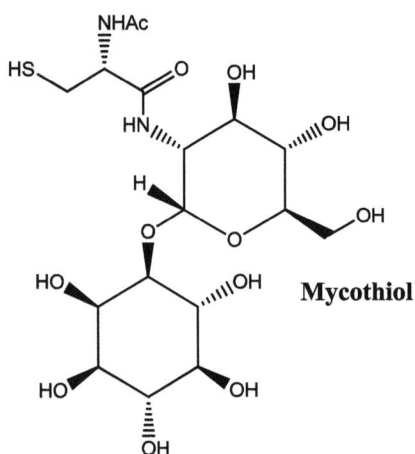

Figure 2: Structure of mycothiol.

DITERPENE

Diaporthein A and B

Two natural pimarane diterpenes diaporthein A and B (Fig. **3**) were isolated from the culture broth of the fungus *Diaporthe* sp. BCC 6140 by Kittakoop and co-workers, which evaluated its anti-TB activity [11,12]. These natural products showed a MIC of 200 μgmL^{-1} and 3.1 μgmL^{-1} respectively, indicating that the carbonyl function in the C-7 position of diaporthein B (Fig. **3**) is critical for the anti-TB activity.

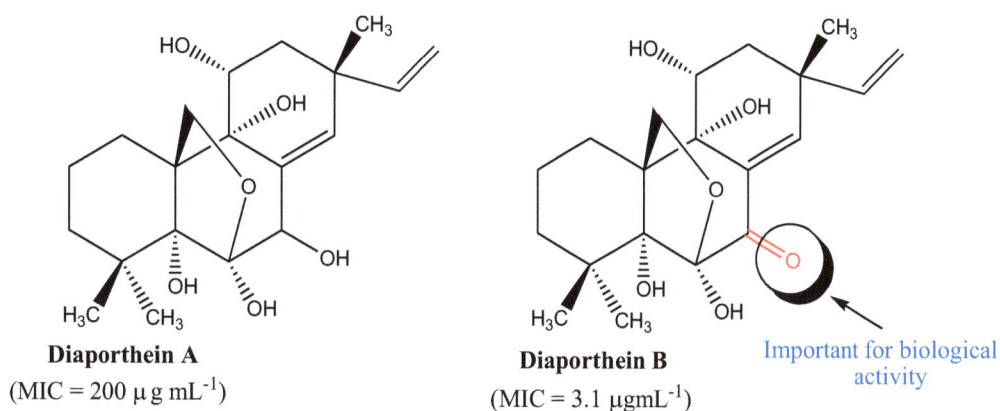

Diaporthein A
(MIC = 200 μ g mL^{-1})

Diaporthein B
(MIC = 3.1 μgmL^{-1})

Important for biological activity

Figure 3: Structure of diaporthein A and B.

MACROLIDE

Pamamycins

Pamamycins are a class of 16-membered macrolide antibiotic first isolated in 1979 from *Streptomyces alboniger* ATCC 12461 possessing potent activity against Gram positive bacterial including MDR strains. For example, pamamycin-607 (Fig. **4**) [13-16] possessed potent activity against *Mycobacterium tuberculosis* with an MIC of 2-4 μgmL^{-1}.

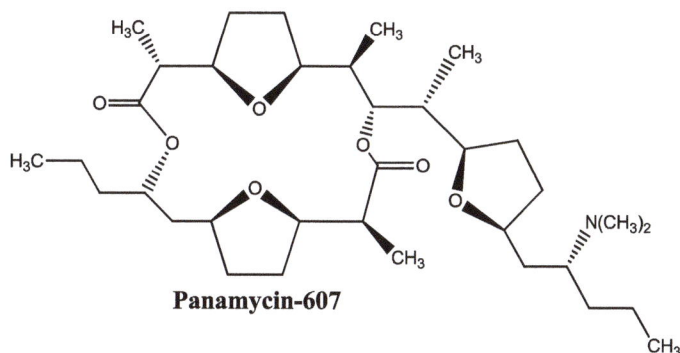

Panamycin-607

Figure 4: Structure of Pamamycin-607.

Thuggacin A

The two new thuggacins [17] were isolated by Jansen and co-workers from the myxobacterium *Sorangium cellulosum*, which also made several studies, such as structure elucidation, conformation analysis, biosynthesis, anti-TB evaluation, and preliminary studies on the mechanism of action. The thuggacin A (Fig. 5) was tested against strain *Mycobacterium tuberculosis* H37RV, and it inhibited the growth at a concentration of 8 µgmL^{-1}.

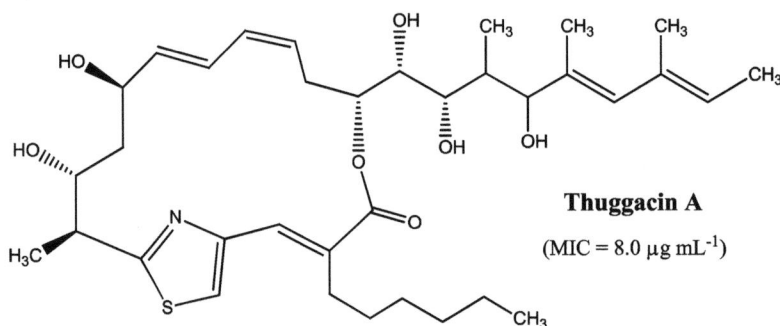

Figure 5: Structure of thuggacin A.

NAPHTHOQUINONES

Preussomerins

The natural product preussomerin **6** (Fig. **6**) was isolated with others compounds from the lichenicolous fungus *Microsphaeropis* sp. BCC 3050 being isolated from a lichen sample, *Dirinaria applanata,* collected from Phu Tee-Suan-Sai forest in Loei province, Northeastern Thailand. The evaluation of antimycobacterial activity of preussomerin **6** was made by Isaka and coworkers, which showed a MIC value of 3.12 µg/mL [18].

Kittakoop and co-workers [19] at BIOTEC have identified two deoxypreussomerin derivatives, palmarumycins JC1 **7** and JC2 **8** (Fig. **7**) from dried *D. ehretioides* fruits. However, they propose that the isolated preussomerins were not metabolites of the plant D. ehretioides, but they might be from fungal epiphytes or endophytes, because this class of compound is commonly found in fungal metabolites. The anti-TB activity displayed a MIC of 6.25 µgmL^{-1} for the compound **7**, however the epoxy **8** was inactive, indicating that the oxidation of the hydroxyl group to ketone and the epoxy replaced by hydroxyl group are important for the biological activity.

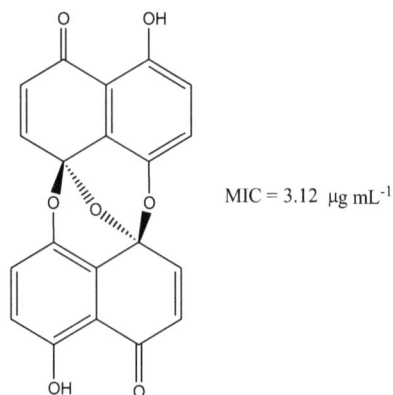

MIC = 3.12 µg mL^{-1}

Figure 6: Structure of preussomerin **6**.

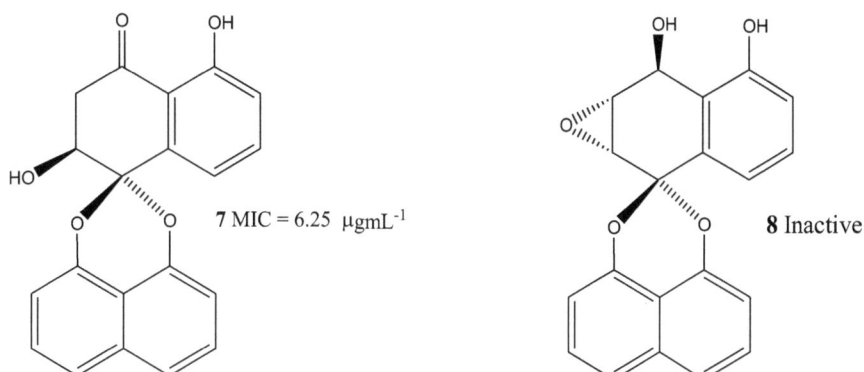

7 MIC = 6.25 µgmL^{-1}

8 Inactive

Figure 7: Structure of palmarumycins JC1 **7** and JC2 **8.**

PEPTIDES

Enniatins

Enniatins (Fig. **8**) are macrolides, which possessed antibiotic, phytotoxic and insecticidal activities, as well as they are able to inhibited acyl-CoA cholesterol acyltransferase (ACAT). This 18-member cyclodepsipeptide class is produced by different *Fusarium* species. Isaka and co-workers [20,21] have isolated, elucidated and tested several compounds of this class from the Thailand BIOTEC Culture Collection (BCC), which displayed potent anti-TB activity with MIC values of 1.56-12.5 µg/mL (Fig. **8**).

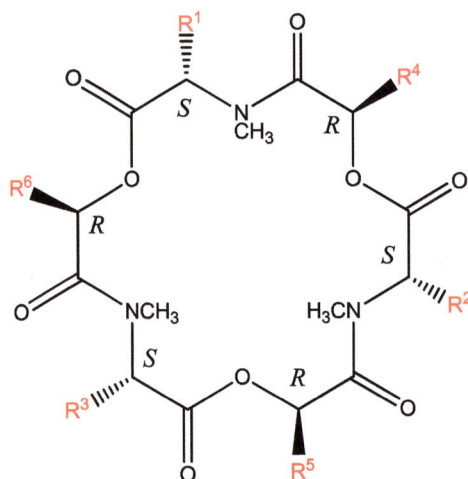

Compounds	R¹	R²	R³	R⁴	R⁵	R⁶	MIC (μg/mL)
Enniatin B	*i*-Pr	*i*-Pr	*i*-Pr	*i*-Pr	*i*-Pr	*i*-Pr	3.12
Enniatin B₄	*i*-Bu	*i*-Pr	*i*-Pr	*i*-Pr	*i*-Pr	*i*-Pr	3.12
Enniatin C	*i*-Bu	*i*-Bu	*i*-Bu	*i*-Pr	*i*-Pr	*i*-Pr	6.25
Enniatin G	*i*-Bu	*i*-Bu	*i*-Pr	*i*-Pr	*i*-Pr	*i*-Pr	6.25
Enniatin H	*i*-Pr	*i*-Pr	*i*-Pr	*s*-Bu(3*s*)	*i*-Pr	*i*-Pr	6.25
Enniatin I	*i*-Pr	*i*-Pr	*i*-Pr	*s*-Bu(3*s*)	*s*-Bu(3*s*)	*i*-Pr	6.25
MK1688	*i*-Pr	*i*-Pr	*i*-Pr	*s*-Bu(3*s*)	*s*-Bu(3*s*)	*s*-Bu(3*s*)	1.56
Enniatin L	*i*-Pr	*i*-Pr	*i*-Pr	*s*-Bu(3*s*OH)	*s*-Pr(2*s*)	*s*-Pr(2*s*)	12.5
Enniatin M₁	*i*-Pr	*i*-Pr	*i*-Pr	*s*-Bu(3*s*OH)	*s*-Bu(3*s*)	*s*-Pr(2*s*)	6.25
Enniatin M₂	*i*-Pr	*i*-Pr	*i*-Pr	*s*-Bu(3*s*OH)	*s*-Pr(2*s*)	*s*-Bu(3*s*)	6.25
Enniatin N	*i*-Pr	*i*-Pr	*i*-Pr	*s*-Bu(3*s*OH)	*s*-Bu(3*s*)	*s*-Bu(3*s*)	3.12

Figure 8: Structure and anti-TB activity of enniatins.

Hirsutellide A

The natural product named hirsutellide A (Fig. **9**) was isolated and elucidated by Kittakoop and co-workers [22] from a cell of the entomopathogenic fungus *Hirsutella kobayasii* BCC 1660. This product showed a MIC with 6-12 μg/mL with no cytotoxic effect toward Vero cells at 50 μg/mL.

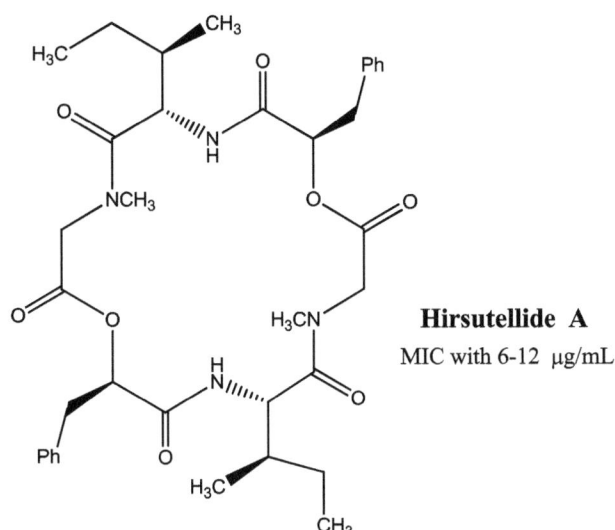

Hirsutellide A
MIC with 6-12 μg/mL

Figure 9: Structure of hirsutellide A.

Nocathiacins

The cyclic thiazolyl peptides (Fig. **10**) are a class of antibiotics known as nocathiacins [23], which was originally isolated from a *Nocardia* sp. (ATCC 202099) fermentation broth extraction. This class has potent activity against Gram-positive bacteria, including antibiotic-resistant clinical pathogens. For example against *Mycobacterium tuberculosis* it displays a MIC of <0.008, however this compound showed some solubility and pharmacokinetics problems.

TRITERPENE

Fusidic Acid

Fusidic acid (Fig. **11**) is a compound derived from the fungus *Fusidium coccineum*, which was originally isolated from monkey faeces. This natural product was developed by Leo Laboratories in Ballerup, Denmark in the 1950-60s as a bacteriostatic antibiotic. Fusic acid has activity against a wide variety of Gram-positive bacteria and a few members of the Gram-negative species with it major activity against staphylococci, including antibiotic resistant strains to, such as methicillin-resistant *Staphylococcus aureus* [24]. This triterpene is also active against *Mybacterium tuberculosis* [25,26] with MIC values ranging between 4 and 32-64 μgmL^{-1}.

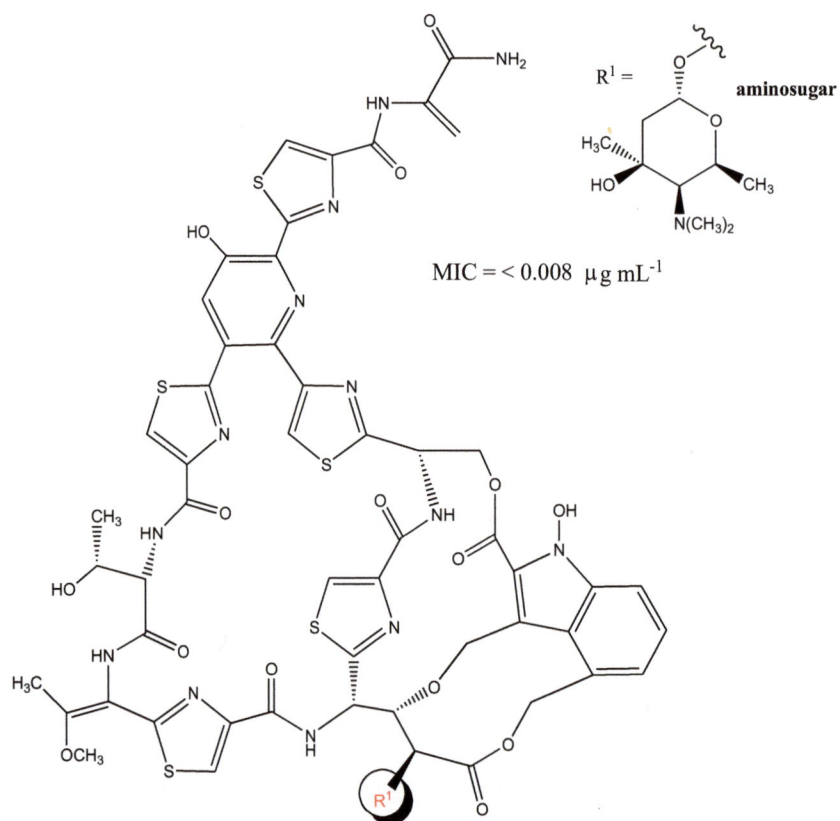

$MIC = < 0.008 \ \mu g \ mL^{-1}$

Figure 10: Structure of the cyclic thiazolyl peptides a class of antibiotics known as nocathiacins.

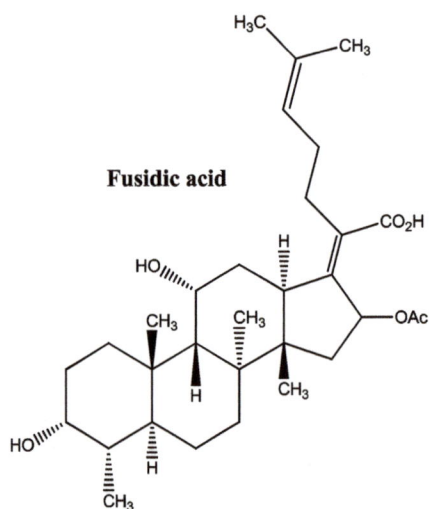

Figure 11: Structure of fusidic acid.

XANTHONE

Phomoxanthones A and B

Isaka and co-workers isolated two unknown Xanthone dimers from the endophytic fungus *Phomopsis* species named phomoxanthones A and B (Fig. **12**) [27], which displayed potent anti-TB activity MIC = 0.5 and 6.25 μgmL^{-1}, respectively. It is important to mention that the deacetyl derivative, produced from **1** by using sulfuric acid in methanol was not active, suggesting the low lipophilicity of this compound when compared to phomoxanthones A and B.

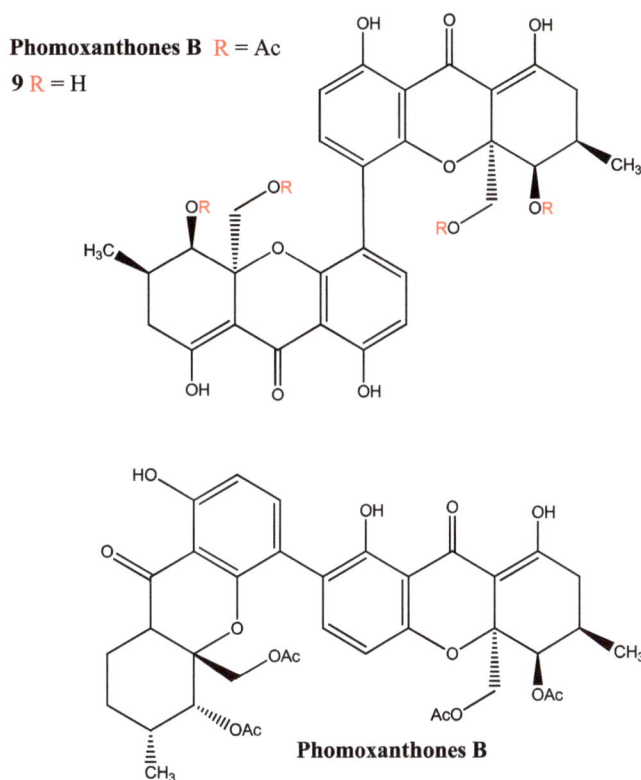

Figure 12: Structure of phomoxanthones A and B.

MISCELLANEOUS

Calpinactam

Tomoda and co-workers isolated from the culture broth of a fungal strain Mortierella alpina FKI-4905 the natural product Calpinactam (Fig. **13**), a new anti-mycobacterial agent, which displayed a MIC of 12.5 µg/mL against *Mycobacterium tuberculosis* [28].

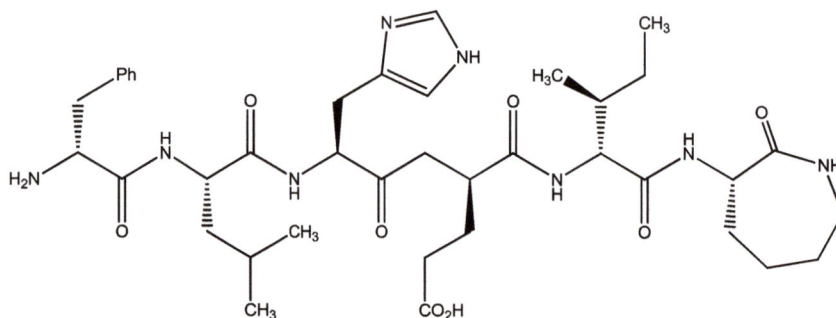

Figure 13: Structure of calpinactam.

Caprazamycin and Pacidamycin

The cell wall biosynthesis has been explored as pharmacological target in the search for new antibiotics since the discovery of penicillin by Fleming in 1929. For example, biosynthesis of peptideoglican and arabinogalactan are essential for the survival of the bacteria and becomes an interesting target in the development of new drugs. In this context it can be mentioned the phospho-*N*-acetylmuramyl-pentapeptide translocase (translocase I), enzyme responsible for catalyzing the first step in the biosynthesis of peptideoglican [29,30]. Several substances have been reported as inhibiting translocase I, among them caprazamycin families [30] and the pacidamycin [31] (Fig. **14**) isolated from *Streptomyces coeruleorubidus* and the culture broth of *Streptomyces sp.* MK730-62F2, respectively.

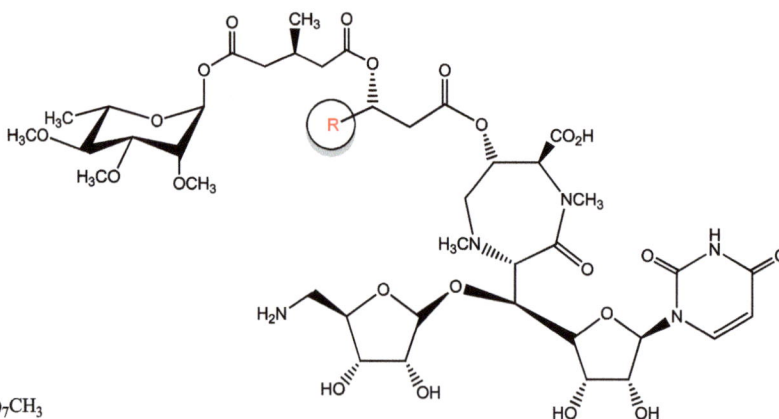

Caprazamycin family
R =

A $CH_3(CH_2)_{11}CH_3$

B $(CH_3)_2CH(CH_2)_9CH_3$

C $CH_2(CH_2)_{10}CH_3$

D $(CH_3)_2CH(CH_2)_8CH_3$

E $CH_3(CH_2)_9CH_3$

F $(CH_3)_2CH(CH_2)_7CH_3$

G $CH_3CH_2CH(CH_3)(CH_2)_7CH_3$

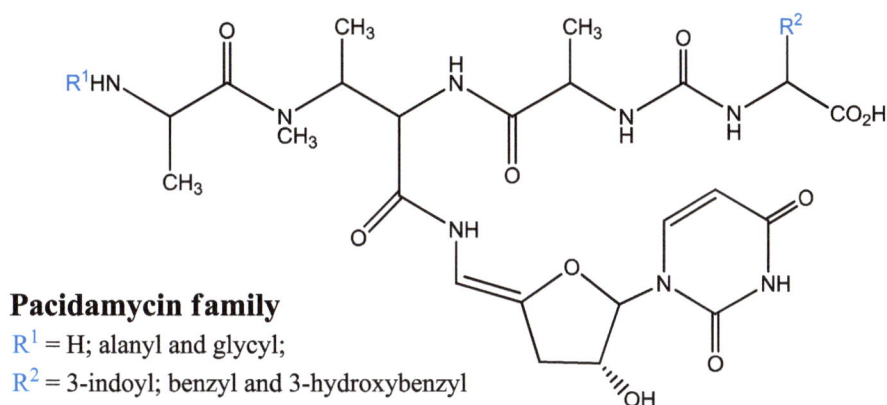

Pacidamycin family

R^1 = H; alanyl and glycyl;

R^2 = 3-indoyl; benzyl and 3-hydroxybenzyl

Figure 14: Structure of caprazamycin and pacidamycin family.

Mycobactins

The class of compounds known as Mycobactins (Fig. **15**) is isolated from mycobacteria including *M. tuberculosis* and *Mycobacterium phlei*. These substances are classified as siderophores (iron carriers), which are iron chelating in general from extracellular media for storage, sequester, and transport iron [32]. For example, mycobacteria has a grave problem of iron acquisition due to the majority form of iron is three (oxidized state), which is very insoluble at physiological pH. An important work in this field is the synthesis and biological evaluation against *Mycobacterium tuberculosis* (MIC = 3.13 µgmL^{-1}) of mycobactin S made by Miller and co-workers [33,34].

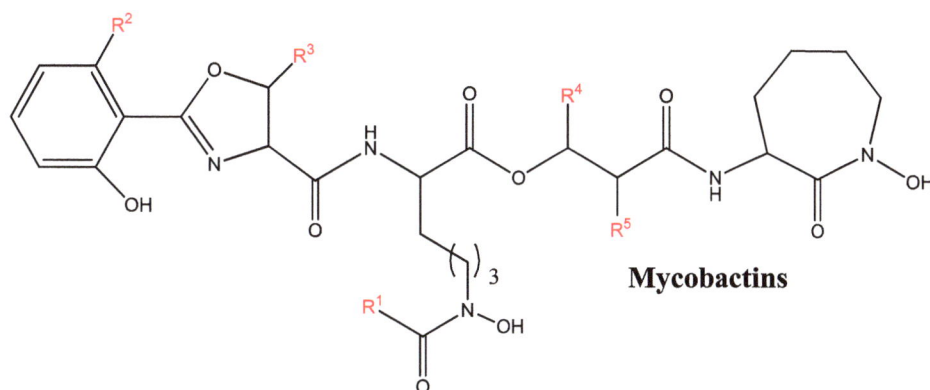

Mycobactins

Mycobactin S = R^1 = $CH_3(CH_2)_{14}$-; $R^2 = R^3 = R^5$ = H; R^4 = CH_3 (*S*)

Figure 15: General structure of mycobactins.

SELECTED ANTI-TB NATURAL PRODUCTS FOUND FROM FUNGI BETWEEN 2011 AND 2012

This section it will highlight select natural products of different class covered between 2011 and 2012, with the respective structure, activity and reference. The selection was based on the potency and other promises perspectives of the compounds (Fig. **16**).

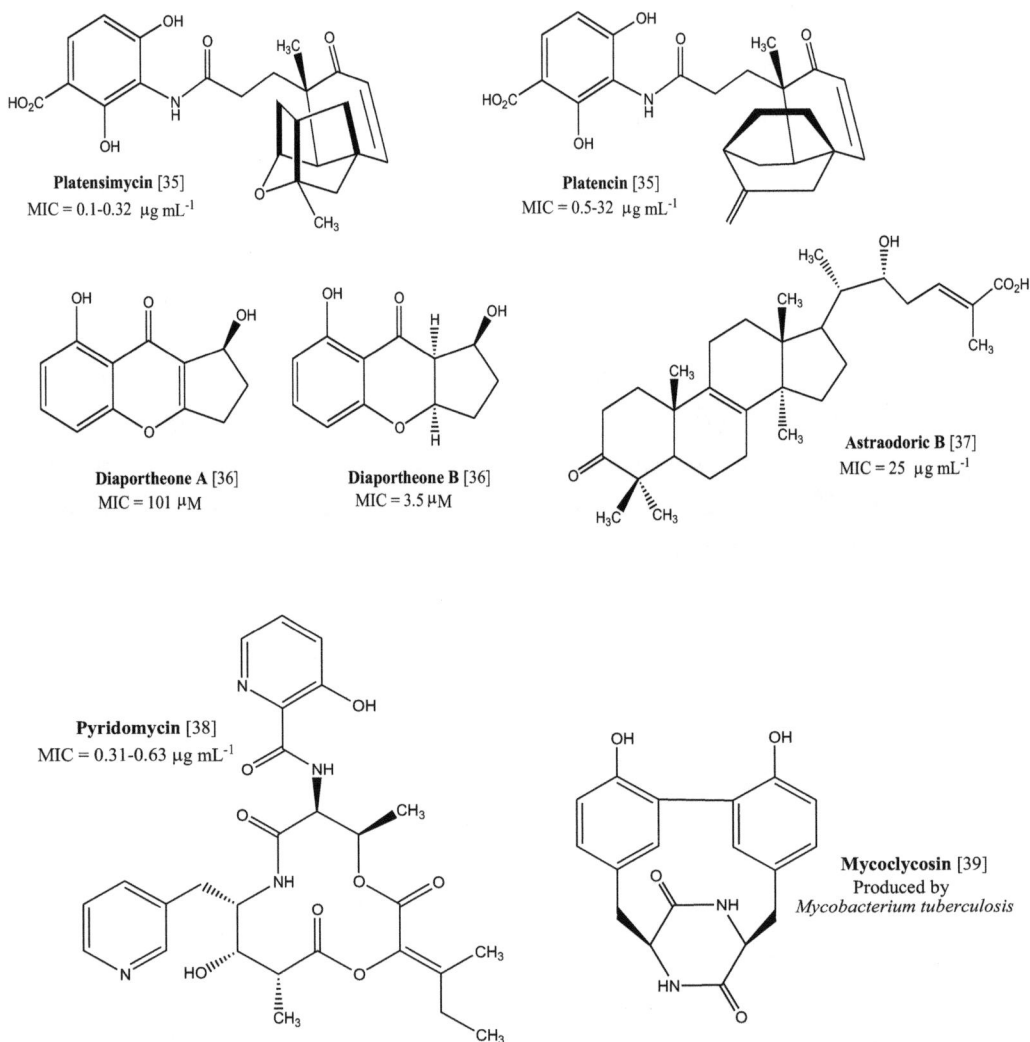

Figure 16: Natural products from fungi found between 2011 and 2012.

ACKNOWLEDGEMENT

None Declared.

CONFLICT OF INTEREST

The author(s) confirm that this chapter content has no conflict of interest.

REFERENCES

[1] De Souza MVN. Promising candidates in clinical trials against multidrug-resistant tuberculosis (MDR-TB) based on natural products. *Fitoterapia* 2009;**80**:453-460.

[2] Isaka M, Rugseree M, Maithip P, Kongsaeree P, Prabpaib S, Thebtaranontha Y. Hirsutellones A-E, antimycobacterial alkaloids from the insect pathogenic fungus Hirsutella nivea BCC 2594. *Tetrahedron* 2005;**61**:5577-5583.

[3] Sakuda S, Zhou ZY, Yamada Y. Structure of a Novel Disulfide of 2-(*N*-Acetylcysteinyl)amido-2-deoxy-α-D-glucopyran-osyl-myo-inositol Produced by Streptomyces sp. *Biosci Biotechnol Biochem* 1994;**58**:1347-8.

[4] Lee S, Rosazza JPN. First Total Synthesis of Mycothiol and Mycothiol Disulfide. *Org Lett* 2004;**6**:365-368.

[5] Newton GL, Leung SS, Wakabayashi JI, Rawat M, Fahey RC.The DinB superfamily includes novel mycothiol, bacillithiol, and glutathione S-transferases. *Biochemistry* 2011;**50**:10751-60.

[6] Sareen D, Newton GL, Fahey RC, Buchmeier NA. Mycothiol is essential for growth of *Mycobacterium tuberculosis* Erdman. *J Bacteriol* 2003;**185**:6736-40.

[7] Sareen D, Newton GL, Fahey RC, Buchmeier NA. Biosynthesis and functions of mycothiol, the unique protective thiol of Actinobacteria. *Microbiol Mol Biol Rev* 2008;**72**:471-94.

[8] Spies HSC, Steenkamp DJ. Thiols of intracellular pathogens. Identification of ovothiol A in *Leishmania* donovani and structural analysis of a novel thiol from *Mycobacterium bovis*. *Eur J Biochem* 1994;**224**:203-13.

[9] Fahey RC. Novel thiols of prokaryotes. *Annu Rev Microbiol* 2001;**55**:333-56.

[10] Blanchard JS, Patel MP. Synthesis of Des-*myo*-Inositol Mycothiol and Demonstration of a Mycobacterial Specific Reductase Activity. *J Am Chem Soc* 1998;**120**:11538-9.

[11] Dettrakul S, Kittakoop P, Isaka M, Nopichai S, Suyarnestakorn C, Tantichareon M, Thebtaranonth Y. Antimycobacterial pimarane diterpenes from the Fungus *Diaporthe* sp. *Bioorg Med Chem Lett* 2003;**13**:1253-5.

[12] De Souza MVN. Plants and Fungal Products with activity against Tuberculosis. *The Scientific World Journal* 2005;**5**:609-628.

[13] Kondo S, Yasui K, Natsume M, Katayama M, Marumo S. Isolation, physico-chemical properties and biological activity of pamamycin-607, an aerial mycelium-inducing substance from Streptomyces alboniger. *J. Antibiot* 1988;**41**:1196-204.

[14]   Lee E, Jeong EJ, Kang, EJ, Lee Taek Sung LT, and Sung Kil Hong, SK. Total Synthesis of Pamamycin-607. *J Am Chem Soc* 2001;**123**:10131-10132

[15]   McCann PA, Pogell BM. Pamamycin: a new antibiotic and stimulator of aerial mycelia formation *J Antibiot* 1979;**32**:673-678.

[16]   Pogell BM. The Pamamycins: developmental autoregulators and antibiotics from *Streptomyces alboniger*. A review and update. *Cell Mol Biol* 1998;**44**:461-3.

[17]   Thuggacins, Macrolide Antibiotics Active against Mycobacterium tuberculosis: Isolation from Myxobacteria, Structure Elucidation, Conformation Analysis and Biosynthesis Steinmetz H, Irschik H, Kunze B, Reichenbach H, Hofle G, Jansen R. *Chem Eur J* 2007; **13**:5822-5832.

[18]   Seephonkai P, Isaka M, Kittakoop P, Palittapongarnpim P, Kamchonwongpaisan S, Tanticharoen M, Thebtaranonth Y. Evaluation of Antimycobacterial, Antiplasmodial and Cytotoxic Activities of Preussomerins Isolated from the Lichenicolous Fungus Microsphaeropsis sp. BCC 3050. *Planta Med* 2000;**68**:45-8.

[19]   Prajoubklanga A, Sirithunyaluga B, Charoenchaib P, Suvannakadb R, Sriubolmasc N, Piyamongkola S, Kongsaereed P, Kittakoop P. Bioactive Deoxypreussomerins and Dimeric Naphthoquinones from Diospyros ehretioides Fruits: Deoxypreussomerins May Not Be Plant Metabolites But May Be from Fungal Epiphytes or Endophytes. *Chemistry & Biodiversity* 2005;**2**:1358-1367.

[20]   Nilanonta C, Isaka M, Chanphen R, Thong-orn N, Tanticharoen M, Thebtaranonth Y. Unusual enniatins produced by the insect pathogenic fungus Verticillium hemipterigenum: isolation and studies on precursor-directed biosynthesis. *Tetrahedron* 2003;**59**:1015-1020.

[21]   Vongvilaia P, Isaka M, Kittakoop P, Srikitikulchai P, Kongsaereea P, Prabpaia S, Thebtaranontha Y. Isolation and Structure Elucidation of Enniatins L, M1, M2, and N: Novel Hydroxy Analogs. *Helv Chim Acta* 2004;**87**:2066-2073.

[22]   Vongvanich N, Kittakoop P, Isaka M, Trakulnaleamsai S, Vimuttipong S, Tanticharoen M, Thebtaranonth Y. Hirsutellide A, a New Antimycobacterial Cyclohexadepsipeptide from the Entomopathogenic Fungus Hirsutella kobayasii. *J Nat Prod* 2002;**65**:1346.

[23]   Pucci MJ, Bronson JJ, Barrett JF, DenBleyker KL, Discotto, LF, Fung-Tomc JC, Ueda Y. Antimicrobial Evaluation of Nocathiacins, a Thiazole Peptide Class of Antibiotics. *Antimicrobial Agents and Chemotherapy* 2004;**48**:3697-3701.

[24]   Collignona P, Turnidge J. Fusidic acid *in vitro* activity. *International Journal of Antimicrobial Agents* 1999;**12**:S45-S58.

[25]   Cantrell CL, Lu T, Fronczek FR, Fischer NH, Adams LB, Franzblau SG. Antimycobacterial Cycloartanes from *Borrichia frutescens*. *J Nat Prod* 1996;**59**:1131-6.

[26]   Hoffner SE, Olsson-Liljequist B, Rydgaard KJ, Svenson SB. Kaellenius G. Susceptibility of mycobacteria to fusic acid. *Eur J Clin Microbiol Infect Dis* 1990;**9**:294-7.

[27]   Isaka M, Jaturapat A, Rukseree K, Danwisetkanjana K, Tanticharoen M, Thebtaranonth Y. Novel Xanthone Dimers from the Endophytic Fungus Phomopsis Species. *J Nat Prod* 2001;**64**:1015-1018.

[28]   Structure and Total Synthesis of Fungal Calpinactam, A New Antimycobacterial Agent Koyama N, Kojima S, Fukuda T, Nagamitsu T, Yasuhara T, Omura S, Tomoda H. *Org Lett* 2010;**12**:432-435.

[29] Souza MVN, Ferreira M, Pinheiro AC, Saraiva MF, Almeida MV, Valle MS. Synthesis and biological aspects of mycolic acids: an important target against *Mycobacterium tuberculosis*. *TSWJ* 2008;**8:**720-51.

[30] Igarashi M, Takahashi Y, Shitara T, Nakamura H, Naganawa H, Miyake T, Akamatsu Y. Caprazamycins, novel lipo-nucleoside antibiotics, from Streptomyces sp.: II. Structure elucidation of caprazamycins. *J Antibiot* 2005;**58**:327-37.

[31] Zhang W, Ostash B, Walsh CT. Identification of the biosynthetic gene cluster for the pacidamycin group of peptidyl nucleoside antibiotics. *Proc natl Acad Sci USA* 2010;**107:**16828-33.

[32] Vergne AF, Walz AJ, Miller MJ. Iron chelators from mycobacteria (1954-1999) and potential therapeutic applications *Nat Prod Rep* 2000;**17**:99-116

[33] Hu J, Miller JM. Total Synthesis of a Mycobactin S, a Siderophore and Growth Promoter of *Mycobacterium Smegmatis*, and Determination of its Growth Inhibitory Activity against *Mycobacterium tuberculosis*. *J Am Chem Soc* 1997;**119**:3462-3468.

[34] Walz AJ, Möllmann U, Miller MJ. Synthesis and studies of catechol-containing mycobactin S and T analogs. *Org Biomol Chem* 2007;**5**:1621-1628.

[35] Martens E, Demain AL. Platensimycin and platencin: promising antibiotics for future application in human medicine. *J Antibiot (Tokyo).* 2011;**64**:705-10.

[36] Swaroop PS, Raut GN, Gonnade RG, Verma P, Gokhale RS, Reddy DS. Antituberculosis agent diaportheone B: synthesis, absolute configuration assignment, and anti-TB activity of its analogues. *Org Biomol Chem* 2012;**10**:5385-94.

[37] Arpha K, Phosri C, Suwannasai N, Mongkolthanaruk W, Sodngam S. Astraodoric acids A-D: new lanostane triterpenes from edible mushroom Astraeus odoratus and their anti-*Mycobacterium tuberculosis* H37Ra and cytotoxic activity. *J Agric Food Chem* 2012;**60**:9834-41.

[38] Hartkoorn RC, Sala C, Neres J, Pojer F, Magnet S, Mukherjee R, Uplekar S, Rottger SB, Altmann, KH, Cole ST. Towards a new tuberculosis drug: pyridomycin - nature's isoniazid. *EMBO Mol Med* 2012;**4**:1032-1042.

[39] Cochrane JR, White JM, Wille U, Hutton CA. Total synthesis of mycocyclosin. *Org Lett* 2012;**14**:2402-5.

CHAPTER 8

Anti-TB Evaluation of Marine Natural Products

Marcus V.N. de Souza[*]

Instituto de Tecnologia em Fármacos – Farmanguinhos, FioCruz – Fundação Oswaldo Cruz, R. Sizenando Nabuco, 100, Manguinhos, 21041-250, Rio de Janeiro, RJ, Brazil

Abstract: The interest of marine natural products in the development of new drugs to treat tuberculosis began in the 1990s with compounds isolated and evaluated in both plant and animal sources becoming an important source of new anti-TB compounds that will be covered in this chapter.

Keywords: Tuberculosis, *Mycobacterium tuberculosis*, natural products, sea, semi-synthesis, synthesis, analogues, treatment, multi-drug-resistant tuberculosis (MDR TB), extensive-drug-resistant tuberculosis (XDR TB), target, mechanism of action, biological evaluation, drug development.

INTRODUCTION

The history of the development of new anti-tuberculosis drugs from natural marine source began in the 1990s with studies of Hamann and Andersen who isolated and evaluated the anti-TB activity of peptide compounds *in vitro* (Fig. **1** and **2**) [1-7]. After that, Hamman and co-workers continued to make important contributions in this field with the isolation, identification and anti-TB evaluation of several natural products belonging to different class, some of them will be discussed in this chapter.

In 1997, Anderson and colleagues also gave an important contribution to the search for new substances with activity against tuberculosis resulting from marine sources [6,7]. They have isolated and evaluated, massetolide A (MIC = 5-10 μg/mL) and viscosin (MIC = 10-20 μg/mL), cyclic depsipeptides isolated from a marine alga and tube worm, respectively (Fig. **2**).

*Adress correspondence to Marcus V.N. de Souza:** Instituto de Tecnologia em Fármacos – Farmanguinhos, FioCruz – Fundação Oswaldo Cruz, R. Sizenando Nabuco, 100, Manguinhos, 21041-250, Rio de Janeiro, RJ, Brazil; E-mail: marcos_souza@far.fiocruz.br

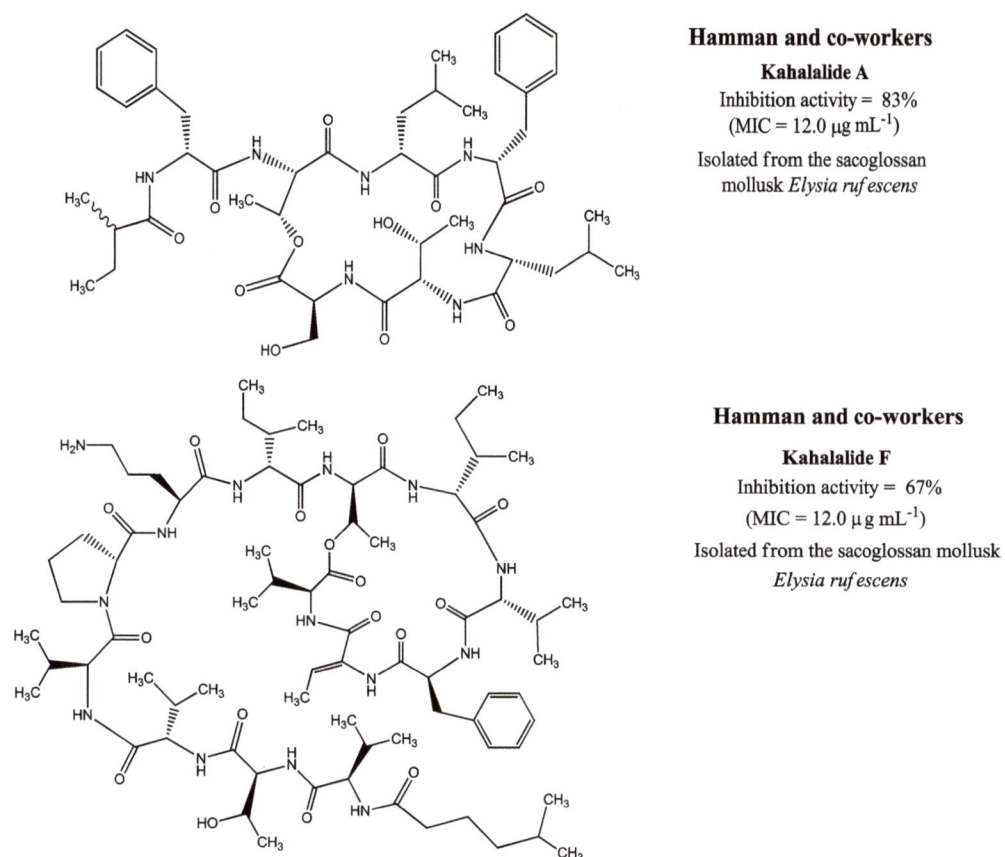

Hamman and co-workers

Kahalalide A

Inhibition activity = 83%

(MIC = 12.0 µg mL^{-1})

Isolated from the sacoglossan
mollusk *Elysia rufescens*

Hamman and co-workers

Kahalalide F

Inhibition activity = 67%

(MIC = 12.0 µg mL^{-1})

Isolated from the sacoglossan mollusk
Elysia rufescens

Figure 1: Structure of kahalalide A and F.

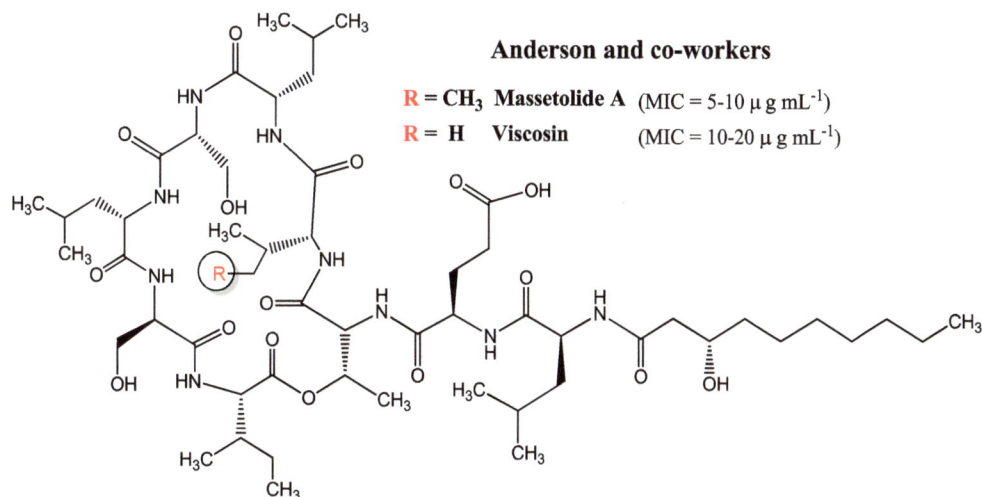

Anderson and co-workers

R = CH$_3$ Massetolide A (MIC = 5-10 µg mL^{-1})

R = H   Viscosin (MIC = 10-20 µg mL^{-1})

Figure 2: Structure of massetolide A and viscosin.

ALKALOIDS

Agelasines

Gundersen and co-workers [8] synthesized the marine natural product agelasine E and several analogues (Fig. **3**) and evaluated them against *Mycobacterium tuberculosis*. This compound, a 7,9-dialkylpurinium salts, was isolated from the marine sponge *Agelas nakamurai*, and it was inactive against this bacteria, however the synthetic *N*-6-methoxy analogues **1** and **2** possess good activity with MIC of 3.13 and 1.56 μgmL^{-1}, respectively.

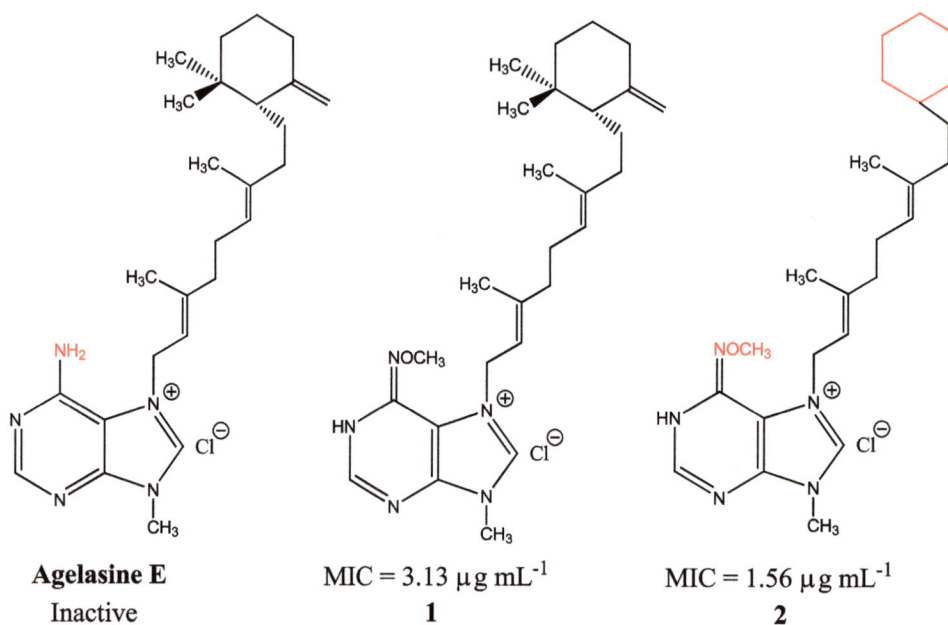

| **Agelasine E** | MIC = 3.13 $\mu g\ mL^{-1}$ | MIC = 1.56 $\mu g\ mL^{-1}$ |
| Inactive | **1** | **2** |

In red: Important positions and / or groups for biological activity.

Figure 3: Structure of agelasine E and analogues.

(+)-Araguspongine C

The red sea specimens of *Xestospongia exigua* [9] possesses diverse biologically significant properties such as vasodilatation [10,11], cytotoxicity [12], antifungal [13] and vasoactive intestinal peptide inhibition [14]. Due to its wide range of biological activities, Orabi and co-workers [15] identified the (+)-araguspongine C, which displayed a promising anti-TB activity with MIC = 3.94 µg/mL [5,15] (Fig. **4**).

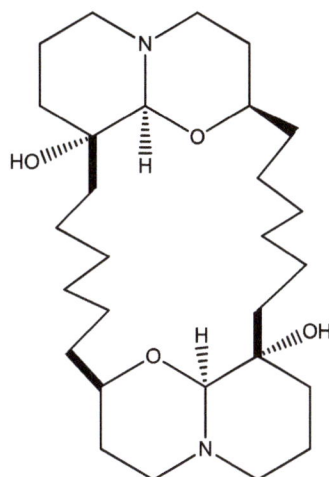

(+)-Araguspongines C
(MIC = 3.94 μ g mL^{-1})

Figure 4: Structure of (+)-araguspongine C.

Australian Non-Verongid Sponge

The enzyme mycothiol S-conjugate amidase (MCA) has several functions such as, remove toxins, alkylating agents, antibiotics and oxidative stress having a critical role in the protection and growth of *Mycobacterium tuberculosis*. In this context, the new alkaloid **3** was one of the first to inhibit this enzyme, which was isolated and identified by Bewley and co-workers from Australian non-verongid sponge (Fig. **5**) [16-18] together with other four new alkaloids, which also displayed inhibition against MCA. Due to its promising perspectives against *Mycobacterium tuberculosis*, the marine natural product **3** was synthesized by Kende and his group in five steps.

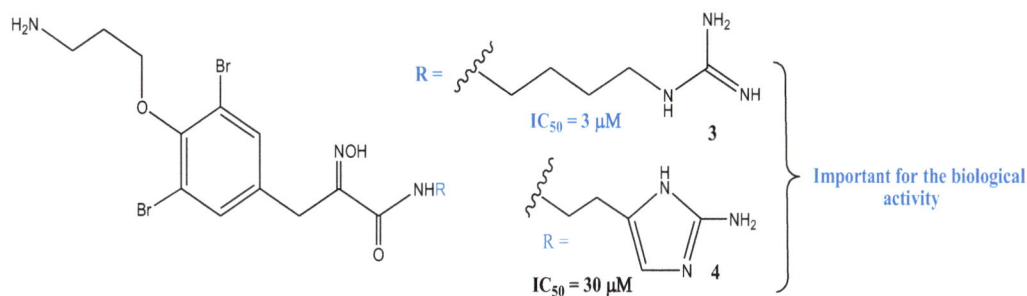

Figure 5: Structure of new alkaloids 3,4 from Australian non-verongid sponge.

Cyclostellettamines

Berlinck and co-workers [19] isolated cyclostellettamines A – F (**5 – 10**) from the sponge *Pachychalina* sp. and cyclostellettamines G - I, K and L (**11 – 15**) obtained by total synthesis (Fig. **6**). These compounds were evaluated against *Mycobacterium tuberculosis* H37Rv, and the isolated cyclostellettamines **6** and **7** (MIC = 4.0 µg mL^{-1}) and the obtained by total synthesis **11** and **15** (MIC = 4.6 µg mL^{-1}). These results suggest the importance of the alkyl-chain size on the distance between the two pyridinium moieties of cyclostellettamines for the activity.

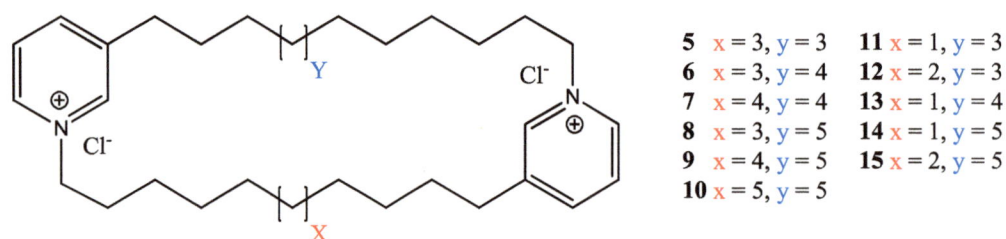

5	x = 3, y = 3	**11**	x = 1, y = 3
6	x = 3, y = 4	**12**	x = 2, y = 3
7	x = 4, y = 4	**13**	x = 1, y = 4
8	x = 3, y = 5	**14**	x = 1, y = 5
9	x = 4, y = 5	**15**	x = 2, y = 5
10	x = 5, y = 5		

Figure 6: Structures of cyclostellettamines A – F (5-10), G - I, K and L (11 – 15).

Ecteinascidins

The class of alkaloid known as Ecteinascidin is commonly isolated from the marine tunicate *Ecteinascidia turbinate* showing potent cytotoxic activity, such as ecteinascidin 743, which is under phase II clinical trials for cancer treatment [20-24]. In the search for new bioactive compounds, Suwanborirux and co-workers isolated and evaluated from Thai tunicate *Ecteinascidia thurstoni* [25] the marine compounds ecteinascidins 770 and 786, which displayed promising anti-TB activity with MIC values of 0.13 and 2.0 µg/mL, respectively (Fig. **7**) [5,25].

Halicyclamine A

Kobayashi and co-workers [26] found a potent anti-TB activity in the marine natural product halicyclamine A (Fig. **8**). This compound was isolated from Indonesian sponge of Haliclona sp. and exhibited activity against *Mycobacterium tuberculosis* under both aerobic and hypoxic condition inducing dormant state. The MIC value of this natural product against *Mycobacterium* H37Rv was 6.25 µgmL^{-1} and the inhibition was in the range of 3.13-6.25 µgmL^{-1}. These results suggests that halicyclamine A would have a different mechanism of action than the first line of TB drugs such as isoniazid, ethambutol, rifampin and the second line drugs such as streptomycin. Another important information is that the growth-inhibitory activity of halicyclamine A was bactericidal, and with isoniazid, ethambutol, rifampin and streptomycin no cross-resistance was observed.

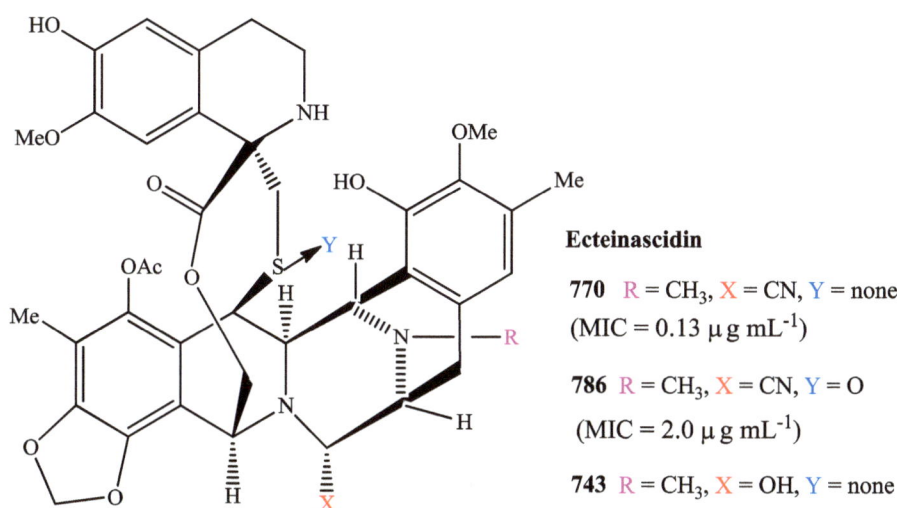

Figure 7: Structure of ecteinascidins **770**, **786** and **743**.

Ecteinascidin

770 R = CH₃, X = CN, Y = none
(MIC = 0.13 µg mL⁻¹)

786 R = CH₃, X = CN, Y = O
(MIC = 2.0 µg mL⁻¹)

743 R = CH₃, X = OH, Y = none

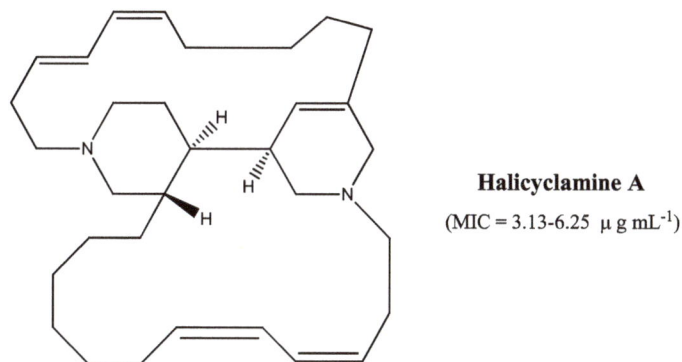

Halicyclamine A
(MIC = 3.13-6.25 µg mL⁻¹)

Figure 8: Structure of halicyclamine A.

Ingenamine G

Ingenamine G (Fig. **9**) and different compounds were isolated from methanol crude extract of the marine sponge *Pachychalina* sp. by Berlinck and co-workers [5,27]. This compound showed a MIC of 8 µg/mL.

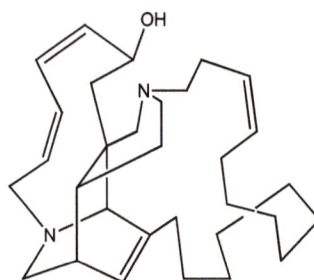

Ingenamine G
(MIC = 8.0 µ g mL⁻¹)

Figure 9: Structure of ingenamine G.

Manzamines

The marine ß-carboline alkalloid class named manzamine is isolated from sponges and exhibits very a large number of pharmacological properties, such as antimalarial, anti-TB, anti-HIV and cytotoxic activity. In this context, several compounds of this family, which display a complex chemical structure, have been evaluated against *Mycobacterium tuberculosis*. Hamman and co-workers isolated and tested new manzanines from Indonesian sponges [28-30]. Considering that, the two new alkaloids called manadomanzamines A and B (Fig. **10**) isolated from Indonesian sponge *Acanthostrongylophora* sp. (Haploscilerida: Petrosiidae) [31]

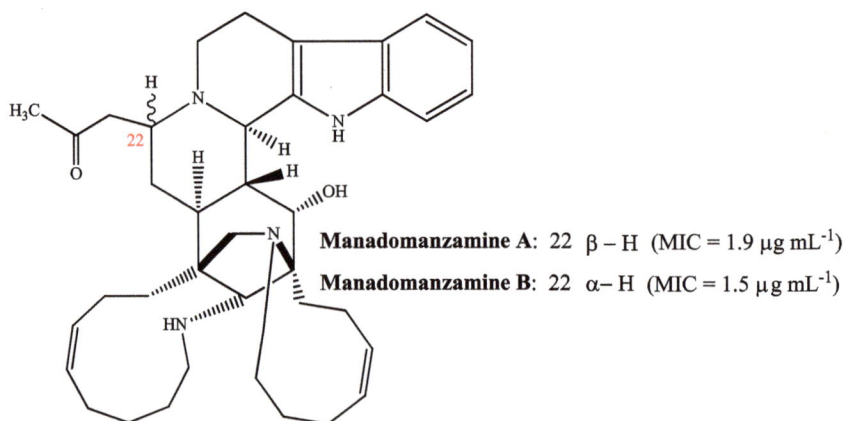

Manadomanzamine A: 22 β – H (MIC = 1.9 µg mL⁻¹)
Manadomanzamine B: 22 α– H (MIC = 1.5 µg mL⁻¹)

Figure 10: Structure of manadomanzamine A and B.

that exhibited strong activity against *M. tuberculosis* with MIC values of 1.9 and 1.5 µg/mL, respectively. These two alkaloids also exhibited significant activity against human immunodeficiency virus (HIV-1) with EC$_{50}$ values of 7.0 and 16.5 µg/mL, respectively and moderate activity against several AIDS opportunistic infections [31,5].

Other manzamines have also been isolated and evaluated by Hamman and co-workers, which demonstrated potent anti-TB activity establishing some SAR information (Fig. **11**).

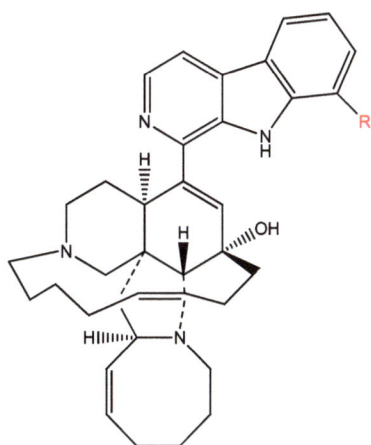

R = H   MIC = 1.53 µg/mL
R = OH MIC = 0.91 µg/mL

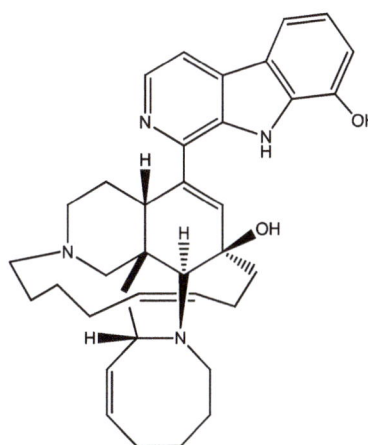

MIC = 3.13 µg/mL

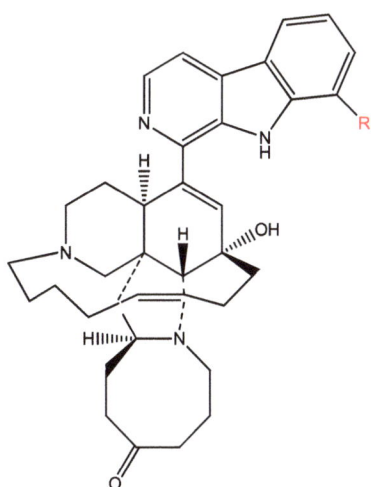

R = H   MIC = 3.76 µg/mL
R = OH MIC = 2.56 µg/mL

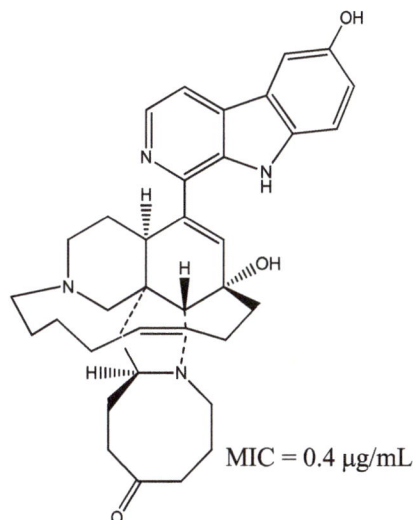

MIC = 0.4 µg/mL

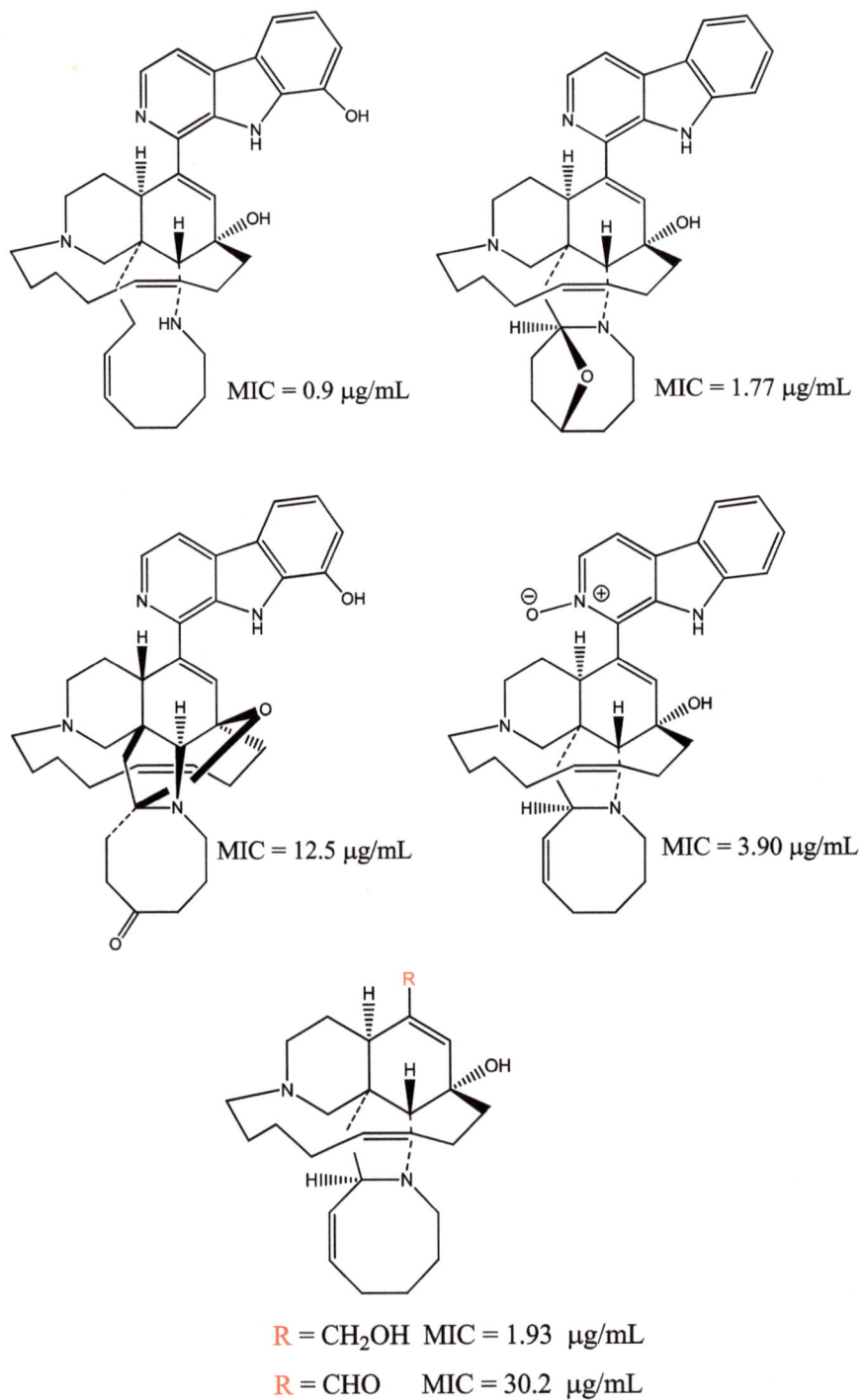

MIC = 0.9 μg/mL

MIC = 1.77 μg/mL

MIC = 12.5 μg/mL

MIC = 3.90 μg/mL

R = CH₂OH MIC = 1.93 μg/mL

R = CHO   MIC = 30.2 μg/mL

Figure 11: Manzamine class aganist *M. Tuberculosis*.

West Indian Corals Gorgonian Octocoral *Pseudopterogorgia Elisabethae*

The alkaloids pseudopteroxazole, homopseudopteroxazole and *seco*-pseudopteroxazole (Fig. **12**) were isolated from an extract of the West Indian corals gorgonian octocoral *Pseudopterogorgia elisabethae* Bayer (order Gorgonacea, family Gorgoniidae, phylum Cnideria) from the waters near San Andréas Islands, Colombia. This work was conducted by Rodrigues and co-workers, which also evaluated the anti-TB activity of these marine natural products, which displayed a MIC of 12.5 µg/mL, which induced at this concentration 97, 88, and 66% inhibition of *Mycobacterium tuberculosis* H37Rv, respectively [32]. From this extract Rodrigues and co-workers also isolated and evaluated other natural product against this disease, such as the diterpenes erogorgiaene and 7-hydroxyerogorgiaene, which displayed MIC = 12.5 µg/mL (96% inhibition) and 6.25 µg/mL (77% inhibition), respectively, which indicated that the oxazole moiety is not essential for activity. Finally, elisapterosin B [33-35] and cumbiasin A and B [36] (Fig. **12**) were also isolated from this extract and evaluated against *Mycobacterium tuberculosis,* however in the case of the compounds elisabethin A and colombiasin A its anti-TB activity have not yet been published [37].

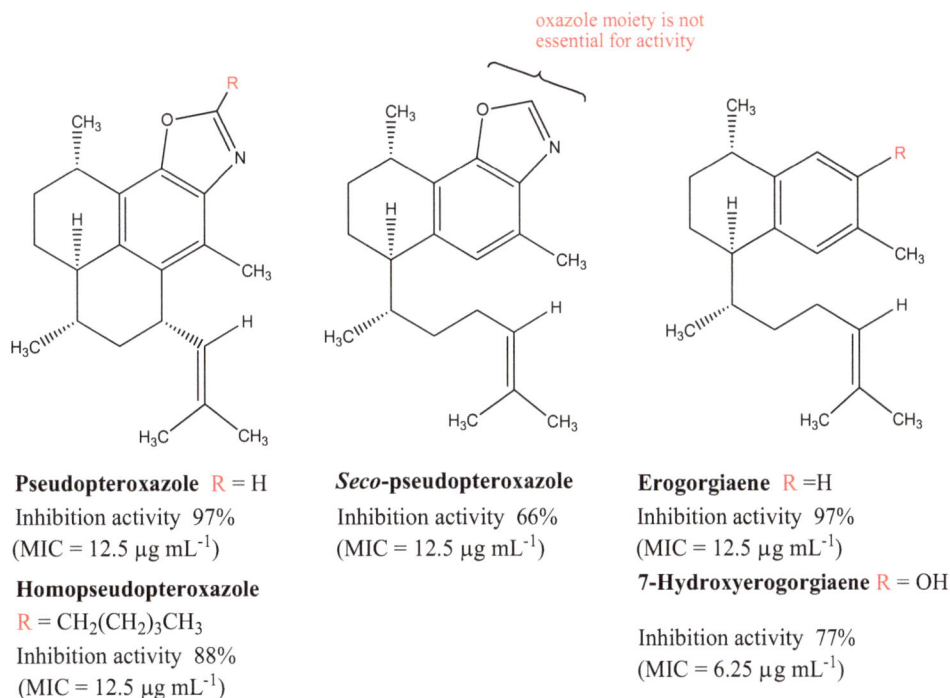

Pseudopteroxazole R = H
Inhibition activity 97%
(MIC = 12.5 µg mL^{-1})

Homopseudopteroxazole
R = CH$_2$(CH$_2$)$_3$CH$_3$
Inhibition activity 88%
(MIC = 12.5 µg mL^{-1})

***Seco*-pseudopteroxazole**
Inhibition activity 66%
(MIC = 12.5 µg mL^{-1})

Erogorgiaene R =H
Inhibition activity 97%
(MIC = 12.5 µg mL^{-1})

7-Hydroxyerogorgiaene R = OH

Inhibition activity 77%
(MIC = 6.25 µg mL^{-1})

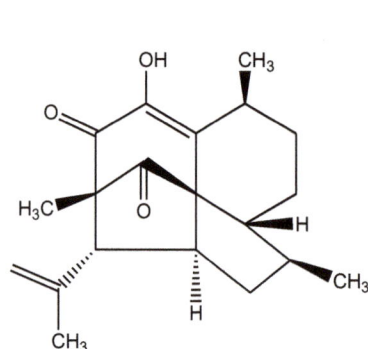

Elisapterosin B
(MIC = 12.3 µg mL^{-1})

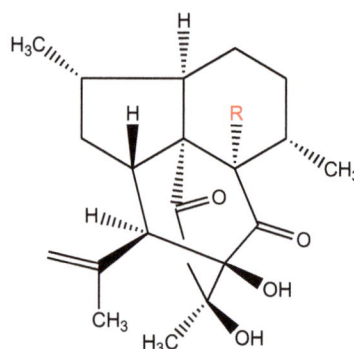

Cumbiasin A R = H   (MIC = 6.25 µg mL^{-1})
Cumbiasin B R = OH   (MIC = 12.5 µg mL^{-1})

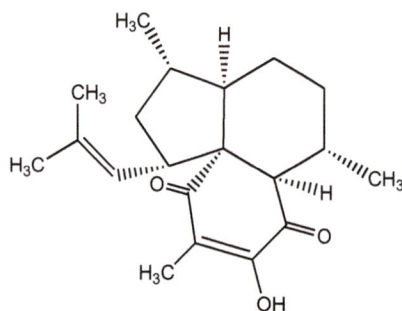

Elisabethin A

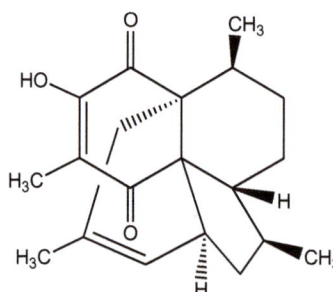

Colombiasin A

MIC have not yet been determinated

Figure 12: Structures of compounds isolated by Rodrigues and co-workers from the West Indian corals gorgonian octocoral *Pseudopterogorgia elisabethae*.

TERPENES

Diterpenes

Axisonitrile-3

The natural product axisonitrile-3 (Fig. **13**) was the best anti-TB compound, which was evaluated from different natural products representative of different classes, such as terpenes, aliphatics, aromatics, alkaloids and sterols [38,5]. This work was conducted by Konig and co-workers, which isolated axisonitrile-3 from the sponge *Acanthella klethra* (MIC = 2.0 µg/mL) with no toxicity to Vero cells at concentrations <200 µg/mL.

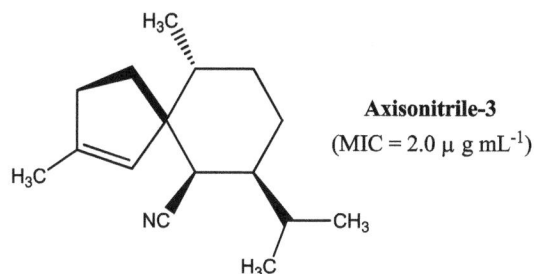

Axisonitrile-3
(MIC = 2.0 μ g mL^{-1})

Figure 13: Structure of axisonitrile-3.

Cyanthiwigin (C)

From Jamaican sponge *Mymekioderma styx* [39,40], Hamman and co-workers isolated and evaluated twenty-seven diterpenes called cyanthiwigins. The natural product known as cyanthiwigin (C) [5,41] was the most active against *Mycobacterium tuberculosis* with 50% of inhibition at 6.25 μg/mL (Fig. **14**).

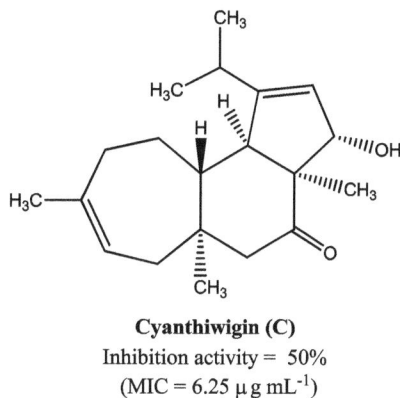

Cyanthiwigin (C)
Inhibition activity = 50%
(MIC = 6.25 μ g mL^{-1})

Figure 14: Structure of cyanthiwigin (C).

SESQUITERPENE

Aureol

The known sesquiterpene aureol **19**, 6'-chloroaureol **20**, and aureol acetate **21** was isolated by Hamann and co-workers [42] from the marine sponge *Smenospongia aurea*, which was collected at Discovery Bay (Jamaica) (Fig. **15**). The aureol was used to produce two new aureole derivatives **22** and **23** in one step. The evaluation against *Mycobacterium tuberculosis* indicated that the thiocarbamate moiety was important to increase the potency of this class of compounds (Fig. **15**).

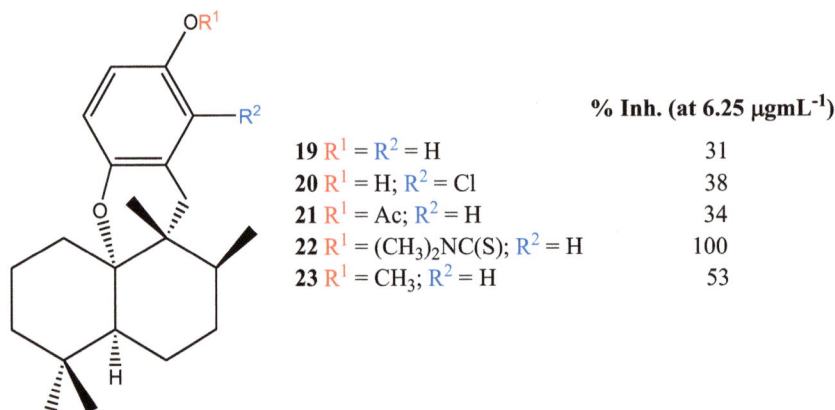

		% Inh. (at 6.25 μgmL^{-1})
19 R^1 = R^2 = H		31
20 R^1 = H; R^2 = Cl		38
21 R^1 = Ac; R^2 = H		34
22 R^1 = (CH$_3$)$_2$NC(S); R^2 = H		100
23 R^1 = CH$_3$; R^2 = H		53

Figure 15: Structures of aureole derivatives.

SESTERPENES

Thai sponge B *Brachiaster* sp

Plubrukarn and co-workers have isolated and tested different sesterpenes from Thai sponge B *Brachiaster* sp against *M. tuberculosis* (H37Rv), such as 12-deacetoxyscalarin 19-acetate and the manoalide 25-acetate (Fig. **16**) with MIC values of 4 and 7 μg/mL, respectively [43,5].

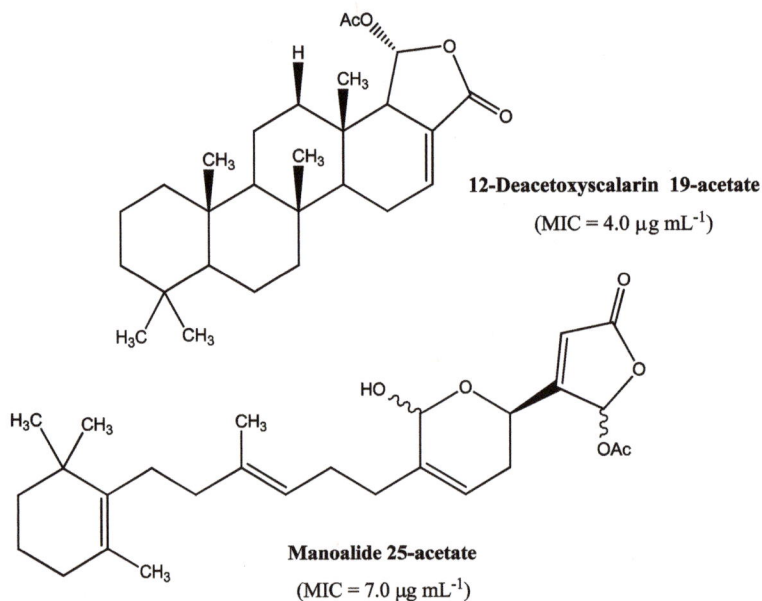

12-Deacetoxyscalarin 19-acetate

(MIC = 4.0 μg mL^{-1})

Manoalide 25-acetate

(MIC = 7.0 μg mL^{-1})

Figure 16: Structures of 12-deacetoxyscalarin 19-acetate and the manoalide 25-acetate.

STEROLS

Linesterol and Nephalsterol B and C

Hamann and his group also evaluated the anti-TB activity of marine sterols. In this context it can be mentioned the C-19 hydroxysteroids litosterol, nephalsterol B and C that were isolated from red sea *Nepthea* sp (Fig. **17**) [44-46]. The natural product litosterol and nephalsterol C had MICs of 3.13 and 12.5 µg/mL inhibiting 90 and 96% of the growth of *M. tuberculosis* (H_{37}Rv) respectively. However, nephalsterol B inhibited only 69% at the same concentration, which indicated that C-7 hydroxylation could reduce the activity. When C-7 hydroxyl was blocked by an acetate group as in the case of nephalsterol C or when it was absent as in litosterol, an improvement of the biological activity was observed [5].

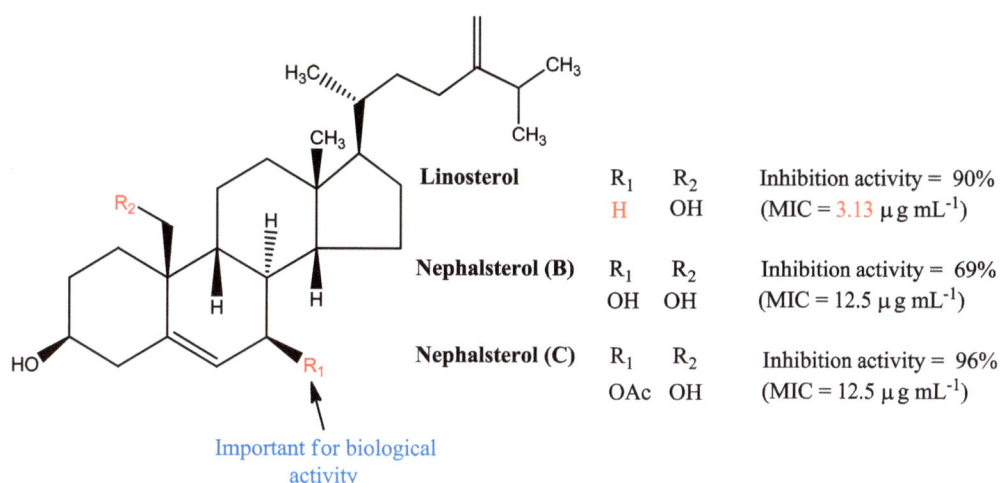

	R$_1$	R$_2$	
Linosterol	H	OH	Inhibition activity = 90% (MIC = 3.13 µg mL^{-1})
Nephalsterol (B)	OH	OH	Inhibition activity = 69% (MIC = 12.5 µg mL^{-1})
Nephalsterol (C)	OAc	OH	Inhibition activity = 96% (MIC = 12.5 µg mL^{-1})

Important for biological activity

Figure 17: Structure of linesterol and nephalsterol B and C.

Saringesterol

Another contribution in this class of compounds was made by Timmermann and co-workers, which isolated from the Chilean brown algae *Lessonia nigrescens Bory* (*Phaeophyta, Laminariales*) the phytosterol saringosterol (Fig. **18**) [5,47]. This natural product showed potent antitubercular activity against the H37Rv strain of *M. tuberculosis*. The 24*S* epimer of saringesterol presented MIC values of 0.125 µg/mL, eight times more active than their epimer 24*R* (1.0 µg/mL), indicating the importance of the hydroxyl position for biological activity.

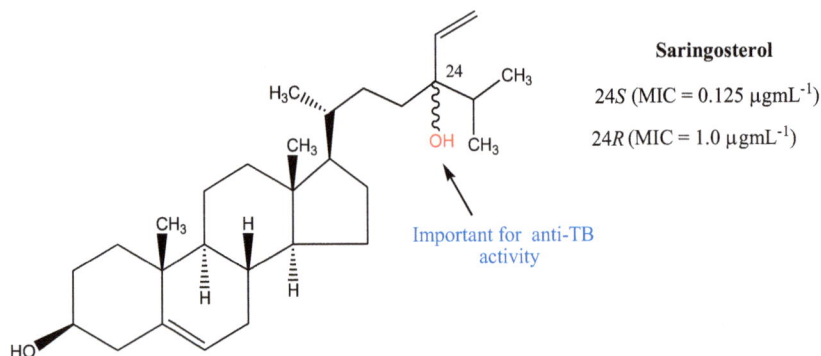

Saringosterol

24*S* (MIC = 0.125 µgmL⁻¹)

24*R* (MIC = 1.0 µgmL⁻¹)

Important for anti-TB activity

Figure 18: Structure of saringosterol.

SELECTED ANTI-TB MARINE NATURAL PRODUCTS FOUND BETWEEN 2011 AND 2013

This section it will highlight select natural products of different class covered between 2011 and 2013, with the respective structure, activity and reference. The selection was based on the potency and other promises perspectives of the compounds (Fig. **19**).

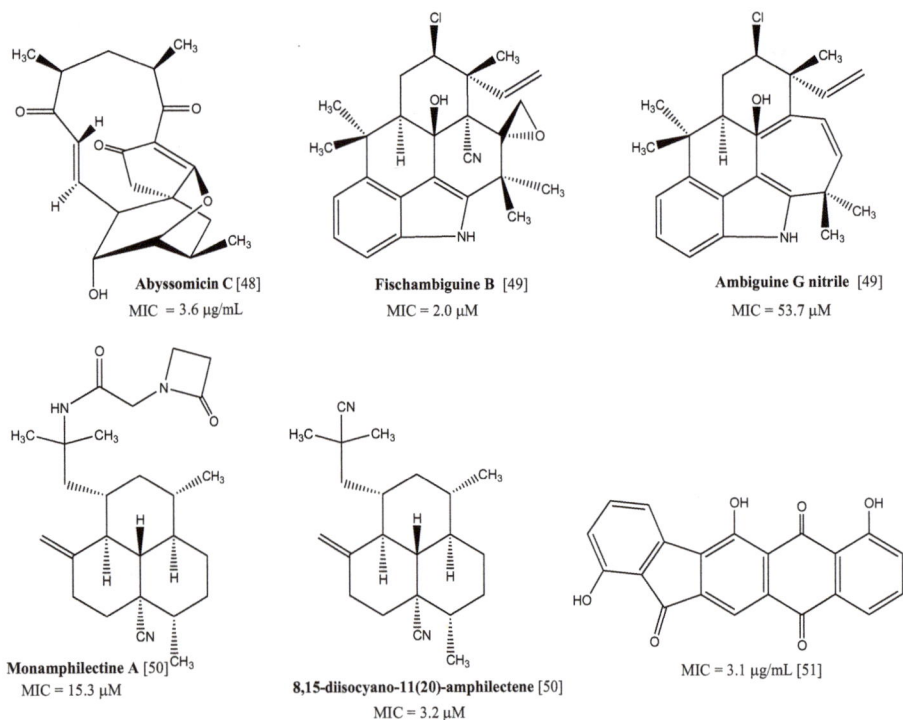

Abyssomicin C [48]
MIC = 3.6 µg/mL

Fischambiguine B [49]
MIC = 2.0 µM

Ambiguine G nitrile [49]
MIC = 53.7 µM

Monamphilectine A [50]
MIC = 15.3 µM

8,15-diisocyano-11(20)-amphilectene [50]
MIC = 3.2 µM

MIC = 3.1 µg/mL [51]

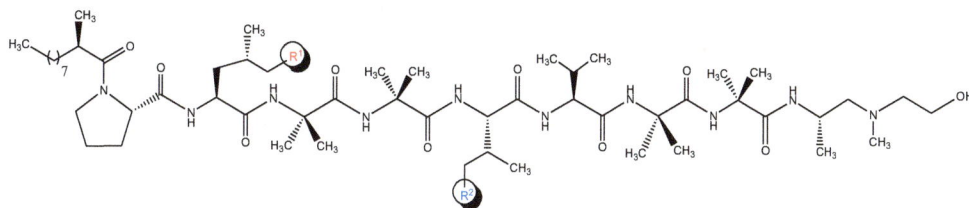

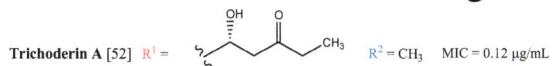

Trichoderin A [52]   R¹ =   R² = CH₃   MIC = 0.12 µg/mL

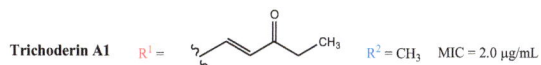

Trichoderin A1   R¹ =   R² = CH₃   MIC = 2.0 µg/mL

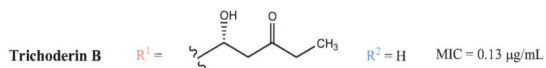

Trichoderin B   R¹ =   R² = H   MIC = 0.13 µg/mL

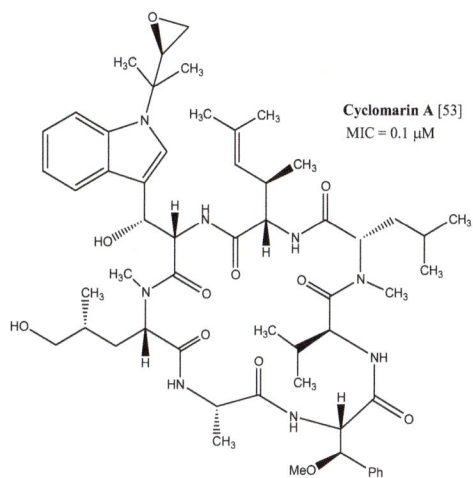

Cyclomarin A [53]
MIC = 0.1 µM

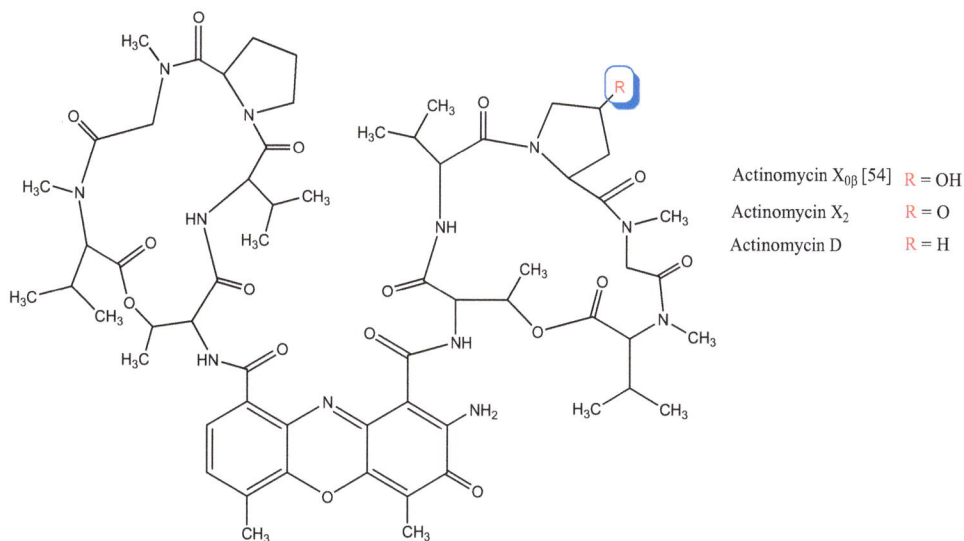

Actinomycin X₀β [54]   R = OH
Actinomycin X₂   R = O
Actinomycin D   R = H

MIC = 16 μg/mL [55]

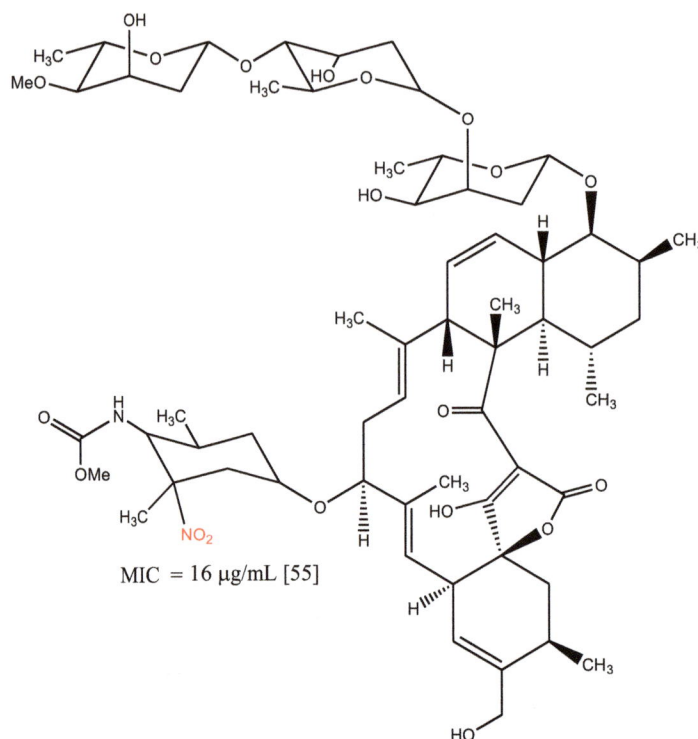

Figure 19: Anti-TB natural products found from fungi between 2011 and 2013.

ACKNOWLEDGEMENT

None Declare

CONFLICT OF INTEREST

The author(s) confirm that this chapter content has no conflict of interest.

REFERENCES

[1]　Hamann MT Scheuer PJ Kahalalide F. A bioactive depsipeptide from the sacoglossan mollusk Elysia rufescens and the green alga *Bryopsis sp. J Am Chem Soc* 1993;**115:**5825-6.

[2]　Hamann MT, Otto CS, Scheuer PJ Dunbar DC. Kahalalides: Bioactive Peptides from a Marine Mollusk *Elysia rufescens* and Its Algal Diet *Bryopsis* sp. *J Org Chem* 1996;**61:**6594-6600.

[3]　Bonnard I, Manzanares I, Rinehart KL. Stereochemistry of Kahalalide F. *J Nat Prod* 2003;**66:**1466-70.

[4]   Bourel-Bonnet L, Rao KV, Hamann MT, Ganesan A. Solid-Phase Total Synthesis of Kahalalide A and Related Analogues. *J Med Chem* 2005;**48**:1330-5.

[5]   De Souza MVN. Marine Natural Products Against Tuberculosis. *The Scientific World Journal* 2006;**6**:847-861.

[6]   Gerard J, Lloyd R, Barsby T, Haden P, Kelly MT, Andersen RJ. Massetolides A–H, Antimycobacterial Cyclic Depsipeptides Produced by Two Pseudomonads Isolated from Marine Habitats. *J Nat Prod* 1997;**60**:223-9.

[7]   Copp BR. Antimycobacterial natural products. *Nat Prod Rep* 2003;**20**:535-57.

[8]   Bakkestuen AK, Gundersen LL, Petersen D, Utenova BTVA. Synthesis and antimycobacterial activity of agelasine E and analogs. *Org Biomol Chem* 2005;**3**:1025–1033.

[9]   Rao J, Desaiah D, Vig P, Venkateswarlu Y. Marine biomolecules inhibit rat brain nitric oxide synthase. *Toxicology* 1998;**129**:103-110.

[10]   Gafni J, Munsch J, Lam T, Catlin M, Costa L, Molinski T, Pessah I. Xestospongins: potent membrane permeable blockers of the inositol 1,4,5-trisphosphate receptor. *Neuron* 1997;**19**:723-33.

[11]   De Smet P, Parys J, Callewaert G, Weidema A, Hill E, De Smet H, Erneux C, Sorrentino V, Missiaen L. Xestospongin C is an equally potent inhibitor of the inositol 1,4,5-trisphosphate receptor and the endoplasmic-reticulum Ca^{2+} pumps. *Cell Calcium* 1999; **26**:9-13.

[12]   Pettit G, Orr B, Herald D, Doubek D, Tackett L, Schmidt J, Boyd M, Pettit R, Hooper J. Isolation and X-ray crystal structure of racemic Xestospongin D from the Singapore marine sponge *Niphates sp¹*. *Bioorg Med Chem Lett* 1996;**6**:1313-18.

[13]   Moon S, MacMillan J, Olmstead M, Ta T, Pessah I, Molinski T. (+)-7S-Hydroxyxestospongin A from the Marine Sponge *Xestospongia* sp. and Absolute Configuration of (+)-Xestospongin D. *J Nat Prod* 2002;**65**:249-54.

[14]   Vassas A, Bourdy G, Paillard J, Lavayre J, Pais M, Quirion J, Debitus C. Naturally Occurring Somatostatin and Vasoactive Intestinal Peptide Inhibitors. Isolation of Alkaloids from Two Marine Sponges. *Planta Med* 1996;**62**:28-30.

[15]   Orabi KY, El Sayed KA, Hamann MT, Dunbar DC, Al Said MS, Higa T, Kelly M. Araguspongines K and L, New Bioactive Bis-1-oxaquinolizidine *N*-Oxide Alkaloids from Red Sea Specimens of *Xestospongia exigua*. *J Nat Prod* 2002;**65**:1782-5.

[16]   Nicholas GM, Newton GL, Fahey RC, Bewley CA. Novel Bromotyrosine Alkaloids: Inhibitors of Mycothiol *S*-Conjugate Amidase *Org Lett* 2001;**3**:1543-5.

[17]   Fetterolf B, Bewley CA. Synthesis of a bromotyrosine-derived natural product inhibitor of mycothiol-*S*-conjugate amidase. *Bioorg Med Chem Lett* 2004;**14**:3785-8.

[18]   Nicholas GM, Eckman LL, Newton GL, Fahey RC, Ray S, Bewley CA. Inhibition and kinetics of *mycobacterium tuberculosis* and *mycobacterium smegmatis* mycothiol-*S*-conjugate amidase by natural product inhibitors. *Bioorg Med Chem Lett* 2003;**11**:601-8.

[19]   De Oliveira JHHL, Seleghim MHR, Timm C, Grube A, Köck M, Nascimento GGF, Martins ACT, Silva EGO, Ana De Souza AO, Minarini PRR, Galetti FCS, Silva CL, Hajdu E, Berlinck RGS. Antimicrobial and Antimycobacterial Activity of Cyclostellettamine Alkaloids from Sponge Pachychalina sp. *Mar Drugs* 2006;**4**:1-8.

[20]   Izbicka E, Lawrence R, Raymond E, Eckhardt G, Faircloth G, Jimeno J, Clarck G, Von Hoff DD. *In vitro* antitumor activity of the novel marine agent, Ecteinascidin-743 (ET-743, NSC-648766) against human tumors explanted from patients. *Ann Oncol* 1998;**9**:981-7.

[21]   Ghielmini M, Colli E, Erba E, Bergamasci D, Pampallona S, Jimeno J, Faircloth G, Sessa C. *In vitro* schedule-dependency of myelotoxicity and cytotoxicity of Ecteinascidin 743 (ET-743). *Ann Oncol* 1998;**9**:989-93.

[22]   Hendriks, H.R., Fiebig, H.H., Giavazzi, R., Langdon, S.P., Jimeno, J.M., and Faircloth, G.T. High antitumour activity of ET743 against human tumour xenografts from melanoma, non-small-cell lung and ovarian cancer. *Ann Oncol* 1999;**10**:1233-40.

[23]   Jin S, Gorfajn B, Faircloth G, Scotto K. Ecteinascidin 743, a transcription-targeted chemotherapeutic that inhibits MDR1 activation. *Proc Natl Acad Sc. USA* 2000;**97**:6775-9.

[24]   Takebayashi Y, Pourquier P, Zimonjic DB, Nakayama K, Emmer S, Ueda T, Urasaki Y, Kanzaki A, Akiyama S, Popescu N, Kraemer KH, Pommier Y. Antiproliferative activity of ecteinascidin 743 is dependent upon transcription-coupled nucleotide-excision repair. *Nat Med* 2001;**7**:961-6.

[25]   Suwanborirux K, Charupant K, Amnuoypol S, Pummangura S, Kubo A, Saito N. Ecteinascidins 770 and 786 from the Thai Tunicate *Ecteinascidia thurstoni J Nat Prod* 2002;**65**:935-7.

[26]   Arai M, Sobou M, Vilchéze C, Baughn A, Hashizume H, Pruksakorn P, Ishida S, Matsumoto M, Jacobs Jr. WR, Kobayashi M. Halicyclamine A, a marine spongean alkaloid as a lead for anti-tuberculosis agent. *Bioorg & Med Chem* 2008;**16**:6732–6736.

[27]   De Oliveira JHH, Grube A, Kock M, Berlinck RGS, Macedo ML, Ferreira AG, Hajdu E. Ingenamine G and Cyclostellettamines G–I, K, and L from the New Brazilian Species of Marine Sponge *Pachychalina* sp. *J Nat Prod* 2004;**67**:1685-9.

[28]   Yousaf M, El Sayed KA, Rao KV, Lim CW, Hu JF, Kelly M, Frazblau SG, Zhang F, Peraud O, Hill R, Hamann MT. 12,34-Oxamanzamines, novel biocatalytic and natural products from manzamine producing Indo-Pacific sponges. *Tetrahedron* 2002;**58**:7397-02.

[29]   Rao KV, Donia MS, Peng J, Garcia-Palomero E, Alonso D, Martinez A, Medina M, Franzblau SG, Tekwani BL, Khan SI, Wahyuono S, Willett KL, Hammann MT. Manzamine B and E and ircinal A related alkaloids from an Indonesian Acanthostrongylophora sponge and their activity against infectious, tropical parasitic, and Alzheimer's diseases. *J Nat Prod* 2006;**69**:1034-40.

[30]   Rao KV, Santarsiero BD, Mesecar AD, Schinazi RF, Tekwani BL, Hamann MT. New Manzamine Alkaloids with Activity against Infectious and Tropical Parasitic Diseases from an Indonesian Sponge. *J Nat Prod* 2003;**66**:823-8.

[31]   Peng J, Hu JF, Kazi AB, Li Z, Avery M, Peraud O, Hill RT, Franzblau SG, Zhang F, Schinazi RF, Wirtz SS, Tharnish P, Kelly M, Wahyuono S, Hamann MT. Manadomanzamines A and B: A Novel Alkaloid Ring System with Potent Activity against Mycobacteria and HIV-1. *J Am Chem Soc* 2003;**125**:13382-6.

[32]   Rodriguez AD. Ramirez C. Serrulatane Diterpenes with Antimycobacterial Activity Isolated from the West Indian Sea Whip *Pseudopterogorgia elisabethae*. *J Nat Prod* 2001;**64**:100-2.

[33]   Rodríguez II, Rodríguez AD. Homopseudopteroxazole, a new antimycobacterial diterpene alkaloid from Pseudopterogorgia elisabethae. *J Nat Prod* 2003;**66**:855-7.

[34]   Rodriguez AD, Gonzalez E, Huang SD. Unusual Terpenes with Novel Carbon Skeletons from the West Indian Sea Whip *Pseudopterogorgia elisabethae* (Octocorallia). *J Org Chem* 1998;**63**:7083-91.

[35]   Rodríguez AD, Ramírez C, Rodríguez II, Barnes CL. Novel terpenoids from the West Indian sea whip Pseudopterogorgia elisabethae (Bayer). Elisapterosins A and B: rearranged diterpenes possessing an unprecedented cagelike framework. *J Org Chem* 2000;**65**:1390-8.

[36]   Rodriguez AD, Ramirez C, Shi YP. The Cumbiasins, Structurally Novel Diterpenes Possessing Intricate Carbocyclic Skeletons from the West Indian Sea Whip *Pseudopterogorgia elisabethae* (Bayer). *J Org Chem* 2000;**65**:6682-7.

[37]   Rodriguez AD, Ramirez C. A Marine Diterpene with a Novel Tetracyclic Framework from the West Indian Gorgonian Octocoral *Pseudopterogorgia elisabethae*. *Org Lett* 2000;**2**:507-10.

[38]   Konig GM, Wright AD, Franzblau SG. Assessment of Antimycobacterial Activity of a Series of Mainly Marine Derived Natural Products. *Planta Med* 2000;**66**:337-42.

[39]   El Sayed PJ, Walsh K, Weedman V, Bergthold JD, Lynch J, Lieu KL, Braude IA, Hamann MT. The new bioactive diterpenes cyanthiwigins E–A from the Jamaican sponge *Myrmekioderma styx*. *Tetrahedron* 2002;**58**:7809-19.

[40]   Peng J, Kasanah N, Stanley CE, Chadwick J, Fronczek FR, Hamann MT.Microbial metabolism studies of cyanthiwigin B and synergetic antibiotic effects. *J Nat Prod* 2003;**69**:727-30.

[41]   Sennett SH, Pomponi SA, Wright AE. Diterpene Metabolites from Two Chemotypes of the Marine Sponge Myrmekioderma styx. *J Nat Prod* 1992;**55**:1421-9.

[42]   New Antiinfective and Human 5-HT2 Receptor Binding Natural and Semisynthetic Compounds from the Jamaican Sponge *Smenospongia aurea*. Hu JF, Schetz JA, Kelly M, Peng JN, Ang KKH, Flotow H, Leong CY, Ng SB, Buss AD, Wilkins SP, Hamann MT, *J Nat Prod* 2002;**65**:476-480.

[43]   Wonganuchitmeta S, Yuenyongsawad S, Keawpradub N, Plubrukarn A. Antitubercular Sesterterpenes from the Thai Sponge *Brachiaster* sp. *J Nat Prod* 2004;**67**:1767-0.

[44]   Sayed KA, Bartyzel P, Shen X, Perry TL, Zjawiony JK, Hamann MT. Marine Natural Products as Antituberculosis Agents. *Tetrahedron* 2000;**56**:949-53.

[45]   Iguchi K, Saitoh S, Yamada Y. Novel 19-oxygenated sterols from the Okinawan soft coral litophyton viridis. *Chem Pharm Bull* 1989;**37**:2553-4.

[46]   Liu J, Zeng L, Wu D. (1992) *Gaodeng Xuexiao Huaxue Xuebao* **13**, 341; *Chem. Abstr. 117*, 230411y.

[47]   Wachter GA, Franzblau SG, Montenegro G, Hoffmann JJ, Maiese WM, Timmermann BN. Inhibition of *Mycobacterium tuberculosis* Growth by Saringosterol from *Lessonia nigrescens*. *J Nat Prod* 2001;**64**:1463-4.

[48]   Freundlich JS, Lalgondar M, Wei JR, Swanson S, Sorensen EJ, Rubin EJ, Sacchettini JC. The abyssomicin C family as *in vitro* inhibitors of *Mycobacterium tuberculosis*. *Tuberculosis* 2010;**90**:298–300.

[49]   Mo S, Krunic A, Santarsiero, BD, Franzblau SG, Orjala J. Hapalindolerelated alkaloids from the cultured cyanobacterium Fischerella ambigua, *Phytochemistry* 2010;71:2116-2123.

[50] Avilés E, Rodríguez AD. Monamphilectine A, a potent antimalarial-lactam from marine sponge Hymeniacidon sp: isolation, structure, semisynthesis, and bioactivity. *Org Lett* 2010;**12**:5290-93.

[51] Sturdy M, Krunic A, Cho S, Franzblau SG, Orjala J. Eucapsitrione, an anti- *Mycobacterium tuberculosis* anthraquinone derivative from the cultured freshwater cyanobacterium *Eucapsis sp. J Nat Prod* 2010;**73**:1441-1443.

[52] Pruksakorn P, Arai M, Kotoku N, Vilchèze C, Baughn AD, Moodley P, Jacobs WR Jr, Kobayashi M. Trichoderins, novel aminolipopeptides from a marine sponge-derived Trichoderma sp., are active against dormant mycobacteria. *Bioorg Med Chem Lett* 2010;**20**:3658-63.

[53] Schmitt EK, Riwanto M, Sambandamurthy V, Roggo S, Miault C, Zwingelstein C, Krastel P, Noble C, Beer D, Rao SP, Au M, Niyomrattanakit P, Lim V, Zheng J, Jeffery D, Pethe K, Camacho LR. The natural product cyclomarin kills *Mycobacterium tuberculosis* by targeting the ClpC1 subunit of the caseinolytic protease. *Angew Chem Int Ed Engl* 2011;**26**:5889-91.

[54] Chen C, Song F, Wang Q, Abdel-Mageed WM, Guo H, Fu C, Hou W, Dai H, Liu X, Yang N, Xie F, Yu K, Chen R, Zhang L. A marine-derived Streptomyces sp. MS449 produces high yield of actinomycin X2 and actinomycin D with potent anti-tuberculosis activity. *Appl Microbiol Biotechnol* 2012;**95**:919-27.

[55] Chen C, Wang J, Guo H, Hou W, Yang N, Ren B, Liu M, Dai H, Liu X, Song F, Zhang L. Three antimycobacterial metabolites identified from a marine-derived *Streptomyces sp. MS100061. Appl Microbiol Biotechnol.* 2013;**97**:3885-92.

Index

A

2-acetyl-3 methylquinoxaline-1,4-dioxide   113

Actinobacterium Streptomyces griseus   138, 180

Acyl hidrozone compounds   102

Agelasine   198

AIDS   3, 16, 28-9, 38, 65-6, 75, 90, 102, 203

Alkaloids   76, 159, 164, 181, 198, 200, 202, 206

Amikacin   22, 30, 32, 142

Aminoglycosides   138, 180

Amodiaquine   77, 81

Anorexia nervosa   8, 10

Anti-TB compounds   85

Anti-TB drugs   38, 55, 93, 104, 106, 112

Anti-TB evaluation of imidazole   105, 107

Anti-TB proprieties   26, 102, 164, 166

Anti-tuberculosis drugs   46, 49

Antibacterial agents   18, 75, 77, 92

Antibiotic streptomycin   20, 138

Antimalarial drugs   75-6, 81

Antimycobacterial drugs   90

β-D-arabinofuranosyl-1-monophosphoryldecaprenol (DPA)   54-5

Arabinofuranosyl transferases   54-5

Arabinogalactan   50, 52-3, 113, 126, 190

Araguspongine   198-9

Artemisinin   158-9

Artificial pneumothorax   13-14

2-(3-aryl-1-oxo-2-propenyl)-3-methylquinoxaline-1,4-dioxides   113

Aryloxyphenyl cyclopropyl methanones   117

Axisonitrile-3   206-7

B

Bacterial type II   44

P

Q

R

www.ingramcontent.com/pod-product-compliance
Lightning Source LLC
Chambersburg PA
CBHW050835220326

41598CB00006B/366